Veerendra Kumar · Mukta Bhatele
Editors

Proceedings of All India Seminar on Biomedical Engineering 2012 (AISOBE 2012)

Springer

Editors
Veerendra Kumar
Jabalpur Engineering College
Jabalpur, Madhya Pradesh
India

Mukta Bhatele
Computer Science
Gyan Ganga College of Technology
Jabalpur, Madhya Pradesh
India

ISSN 2195-271X ISSN 2195-2728 (electronic)
ISBN 978-81-322-0969-0 ISBN 978-81-322-0970-6 (eBook)
DOI 10.1007/978-81-322-0970-6
Springer New Delhi Heidelberg New York Dordrecht London

Library of Congress Control Number: 2012952004

Printed on acid-free paper

Springer is part of Springer Science+Business Media (www.springer.com)

Preface

The Institution of Engineers (India) came up with the idea of All India Seminar on Biomedical Engineering 2012 (AISOBE 2012) to be held on 3rd and 4th of November 2012. AISOBE 2012 is an attempt to bring forward the latest research in the fields of bio-medical engineering, information technology, and soft computing. Our vision behind organizing this seminar was to provide a platform to bring researchers and practitioners together including engineers, biologists, health professionals and informatics/computer scientists, to create an integrated environment for personnel interest in both theoretical advances and applications of information systems, artificial intelligence, signal processing, electronics and other engineering tools in knowledge areas related to biology and medicine.

Biomedical engineering is the application of engineering principles and design concepts to medicine and biology. This field seeks to close the gap between engineering and medicine: it combines the design and problem-solving skills of engineering with medical and biological sciences to improve healthcare diagnosis, monitoring and therapy.

Thanks to our authors who had submitted papers related to the fields of medicine, computing and image processing all complying with the theme of the seminar.

We were obliged with the presence of renowned medical practitioners who enlightened us with their research in fields like treatment of arachnoid cyst, stereolithography and health monitoring.

We had topics in the field of nanoparticles and nanotechnology and its use in medicine. We had papers about development of medicinal drugs for cancer treatment.

Some papers depicted the use of image processing in the field of biomedical engineering, covering topics like analysis of CT images of bones, analysis of EEG signals, and enhancement of medical image security using digital watermarking, registration, de-noising and compression of medical images.

Numerous papers were related to soft computing, which provided us information about how computing can take advantages from biology by creating computer systems based on human immune system, human cells, etc. Some interesting researches related to genetic algorithm and neural networks were also presented.

We had research papers about wireless sensor networks, MANETs and VANETs, and how these technologies can help in the field of medicine. Some papers were about software used in hospitals and in the field of medicine.

We also enjoyed the presence of few inter-disciplinary research topics from the field of information technology, which are providing their services to the fields of medicine and engineering.

Acknowledgment

AISOBE 2012 is a result of a collective and collaborative endeavor of many individuals and organizations. This acknowledgment is an attempt at thanking all of those who have made it possible.

First and foremost our heartiest thanks to The Institution of Engineers (India) (IEI) for hosting and organizing this seminar and praiseworthy effort of all the members of IEI and office staff at Jabalpur Local Centre (JLC).

We sincerely thank all the authors who were part of this seminar and enlightened us with their work related to theme of the seminar. We are thankful to the management and faculty members at Jabalpur Engineering College, Jabalpur, for their support. We are also grateful to Er. D. C. Jain, Mr. Rajneet Jain, Dr. Maneesh Choubey and all faculty members of Gyan Ganga Group of Institutes Jabalpur. Similarly we are grateful to Shri Ram Group of institutes, Jabalpur for their support.

We would like to thank Dr. I. K. Bhat, Dr. A. D. Bhat, Dr. A. M. Kuthe, Dr. R. K. Shrivastava, Dr. K. Pandesar, Dr. Puneet Tandon, Dr. Rajesh Dhiravani, Dr. Jitendra Jamdar, Dr. Pushpraj Bhatele, Dr. Parimal Swamy, Dr. Arun Sharma, Dr. Tapas Chakma, Dr. H. K. T. Raza, Dr. Y. R. Yadav and Dr. D. P. Lokwani for reviewing the papers. We would also like to thank the management and doctors at Jabalpur Hospital Pvt Ltd, Jamdar Hospital Pvt Ltd and Apex Hospital, Jabalpur.

We express our gratitude toward Mr. S. L. Garg, FIE President, Dr. R. K. Dave, Mr. Suneel Grover, Mr. V. K. Gupta, Dr. M. Selot and Mr. K. C. Sethi, who are respected members of our National Advisory Committee and to Er. Rakesh Rathore, Er. Raman Mehta and Er. P. S. Naidu, who are respected members of Executive Committee JLC, IEI. We are also very grateful to Dr. Veerendra Kumar, Convener and Er. Mukta Bhatele, Organizing Secretary, AISOBE 2012.

We appreciate Springer India Pvt Ltd, especially Mr. Yumnam Ojen Singh and his team at Springer for publishing presented papers in *Proceedings of All India Seminar on Biomedical Engineering 2012 (AISOBE 2012).*

Finally, we would like to thank everyone who attended the seminar and made it success, and it is very likely that we had missed some names; therefore, we are grateful to everyone who has directly or indirectly catered to this seminar.

Contents

Expert List

National Advisory Committee

Chairman

Mr. S. L. Garg, FIE President, IEI

Co-Chairman

Dr. R. K. Dave, FIE Chairman, ICC, IEI
Mr. Suneel Grover, Member, ICC, IEI
Mr. V. K. Gupta, Member, ICC, IEI
Dr. M. Selot, Member, ICC, IEI
Mr. K. C. Sethi, Member, ICC, IEI

Convener

Dr. Veerendra Kumar

Organizing Committee

Chairman

Mr. Rakesh Rathore, FIE, Chairman, JLC, IEI

Organising Secretary

Er. Mukta Bhatele

Honorary Secretary

Mr. Raman Mehta, FIE

Joint Org. Secy

Er. P. S. Naidu, FIE

Members

Mr. N. K. Mehta, Mr. S. K. Tiwari, Mr. Laxman Das, Mr. B. S. Baghel, Mr. R. K. Chouksey, Mr. V. K. Sahu, Mr. M. K. Raghuvanshi, Mr. K. K. Jain, Dr. I. K. Khanna, Mr. V. K. Birthire, Mr. V. K. Pandya, Dr. P. S. Bundella, Col R. S. Malhotra

Editor-in-Chief

Dr. Veerendra Kumar

Editors

Dr. Mukta Bhatele
Dr. J. S. Yadav
Dr. Neetu Bhatia

Technical Committee

Dr. I. K. Bhat
Dr. A. D. Bhat
Dr. A. M. Kuthe
Dr. R. K. Shrivastava
Dr. K. Pandesar
Dr. Puneet Tandon
Dr. Rajesh Dhiravani
Dr. Jitendra Jamdar
Dr. Pushpraj Bhatele
Dr. Tapas Chakma
Dr. H. K. T. Raza
Dr. Y. R. Yadav
Dr. D. P. Lokwani
Prof. (Dr.) D. C. Chaurasia

Special Invitees

Dr. N. R. Bandyopadhyay
Dr. U. Chandrasekhar
Dr. Pradeep Chaturvedi
Dr. G. S. Yadava
Lt. Gen. (Dr.) V. J. Sundaram
Prof. (Dr.) T. S. Kamal
Mr. P. K. Maity
Mr. A. K. Saxena
Prof. S. Radhakrishnan
Dr. Sanjeev Banerjee
Dr. Parimal Swamy
Dr. Parvez Siddiqui
Dr. Ajay Seth
Dr. Anant Joshi
Dr. Bhavin Jahnkaria
Dr. Sanjay Pandey
Dr. Yugal Mishra
Dr. Chandrashekhar Niyogi
Dr. N. P. Gupta
Dr. Prashant Jain

About the Editors

Prof. Veerendra Kumar is currently the Principal of Jabalpur Engineering College, India. Earlier to this, he was the Dean (Planning and Evaluation) of the college from June 2010 to July 2012. He was also the Head of the Department of Mechanical Engineering from December 2008 to July 2012. He has more than 25 years of experience in teaching and training. Prof. Kumar has recently submitted a Ph.D. thesis on Biomechanics to the National Institute of Technology, Hamirpur, India. He is an M.E. in Machine Design (completed in 1985) from Rani Durgavati Vishwavidyalaya, Jabalpur. In 1982, he completed B.E. in Mechanical Engineering from University of Jabalpur, Jabalpur. His areas of specialization include Biomechanics, Machine Design, Finite Element Method, and Computer Aided Design. Professor Kumar has published a book titled "A Textbook of Industrial Robotics" in 2010 with Dhanpat Rai Publishing Company (P) Limited, New Delhi and 13 papers in international journals. He was Editor of the Proceedings of National Seminar on Role of Information Technology in 21st Century, February 11 and 12, 1999 at Government Engineering College, Jabalpur. He is a Life Member of the Indian Society for Technical Education and the Association for Machines and Mechanisms, and a Member of The Institution of Engineers (India).

Prof. (Mrs) Mukta Bhatele is currently a faculty member in the Computer Science and Engineering Department of Gyan Ganga College and Technology, Jabalpur. She holds B.E. and M.Tech. degrees from Maulana Azad National Institute of Technology (previously Maulana Azad College of Technology), Bhopal. She has more than 17 years of experience as a teacher. She has 10 publications in renowned international journals and numerous publications in national level journals and conferences. She is currently the Honorary Secretary of The Institution of Electronics and Telecommunication Engineers, Jabalpur Centre and a Member of The Institution of Engineers (India).

Stereolithography: A Recent Tool in Diagnosis, Treatment Planning, and Management of Craniofacial Deformities

Rajesh B. Dhirawani

Abstract Medical rapid prototyping (MRP) is defined as the manufacture of dimensionally accurate physical models of human anatomy derived from medical image data using a variety of rapid prototyping (RP) technologies. It has been applied to a range of medical specialties, including oral and maxillofacial surgery [1–7], dental implantology, neurosurgery [8, 9], and orthopedics [10, 11]. The source of image data for 3-dimensional (3D) modeling is principally computed tomography (CT), although magnetic resonance imaging and ultrasound have also been used. Medical models have been successfully built of hard tissue (bone) and soft tissues (blood vessels and nasal passages). MRP was described originally by Mankowich et al. in 1990 [12].

Keywords Stereolithography · Maxillofacial surgery · Dental implantology

Stereolithography

An SL RP system consists of a bath of photosensitive resin, a model-building platform, and an ultraviolet (UV) laser for curing the resin. Figure 1 shows the principle of operation of SL apparatus. A mirror is used to guide the laser focus onto the surface of the resin, where the resin becomes cured when exposed to UV radiation. The mirror is computer controlled, with its movement being guided to cure the resin on a slice-by-slice basis. A model is initially designed with CAD

R. B. Dhirawani (✉)
Director at Jabalpur Hospital & Research Centre, Jabalpur, India

R. B. Dhirawani
Director at Hitkarini Dental College & Hospital, Jabalpur, India

V. Kumar and M. Bhatele (eds.), *Proceedings of All India Seminar on Biomedical Engineering 2012 (AISOBE 2012)*, Lecture Notes in Bioengineering,
DOI: 10.1007/978-81-322-0970-6_1,

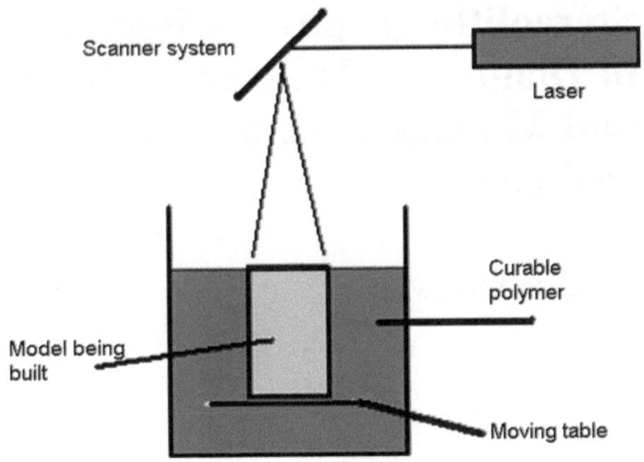

Fig. 1 Diagram showing the principle of operation of an SL system. Winder and bibb. Medical rapid prototyping technologies. J Oral Maxillofac Surg 2005

software in a suitable file format (commonly STL) and transferred to the SL machine for building. The CAD data file is converted into individual slices of known dimensions. This slice data are then fed to the RP machine, which guides the exposure path of the UV laser onto the resin surface. The layers are cured sequentially and bond together to form a solid object beginning from the bottom of the model and building up. As the resin is exposed to the UV light, a thin well-defined layer thickness becomes hardened. After a layer of resin is exposed, the resin platform is lowered within the bath by a small known distance. A new layer of resin is wiped across the surface of the previous layer using a wiper blade, and this second layer is subsequently exposed and cured. The process of curing and lowering the platform into the resin bath is repeated until the full model is complete. The self-adhesive property of the material causes the layers to bond to one another and eventually form a complete, robust, 3D object. The model is then removed from the bath and cured for a further period of time in a UV cabinet Fig. 2. The built part may contain layers, which significantly overhang the layers below. If this is the case, then a network of support structures, made of the same material, is added beneath these overhanging layers at the design stage to add support during the curing process. These support structures, analogous to a scaffold, are removed by hand after the model is fully cured. This is a labor-intensive and time-consuming process. Generally, SL is considered to provide the greatest accuracy and the best surface finish of any RP technology. The model material is robust, slightly brittle, and relatively light, although it is hydroscopic and may physically warp over time (a few months) if exposed to high humidity.

Continued advances in biomodeling can facilitate better diagnosis, treatment planning, and fabrication of implants for craniomaxillofacial surgeries. Clinically, these models are used mainly for craniofacial deformities, reconstructive surgeries, pathologies, and trauma [13]. Biomodels generated by stereolithography (SL) have been confirmed to have a higher accuracy compared with milled models and 3-dimensional (3D) computed tomography (CT) visual models [14, 15].

The technology allows production of highly accurate and realistic replicas of the body structures of an individual. The literature has shown some promising

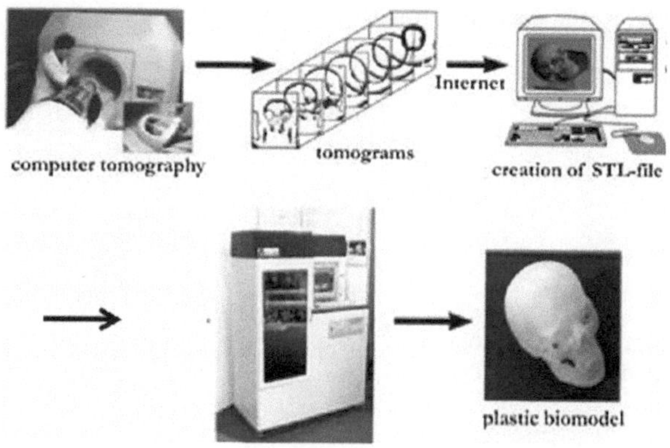

Fig. 2 The pictorial presentation of the complete process of fabrication of a stereolithographic model

results using a stereolithographic model as a guide for reconstruction [16–19]. Facial asymmetry, when obvious, has enormous socio-psychological impact on the affected individuals. It can occur as a consequence of developmental anomalies or disease or after trauma or surgery. Surgical reconstruction is usually indicated in most instances involving a noticeable facial asymmetry. In such surgeries the use of a rapid prototype technique—SL can help yield accurate, esthetic, and desired results.

SL models have the following range of applications:

- To aid production of a surgical implant
- To improve surgical planning
- To act as an orienting aid during surgery
- To enhance diagnostic quality
- To be useful in preoperative simulation
- To achieve patient's agreement prior to surgery
- To prepare a template for resection

The technique of color SL was developed very recently. This technique allows the selective coloring of structures in the 3D solid model. The 3D information of a solid model combined with the extra information from the selective coloring of certain anatomical structures both combine as an ultimate diagnostic and preoperative planning tool [20].

Clinical Applications

Traumatology

Stereolithographic models in trauma cases have proven to be useful in terms of visualizing the bony displacement, facilitating anatomical reduction, minimizing surgical approaches, and saving operating time [14]. Due to surgery simulation it

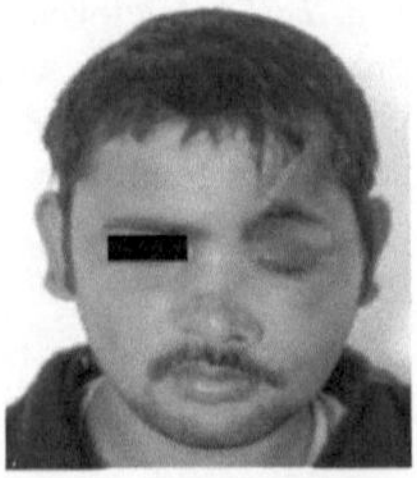

Fig. 3 Pre-operative frontal bone defect

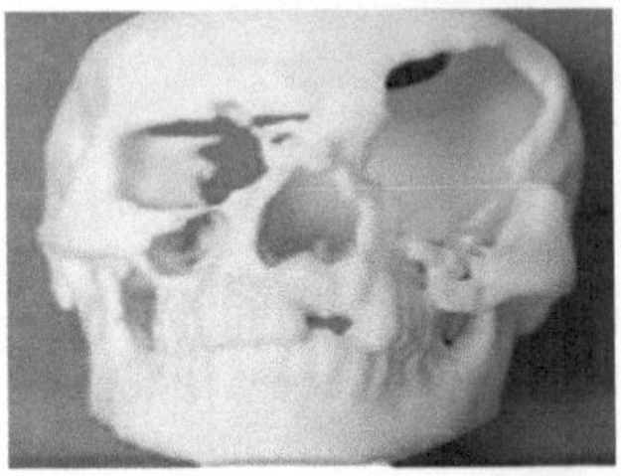

Fig. 4 Stereolithographic model of the patient

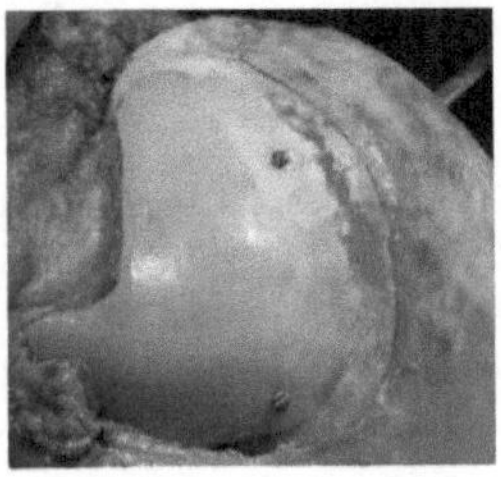

Fig. 5 Intraoperative picture showing fixation of the acrylic implant

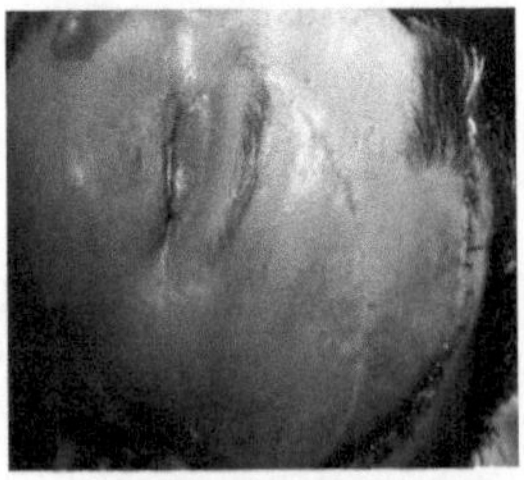

Fig. 6 Intraoperative correction of defect

becomes possible to adjust prefabricated mini- or microplates in the patient as in the preoperative planning. The configuration and bending of the plates also acts as a device for the anatomical reduction of the fragments. However, in case of comminution with very small fragments, surgery simulation with complete reduction on the 3D model is not advisable [21].

A case was done at our center, where the patient had a frontal bone defect due to trauma. A stereolithographic model was fabricated which facilitated in the visualization of defect in 3D, proper assessment of the injury, and aided in the fabrication of acrylic prosthesis to correct the defect (Figs. 3, 4, 5, 6, 7).

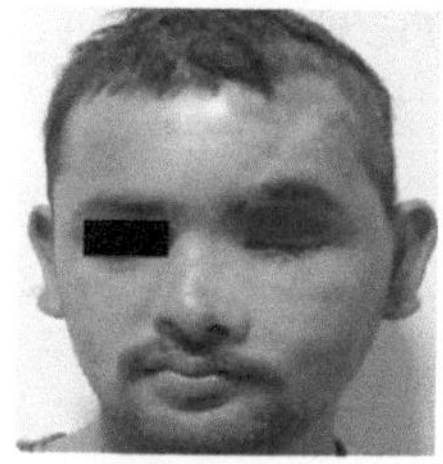

Fig. 7 Postoperative picture showing correction of the deformity and facial symmetry

Tumor Surgery

Preoperative model planning by color SL is useful in ablative surgery of tumors of the craniofacial region. The coloring of the tumor clarifies its relation to surrounding structures and illustrates eventual extension in the adjacent tissue. The main advantages of this technique are visualization of the problem, planning of the surgical approach, and determination of extent of the resection in areas of complex anatomy.

Reconstructive Surgery

Surgery simulation is helpful in primary reconstruction of maxillofacial defects and estimation of the amount of graft required for the reconstruction. Proper placement of the graft in the exact position can be accurately determined. Even plates can be prefabricated to hold the future bone graft. The precise fitting implants facilitate surgery thus saving operating time.

Trauma, cranial bone tumors, and congenital anomalies are the main reasons for craniofacial defects. The main indications for reconstruction of these defects are cosmetic reasons and protection of intracranial structures (Fig. 8).

Advantages

- Plate handling in the operating theater is minimal, thus preserving its strength.
- Decreased exposure time to general anesthesia.
- Decreased blood loss.
- Shorter wound exposure time [22].

Craniofacial Surgery

Craniosynostoses is the term that designates premature fusion of one or more sutures in either the cranial vault or cranial base. The disparity between intra-cranial volume and brain volume may increase intracranial pressure. The goals of

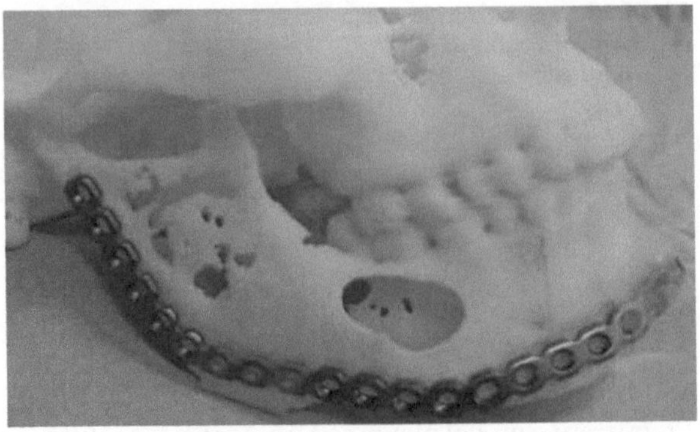

Fig. 8 Stereomodel used for adaptation of titanium plate

surgery of the newborn with a craniosynostosis are twofold: (1) Decompression of the intracranial space (to reduce intracranial pressure, to prevent visual problems, and to permit normal mental development) and (2) Achievement of satisfactory craniofacial form. The different methods of osteotomy for cranial vault remodeling can be simulated on the 3D model. The introduction of SL for cranioplasty of newborns and infants has reduced operating time significantly [22].

Distraction Osteogenesis

Stereomodels have proven to be highly beneficial in cases of distraction osteogenesis. They help in the planning, positioning of the device, placement of the osteotomy cuts, and predicting and visualizing the end results of the treatment. They also help in patient education and better understanding of the treatment procedure.

Conclusion

- The use of 3D models in oral and maxillofacial surgery has significantly improved predictability of clinical outcomes when compared to similar treatments without its use.
- Total operating time is reduced which has the benefit of decreasing the duration of general anesthesia and reducing wound exposure time.
- Assessment of extensive traumatic and pathologic defects in three-dimensions prior to surgical reconstruction.
- The models are useful in the design and fabrication of custom prosthesis and sizing of bone grafts, distraction osteogenesis, and patient education.

References

1. Anderl H, Zur Nedden D, Muhlbauer W et al (1994) CT-guided stereolithography as a new tool in craniofacial surgery. Br J Plast Surg 47:60
2. Arvier JF, Barker TM, Yau YY et al (1994) Maxillofacial biomodelling. Br J Oral Maxillofac Surg 32:276
3. D'Urso PS, Barker TM, Earwaker WJ et al (1999) Stereolithographic biomodelling in cranio-maxillofacial surgery: a prospective trial. J Craniomaxillofac Surg 27:30
4. Eufinger H, Wehmoller M (1998) Individual prefabricated titanium implants in reconstructive craniofacial surgery: clinical and technical aspects of the first 22 cases. Plast Reconstr Surg 102:300
5. Gateno J, Allen ME, Teichgraeber JF et al (2000) An in vitro study of the accuracy of a new protocol for planning distraction osteogenesis of the mandible. J Oral Maxillofac Surg 58:985
6. Sailer HF, Haers PE, Zollikofer CP et al (1998) The value of stereolithographic models for preoperative diagnosis of craniofacial deformities and planning of surgical corrections. Int J Oral Maxillofac Surg 27:327
7. Hughes CW, Page K, Bibb R et al (2003) The custom made orbital floor prosthesis in reconstruction for orbital floor fractures. Br J Oral Maxillofac Surg 41:50
8. Winder RJ, Cooke RS, Gray J et al (1999) Medical rapid prototyping and 3D CT in the manufacture of custom made cranial titanium plates. J Med Eng Tech 23:26
9. Heissler E, Fischer F, Bolouri S et al (1998) Aesthetic and reconstructive surgery: custom-made cast titanium implants produced with CAD/CAM for the reconstruction of cranium defects. Int J Oral Maxillofac Surg 27:334
10. Mankovich NJ, Cheeseman AM, Stoker NG (1990) The display of three-dimensional anatomy with stereolithographic models. J Digit Imaging 3:200
11. Cheung LK, Wong MC, Wong LL (2002) Refinement of facial reconstructive surgery by stereo-model planning. Ann R Australas Coll Dent Surg 16:129
12. Lill W, Solar P, Ulm C et al (1992) Reproducibility of three-dimensional CT-assisted model production in the maxillofacial area. Br J Oral Maxillofac Surg 30:233
13. Klein HM, Schneider W, Alzen G et al (1992) Pediatric craniofacial surgery: comparison of milling and stereolithography for 3D model manufacturing. Pediatr Radiol 22:458
14. Kermer C, Linder A, Friede I et al (1998) Preoperative stereolithographic model planning for primary reconstruction in craniomaxillofacial trauma surgery. J Craniomaxillofac Surg 26:136
15. Holck DEE, Boyd EM, Ng J et al (1999) Benefits of stereolithography in orbital reconstruction. Ophthalmology 106:1214
16. Kernan BT, Wimsatt JA (2000) Use of a stereolithography model for accurate, preoperative adaptation of a reconstruction plate. J Oral Maxillofac Surg 58:349
17. Eppley BL (2002) Craniofacial reconstruction with computer-generated HTR patient-matched implants: use in primary bone tumor excision. J Craniofac Surg 13:650
18. Tada H, Hatoko M, Tanaka A et al (2002) Preshaped hydroxyapatite tricalcium-phosphate implant using three-dimensional computer tomography in the reconstruction of bone deformities of craniomaxillofacial region. J Craniofac Surg 13:287
19. Wong Tung-Yiu, Fang Jing-Jing, Chung Ching-Hung et al (2005) Comparison of 2 methods of making surgical models for correction of facial asymmetry. J Oral Maxillofac Surg 63:200–208
20. Bill J, Reuther J, Dittmann W, Kübler N, Meier J, Pistner H, Wittenberg G (1995) Stereolithography in oral and maxillofacial operation planning. Int J Oral Maxillofac Surg 24:98–103
21. Kärcher H (1992) Three-dimensional craniofacial surgery: transfer from a three-dimensional model (Endoplan) to clinical surgery: a new technique (Graz). J Cranio-Max Fac Surg 20:125–131
22. Lambrecht JT (1989) Planning orthognathic surgery with three dimensional models. Int J Adult Orthodon Orthognath Surg 4:141–144

Image Denoising by Data Adaptive and Non-Data Adaptive Transform Domain Denoising Method Using EEG Signal

Vandana Roy and Shailja Shukla

Abstract This chapter proposes an automatic method for artifact removal and noise elimination from scalp electroencephalogram recordings (EEG). The method is based on transform domain method having combination of data adaptive and non-data adaptive transform domain image denoising method to improve artifact elimination (ocular, high frequency muscle, and electrocardiogram (ECG) artifacts). The elimination of artifact from scalp EEGs is of substantial significance for both the automated and visual examination of underlying brainwave actions. These noise sources increase the difficulty in analyzing the EEG and obtaining clinical information related to pathology. Hence it is crucial to design a procedure to decrease such artifacts in EEG records. The role of a data adaptive transform domain, i.e., ICA to separate the signal from multichannel sources, then non-data adaptive transform, i.e., wavelet is applied to denoise the signal. The proposed methodology successfully rejected a good percentage of artifacts and noise, while preserving almost all the cerebral activity. The "denoised artifact-free" EEG presents a very good improvement compared with recorded raw EEG.

Keywords Artifact removal · Electroencephalogram (EEG) · Wavelet denoising · Independent component analysis (ICA)

V. Roy (✉)
Department of Electronics and Communication, Jabalpur Engineering College, Jabalpur, Madhya Pradesh, India
e-mail: vandana.roy20@gmail.com

S. Shukla
Department of Computer Science Engineering, Jabalpur Engineering College, Jabalpur, Madhya Pradesh, India

V. Kumar and M. Bhatele (eds.), *Proceedings of All India Seminar on Biomedical Engineering 2012 (AISOBE 2012)*, Lecture Notes in Bioengineering,
DOI: 10.1007/978-81-322-0970-6_2, © Springer India 2013

Introduction

The electrical activity produced by the brain is recorded by the electroencephalogram (EEG) using several electrodes placed on the scalp. Signal characteristics vary from one state to another, such as wakefulness/sleep or normal/pathological. EEG is the multivariate time series data measured using multiple sensors positioned on the scalp that imitates electrical potential produced by behaviors of brain and is a record of the electrical potentials created by the cerebral cortex nerve cells. There are two categories of EEG based on where the signal is obtained in the head: scalp or intracranial. Scalp EEG being the main focus of the research, uses small metal discs, also called electrodes, which are kept on the scalp with good mechanical and electrical touch. Intracranial EEG is obtained by special electrodes placed in the brain during a surgery. The electrodes should be of low impedance in order to record the exact voltage of the brain neuron. The variations in the voltage difference among electrodes are sensed and amplified before being transmitted to a computer program [1]. Classically, five major brain waves can be distinguished by their frequency ranges: delta (δ) 0.5–4 Hz, theta (θ) 4–8 Hz, alpha (α) 8–13 Hz, beta (β) 13–30 Hz and gamma (γ) 30–128 Hz. The informative cortically generated signals are contaminated by extra-cerebral artifact sources: ocular movements, eye blinks, electrocardiogram (ECG), muscular artifacts. Generally, the mixture between brain signals and artifactual signals is present in all sensors, although not necessarily in the same proportions (depending on the spatial distribution). Moreover, the EEG recordings are also affected by other unknown basically random signals (instrumentation noise, other physiological generators, external electromagnetic activity, etc.) which can be modeled as additive random noise. These phenomena make difficult the analysis and interpretation of the EEGs, and a first important processing step would be the elimination of the artifacts and noise. Several methods for artifact elimination were proposed. Most of them consist of two main steps: artifact extraction from the multichannel recorded signals, generally using some signal separation methods, followed by signal classification. Our goal is to contribute to EEG artifact rejection by proposing an original and more complete automatic methodology consisting of an optimized combination of several signal processing and data analysis techniques [2].

This chapter is organized as follows: Supporting Literature briefs the supporting literature, Data Adaptive Transform Domain Image Denoising Method: ICA states the data adaptive transform domain method to separate the signals from multichannel sources, then Non Data Adaptive Transform Domain Based Denoising (Wavelet denoising) gives details of non-data adaptive transform domain method to denoise the signal to remove artifacts. This method assumes that EEG contains two classes namely, artifact and non- artifact signal, and then it calculates the optimum threshold separating these two classes. Proposed Method is dedicated to our present approach to denoise the signal and Experimental Results presents the main results in Sect. 6.

Supporting Literature

EEG Signals: The nervous system sends commands and communicates by trains of electric impulses. When the neurons of the human brain process information they do so by changing the flow of electrical current across their membranes. These changing currents (potential) generate electric fields that can be recorded from the scalp. Studies are interested in these electrical potentials but they can only be received by direct measurement. This requires a patient to undergo surgery for electrodes to be placed inside the head. This is not acceptable because of the risk to the patient. Researchers therefore collect recordings from the scalp receiving the global descriptions of the brain activity. Because the same potential is recorded from more than one electrode, signals from the electrodes are supposed to be highly correlated. These are collected by the use of an electroencephalograph and are called EEG signals. Understanding the brain is a huge part of Neuroscience, and the development of EEG was for the explanation of such a phenomenon. The morphology of EEG signals has been used by researches and in clinical practice to:

- Diagnose epilepsy and see what type of seizures is occurring.
- Produce the most useful and important test in conforming a diagnosis of epilepsy.
- Check for problem with loss of consciousness or dementia.
- Help find out a person's chance of recovery after change in consciousness.
- Find out whether a person is in coma or is brain dead.
- Study sleep disorder such as narcolepsy.
- What brain activity occurs while a person is receiving general anesthesia during brain surgery.
- Help find out whether a person has a physical problem (in the brain, spinal cord, or nervous system) or a mental health problem.

The signals must therefore present a true and clear picture of brain activities. Being a physical system, recording electrical potentials present EEG with problems; all neurons, including those outside the brain, communicate using electrical impulses. These non-cerebral impulses are produced from:

- Eye movement and blinking—Electrooculogram (EOG)
- Cardiac movement—Cardiograph (ECG/EKG)
- Muscle movement—Electromyogram (EMG)
- Chewing and sucking movement—Glassokinetic
- The power lines.

EEG recordings are therefore a combination of these signals called artifacts or noise and the pure EEG signal defined mathematically as in Eq. (1):

$$E(t) = S(t) + N(t) \tag{1}$$

where,

S is pure EEG signal,

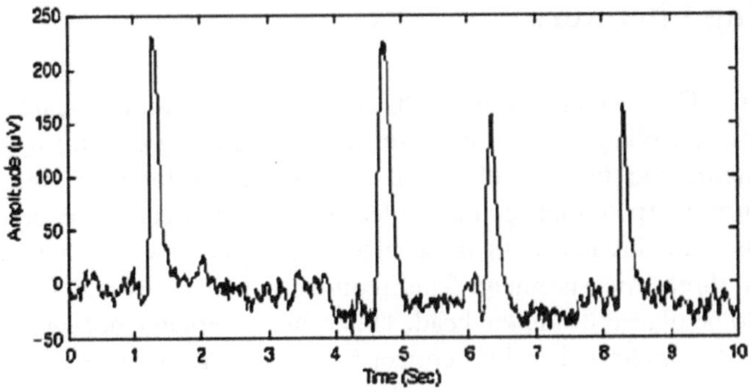

Fig. 1 EEG contaminated with EOG producing spikes

N is the noise and
E represents the recorded signal.

The presence of these noises introduces spikes which can be confused with neurological rhythms. They also mimic EEG signals overlying these signals resulting in signal distortion (Fig. 1). Correct analysis is therefore impossible, resulting in misdiagnosis in the case of some patients. Noise must be eliminated or attenuated.

The method of cancellation of the contaminated segments, although practice can lead to considerable information loss, thus other methods such as principal component analysis (PCA) and more recently ICA and WT have been utilized [3].

Data Adaptive Transform Domain Image Denoising Method: ICA

Definitions of ICA: We can define the ICA as it is a random vector X which consists of finding a linear transform as in Eq. (2):

$$X = AS \tag{2}$$

so that the components s_i are as independent as possible w.r.t. some maximum function that measures independence. This definition is known as a general definition where no assumptions on the data are made. Independent component analysis (ICA) is the decomposition of a random vector in linear components which are "as independent as possible". Here, 'independence' should be understood in its strong statistical sense: it goes beyond second order decorrelation and thus involves the non-gaussianity of the data. The ideal measure of independence is the higher order cumulants like kurtosis and mutual information.

In addition to the basic assumption of statistically independence, by imposing the following fundamental restrictions, the noise free ICA model can be defined if:

1. All the independent components S_i, with the possible exception of one component, must be non-Gaussian
2. The number of observed linear mixtures m must be at least as large as the number of independent components n, i.e., $m > p$
3. The matrix A must be of full column rank.

We can invert the mixing matrix as in Eq. (3):

$$S = A^{-1} X \tag{3}$$

Thus, to estimate one of the independent components, we can consider a linear combination of X_i Let us denote this by Eq. (4):

$$Y = b^T X = b^T AS \tag{4}$$

Hence, if b were one of the rows of A^{-1}, this linear combination $b^T X$ would actually equal one of the independent components. But in practice we cannot determine such 'b' exactly because we have no knowledge of matrix A, but we can find an estimator that gives a good approximation. In practice there are two different measures of non-Gaussianity.

Kurtosis

The classical measure of non-Gaussianity is kurtosis or the fourth order cumulant. It is defined by Eq. (5)

$$\text{Kurt}\,(y) = E\{y^4\} - 3(E\{y^2\})^2 \tag{5}$$

As the variable y is assumed to be standardized we can say in Eq. (6) as:

$$\text{Kurt}\,(y) = E\{\,y4\} - 3 \tag{6}$$

Hence the kurtosis is simply a normalized version of the fourth moment E{y4}. For the Gaussian case the fourth moment is equal to 3 and hence kurt (y) = 0. Thus, for Gaussian variable kurtosis is zero but for non-Gaussian random variable it is nonzero [4, 5].

Non-Data Adaptive Transform Domain-Based Denoising (Wavelet Denoising)

We know that Fast ICA are expected to correspond to artifacts only, on the other hand, some brain action might escape to these gathered signals. The purpose of conventional filtering is to process raw EEG data x(t) to eliminate 50 Hz line noise, baseline values, artifacts inhabiting very low frequencies and high frequency sensor noise v(t), and this phase may include mixture of different existing notch, lowpass, and/or highpass filters. As artifacts have a frequency overlap with the brain signals, the conventional filtering technique cannot be utilized, and therefore this paper focuses on using Wavelet Denoising to explore brain activity from gathered independent components [1].

Image signal and noise signal by the wavelet transform have different characteristics:

1. In the wavelet transform, the noise energy reduces rapidly as scale increases, but the image signal does not reduce rapidly.
2. Noise is not highly relevant at different scales of the wavelet transform. But the wavelet transform of image signal generally has a strong correlation, the scale of the adjacent local maxima almost appear in the same position and have the same symbol.

The two above-mentioned points will separate image signal and noise signal, that is to say they are the base of image denoising [6].

Wavelet Domain-Based Denoising Algorithm

An image is often corrupted by noise in its acquisition or transmission. Wavelet provides an appropriate basis for separating noisy signal from image signal. The motivation is that as the wavelet transform is good at energy compaction, small coefficient is more likely due to noise and large coefficient due to important signal features. These small coefficients can be threshold without affecting the significant features of the images.

The problem that arises is how to find an optimal threshold such that the mean squared error between the signal and its estimate is minimized. The wavelet decomposition of an image is done as the image is split into 4 subbands, namely the HH, HL, LH, and LL subbands as shown in Fig. 2. The HH subband gives the diagonal details of the image; the HL subband gives the horizontal features while the LH subband represents the vertical structures. The LL subband is the low resolution residual consisting of low frequency components and it is this subband which is further split at a higher level of decomposition as shown in Fig. 2 [7].

The low pass filters represent the “approximation” of the signal or its dc component and the high pass filters represent the “details” or its high frequency

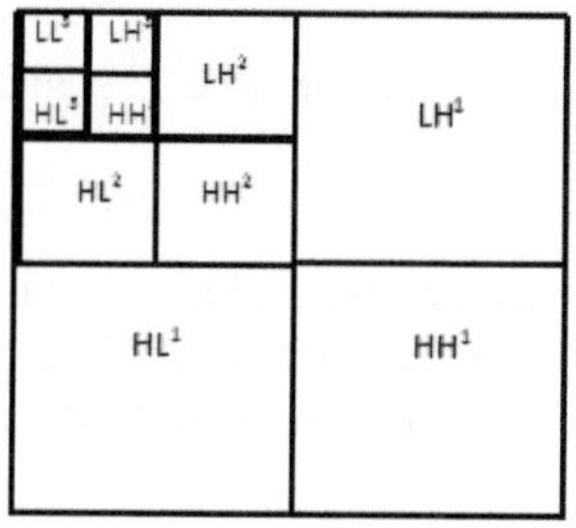

Fig. 2 Wavelet decomposition: 1, 2, 3 decomposition levels, *H* high frequency bands, *L* low frequency bands

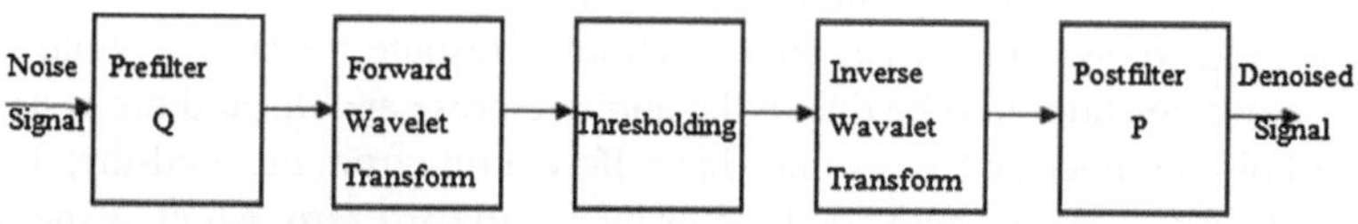

Fig. 3 Denoising by wavelet domain

components. The successive analysis of the low pass component only is called wavelet decomposition, (Fig. 1b), whereas the analysis of both the low and high pass components is called wavelet packet decomposition; the existence of small coefficients is more likely to be due to the noise contamination, whereas the large coefficients contain significant image details. Hence, the small magnitude coefficients may be thresholded without affecting the large ones and therefore the quality of the image [8].

The investigations show that themethod for denoising differs only in the selection of the wavelets and their decomposition levels [6].

The algorithm has the following steps:

1. Calculate the DWT of the image.
2. Threshold the wavelet coefficients (Threshold may be universal or subband adaptive).
3. Compute the IDWT to get the denoised estimate.

Wavelet transform of noisy signal should be taken first and then thresholding function is applied on it. Finally the output should be undergone inverse wavelet transformation to obtain the estimate x as shown in Fig. 3.

The DWT of any signal sample is given by Eq. (7)

$$S_{\mathrm{DWT}}(j,k) = \sum_{n=0}^{N-1} S_{nj,k}\, w_n, \quad a = 2^j,\ \tau = k2^j \tag{7}$$

S_n s(nT) Signal samples
$j,k\ W_n$ nth sample of kth sifted version of a 2^j scaled discrete wavelet
N number of signal samples.

There are four thresholds frequently used, i.e., hard threshold, soft threshold, semi-soft threshold, and semi-hard threshold. The hard-thresholding function keeps the input if it is larger than the threshold, otherwise, it is set to zero. It is described as in Eq. (8)

$$\begin{aligned} f_h(x) &= x \quad \text{if}\, x \geq \lambda \\ &= 0 \quad \text{otherwise} \end{aligned} \tag{8}$$

The hard-thresholding function chooses all wavelet coefficients that are greater than the given threshold $\lambda\ \psi$ and sets the others to zero. The threshold λ is chosen according to the signal energy and the noise variance 2σ. If a wavelet coefficient is greater than λ, we assume that as significant and attribute it to the original signal. Otherwise, we consider it to be due to the additive noise and discard the value. The soft-thresholding function has a somewhat different rule from the hard-thresholding function. It shrinks the wavelet coefficients by $\lambda\ \psi$ toward zero, which is the reason why it is also called the wavelet shrinkage function. It is explained in Eq. (9) as:

$$\begin{aligned} f_s(x) &= x - \lambda \quad \text{if} x > \lambda \\ &= 0 \quad \text{if} x < \lambda \\ &= x + \lambda \quad \text{if} x \leq -\lambda \end{aligned} \tag{9}$$

The soft-thresholding rule is chosen over hard-thresholding, as the soft-thresholding method yields more visually pleasant images over hard-thresholding.

Then finally IDWT is calculated by Eq. (10)

$$s_n = \frac{1}{N} \sum_{j=0}^{log_2 N} \sum_{k=0}^{int(N/2^{j+1})} S_{j,k} j, kw_n \tag{10}$$

where
$j,\ kw_n$ nth sample of kth sifted version of a 2^j scaled discrete wavelet
J,k row index
n column index [8].

In our work we have used OTSU'S thresholding to denoise the image which chooses the threshold in such a way that all variances available in black and white pixels in the same signal are minimized.

level = graythresh (I) computes a global threshold (level) that can be used to convert an intensity image into a binary image with im2bw. level is a normalized intensity value that lies in the range [0, 1].

The graythresh function uses Otsu's method, which chooses the threshold to minimize the intraclass variance of the black and white pixels.

Multidimensional arrays are converted automatically in to 2D arrays using reshape. The graythresh function ignores any nonzero imaginary part of I.

[level EM] = graythresh (I) returns the effectiveness metric, EM, as the second output argument. The effectiveness metric is a value in the range [0 1] that indicates the effectiveness of the thresholding of the input image. The lower bound is attainable only by images having a single gray level, and the upper bound is attainable only by two-valued images.

Proposed Method

In this chapter we have taken the pure EEG signals having four samples that are then mixed with noise. The signal is processed with ICA and then further with wavelet denoise. ICA is applied so as to separate the signals from a multichannel source of signals and then wavelet denoising to remove noise from an independent component of the signal; we find that the final signal shows better artifacts removal as compared to simple filtering methods. The complete process is explained in the following algorithm:

Algorithm

1. Plot the EEG signal that is mixed with noise with respect to *j* and *k*.
2. Apply conventional filtering through Kurtosis that is defined by Eq. (5):

$$\mathrm{Kurt}(y) = E\{y^4\} - 3\left(E\{y^2\}\right)^2$$

3. Let the original signal be defined by X, then basic ICA model is expressed by Eq. (11)

$$X = AS + N \tag{11}$$

where,

A mixing matrix
S independent component
N noise added

4. To denoise the image using ICA we have to process the image. The preprocessing consists of two steps:

a. Centering: the signal is first centered, i.e., we substract the image mean from the noisy image. It is expressed mathematically as in Eq. (12):

$$X \leftarrow X - E\{X\} \tag{12}$$

b. Whitening: in whitening we remove the second order statistical dependence in the data, i.e., the whitened data have unit variance and they are uncorrelated. Let Z be zero mean random vector, then in terms of covariance matrix we can write

$$\mathrm{E}\left\{\mathrm{ZZ}^{\mathrm{T}}\right\} = \mathrm{I} \tag{13}$$

where I is identity matrix.
Finally whitened data Z is expressed by Eq. (14):

$$\mathrm{Z} = \mathrm{D}^{-1/2}.\mathrm{E}^{\mathrm{T}}.\mathrm{X} \tag{14}$$

where E is matrix whose columns are unit norm eigenvectors of covariance matrix.

$$\mathrm{C_X} = \mathrm{E}\left\{\mathrm{XX}^{\mathrm{T}}\right\} \tag{15}$$

D is diagonal matrix of eigenvalues of $\mathrm{C_X}$

5. Using the demixing matrix obtained above we obtain the mixing matrix A by the equation

$$\mathrm{A} = \text{ pseudoinverse } (\mathrm{w}) \tag{16}$$

6. Finally denoised image is obtained by the mixing matrix A and the independent component.
7. Then Otsu's thresholding is done and values below a certain threshold are set to zero.
8. This gives the whitened denoisd image. To reconstruct the image from this we add the mean to this image which was substracted earlier and multiply the whitening matrix to obtain the final denoised image.

Experimental Results

This section presents the evaluation of the proposed artifact removal technique. Initially, EEG signals are captured with occurrence of artifacts. Figure 4 shows the four samples of EEG signal that is effected through noise and artifacts. We defined *n* as the number of iterations and to plot our data to number of values to number of iteration we defined *j* and also *j* as the original matrix value of data and k defines the number of blocks available in data. Then Fig. 5 shows the result using ICA so as to find the independent component. Figure 6 is a result of signal after implementation of wavelet denoising on the signals of Fig. 5. From these figures, it has been observed that the proposed artifact removal technique results in better removal of artifacts. This will help in improving the performance of the further processing of this EEG signal.

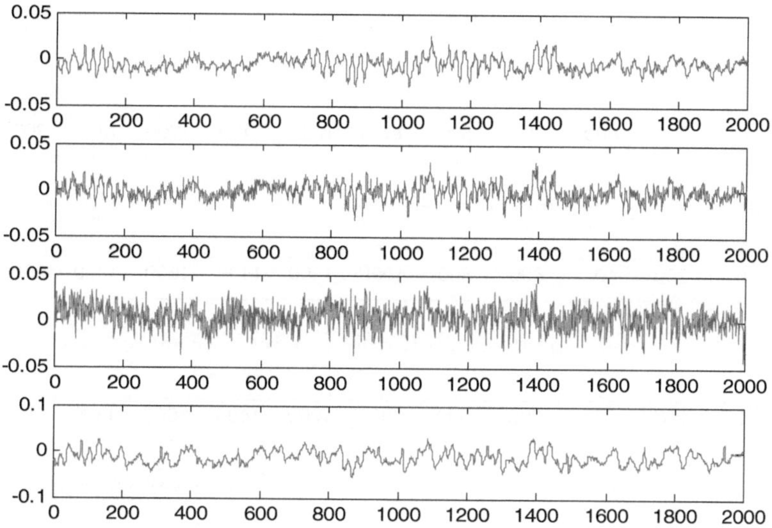

Fig. 4 EEG signal mixed with noise

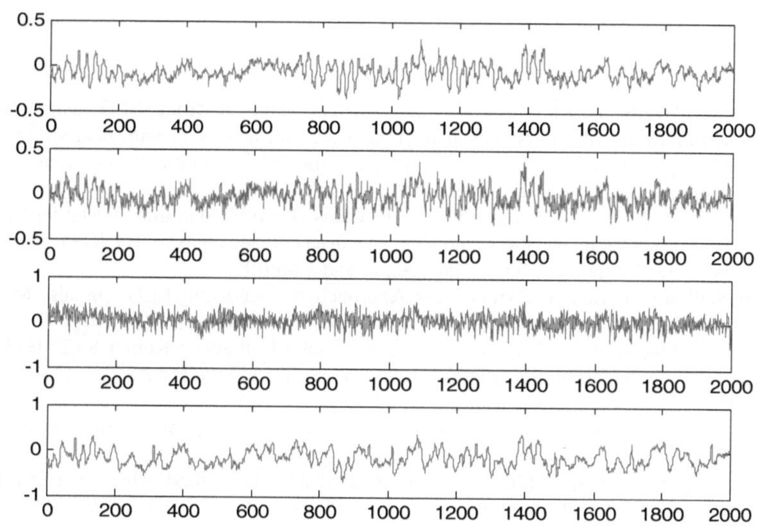

Fig. 5 EEG signal after applying independent component analysis

Here, from Fig. 6 we can conclude that artifacts and noise is removed from the original EEG signal to a great extent because of use of both methods ICA and wavelet denoising, which use Otsu's method for thresholding.

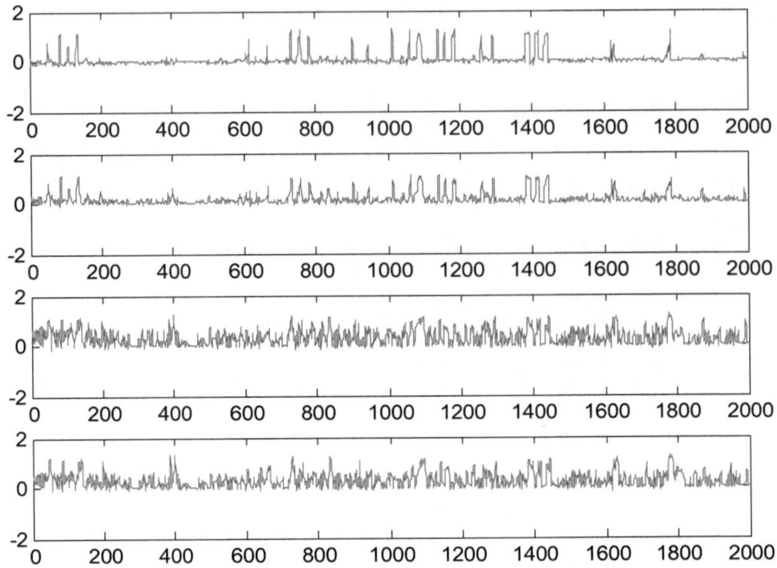

Fig. 6 EEG signal after applying ICA and wavelet denoising

References

1. Geethaa G, Geethalakshmia SN (2012) "Artifact removal from EEG using Spatially constrained independent component analysis and wavelet denoising with otsu's thresholding technique", International conference on communication technology and system design 2011, Procedia Engineering 30 (2012) 1064–1071
2. Romo Vázqueza R, Vélez-Péreza H, Rantab R, Louis Dorrb V, Maquinb D, Maillard L (2011) Blind source separation, wavelet denoising and discriminant analysis for EEG artifacts and noise cancelling, Biomedical Signal Processing and Control
3. Walters-Williams J, LiA Y (2011) New Approach to Denoising EEG Signals: Merger of Translation Invariant Wavelet and ICA. Int J Biometrics Bioinform 5(2):130–149
4. Khaparde A, Madhavilath M, Manasa MBL, Anil Babu P, Pradeep Kumar S (2008) FastICA Algorithm for the Separation of Mixed Images. Wseas Trans Sign Proces 4(5):271–277 ISSN: 1790-5052
5. Hyvarinen A, Oja E (1997) A fast fixed point algorithm for independent component analysis. Neural Comput 9(7):1483–1492
6. Hongqiao1 L, Shengqian W (2009) A new image denoising method using wavelet transform International forum on information technology and applications, vol 1. pp 111–114
7. Gonzalez RC, Elwood's R (1993) Digital Image Processing. Addison-Wesley, MA
8. Ellinas JN, Mandadelis T, Tzortzis A, Aslanoglou L (2004) "Image denoising using wavelets", T.E.I. of Piraeus Applied Research Review, vol IX. no.1 pp 97–109

Flowing Human Blood-Based Transistor

Mukta Bhatele, S. P. Kosta and P. Mor

Abstract For the first time, scientific investigation on the feasibility of "Flowing blood based electronic transistor" is presented. The effect of variables like blood temperature, blood flow rate, distance between the forming probes on the input/output characteristics as well as current gain factor β of the transistor is studied. Emerging applications of human blood electronic circuits toward medical science, specifically cyborg implants, human–machine interface, human disease detection/healing, human health sensors, and digital signal processing are visualized.

Keywords Flowing human blood · Input/output characteristics

Introduction

Human tissue blood electronic circuits have now become an interesting area of research in medical health care science. The Google search on "human blood liquid memristor" [1] presents rather global praiseworthy comments on our chapter **"Human blood liquid memristor"** [2]. The comments narrate the importance of human blood circuitry to cyborg implants/engineering, man–machine interfacing, human disease detection and healing, and artificial brain evolution.

M. Bhatele (✉)
Gyan-Ganga College of Science and Technology, Jabalpur, MP, India
e-mail: mukta_bhatele@rediffmail.com

S. P. Kosta
Charotar University of Science and Technology, Changa, India

P. Mor
Department of Electronics and Physics, Rani Durgawati University, Jabalpur, MP, India

V. Kumar and M. Bhatele (eds.), *Proceedings of All India Seminar on Biomedical Engineering 2012 (AISOBE 2012)*, Lecture Notes in Bioengineering,
DOI: 10.1007/978-81-322-0970-6_3,

Our research team has so far successfully developed [2–5] electronic passive (R, C, and L) and active component diodes along with some simple digital and analog circuits.

In this communication, we report realization of the flowing human blood transistor device. The effect of variables like blood temperature, blood flow rate, distance between the forming probes on the input and output characteristics as well as current gain factor β of the transistor is studied.

Physical Model of Flowing Human Blood-Based Transistor

The experimental setup comprises mechanical and electronic transistor architecture systems as under:

1. **Mechanical system**: Consists of a glass vessel (tank supported by a wooden stand) containing human blood (group B+), from where the blood flows through a capillary tube, which in turn passes through another glass vessel containing water. External water reservoir supplies water at desired temperatures to this vessel. This capillary tube is further extended horizontally through which the blood at desired temperature passes. The blood after passing through this horizontal capillary tube portion proceeds toward the sink vessel where it is collected. The height of the tank controls the blood flow rate (Fig. 1).
2. **Electronic transistor architecture**: The transistor has two diodes in back-to-back configuration, one formed by blood inserted set of two probes 1–2 and second, by blood inserted another set of two probes 3–4. The geometry and distance between forming diodes (set of two probes) as well as spacing between probes 2 and 3 play vital roles in the development of the transistor. The input circuit contains variable voltage power supply along with current measuring multimeter to realize voltage/current (V_{BE}, I_{BE}) between base and ammeter. Similarly, output circuit is realized by another variable voltage supply and resulting current (V_{CE}, I_{CE}), between collector and ammeter. The transistor manifested technically acceptable input and output characteristics of the device including the current gain factor β variation.

The effects of variable parameters of (1) temperature, (2) distance between probes 1–2–3–4, and (3) flow rate (drops/min) of the blood transistor were studied while conducting development of this transistor configuration.

Method of Measurement for Input/Output Characteristics

1. **For Input Characteristics**: Varying voltage V_{BE} between probes 1 and 2 was applied while keeping voltage V_{CE} between probes 3 and 4 constant. During

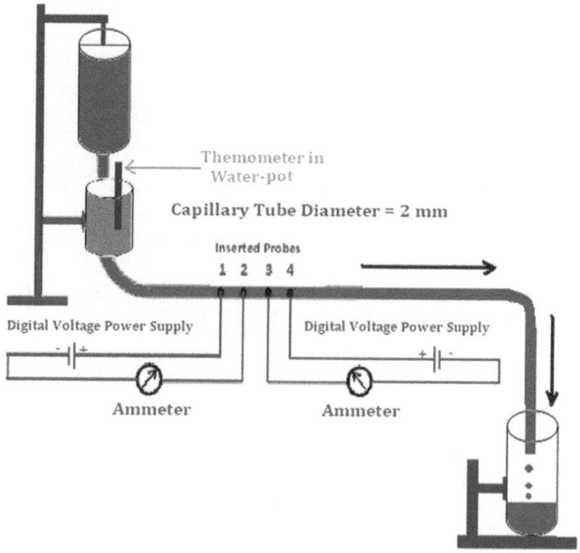

Fig. 1 Experimental setup for blood transistor development

this measurement, we kept fixed distance between inserted probes 1–2–3–4, flow rate constant, and also temperature of water pot. Observations were recorded. Graph 1 depicts a typical input characteristic of the transistor.

2. **For Output Characteristics**: Keeping fixed distance between probes 1–2–3–4, flow rate constant, and constant water pot temperature., varying voltage V_{CE} between probes 3 and 4 was applied while keeping voltage V_{BE} between probes 1 and 2 constant, observations were recorded. Graph 2 depicts typical output characteristics of the transistor.
3. **Effect of varying physical blood parameters**: Process of measurements under 1 and 2 was repeated to study the effect of variable parameters (1) temperature, (2) distance between probes 1–2–3–4, (3) flow rate (drops/min) of the blood transistor was considered while conducting development of this transistor configuration.
4. **On Data repeatability and error possibilities**: The readings for V_{BE}, V_{CE}, I_{BE}, and I_{CE} (after they stabilized) were repeatedly observed and recorded. Under any uncertainties, the readings (magnitude wise) were found to be repeatable within 5–10 %. The readings (depicting magnitudes) sometimes were vibrating but we took precaution and recorded their average. From an error analysis point of view, the accuracy was assured to remain within 10 % (measurement accuracy). By changing the height of the tank the blood flow rate variation was achieved.
5. Keeping brevity of manuscript in view, only representative typical graphs are presented to demonstrate the feasible functioning of the device developed.

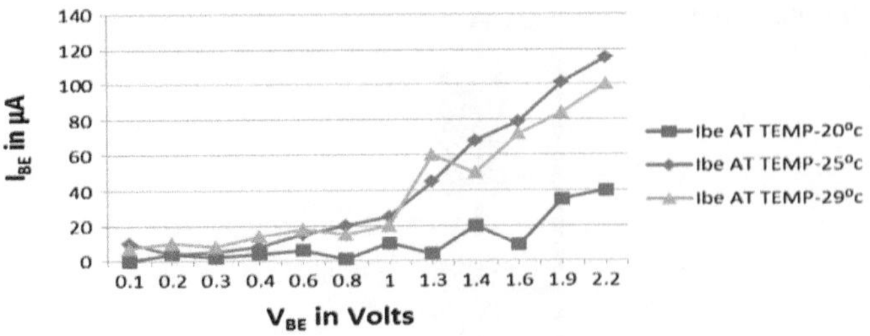

Graph 1 Input characteristics: human blood transistor (*flow mode*) spacing between probes D = 1.1.1.1, 40 drops/min, and V_{CE} = 1.5 V

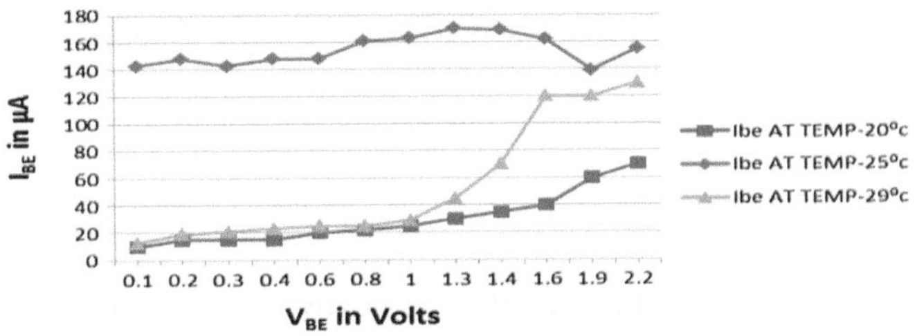

Graph 2 Output characteristics: human blood transistor spacing between probes D = 1.1.1.1, 40 drops/min, V_{BE} = 1.5 V

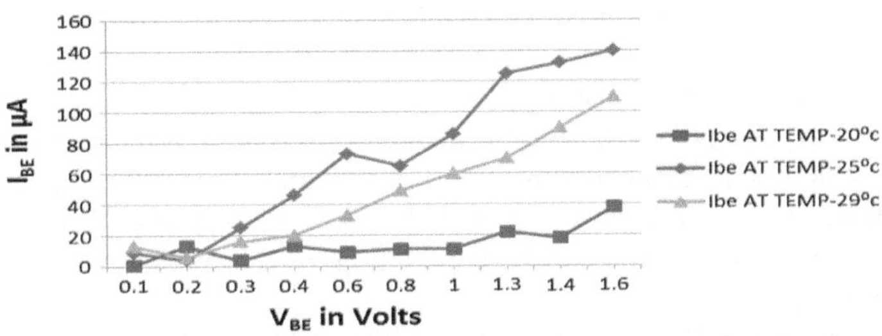

Graph 3 I/P characteristics of transistor spacing between probes D = 1.1.1.1, 40 drops/min, and V_{CE} = 3 V

The Measured Experimental Data with Remarks

The measured data is plotted in the graphs and graphs 1, 2, 3, 4, 5, 6, 7, and 8 depicts input and output characteristics of the transistor.

From the first order of approximation study of Graphs 1, 2, 3, 4, 5, 6, 7, and 8 the following inferences can be drawn:

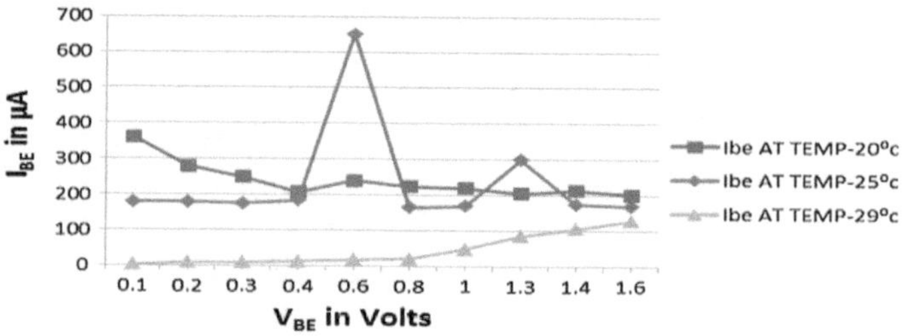

Graph 4 O/P characteristics of transistor (*flow mode*) spacing between probes D = 1.1.1.1, 40 drops/min, and $V_{BE} = 3$ V

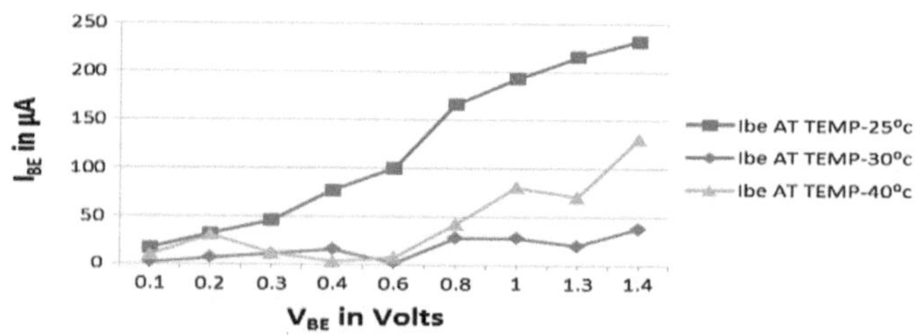

Graph 5 I/P characteristics of transistor spacing between probes D = 1.1.2.1, 60 drops/min, and $V_{CE} = 1.5$ V

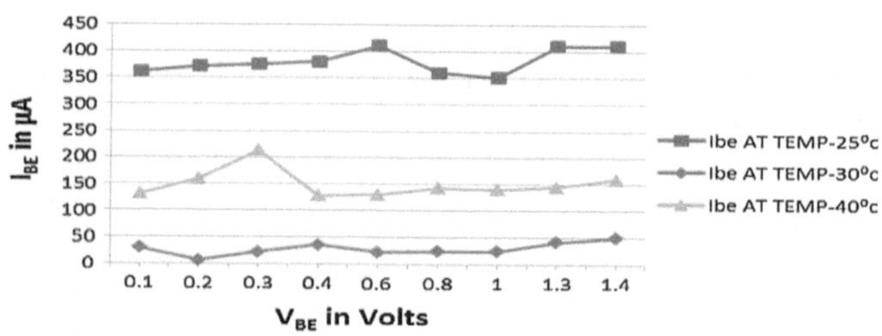

Graph 6 O/P characteristics of transistor spacing between probes D = 1.1.2.1, 60 drops/min, and $V_{BE} = 1.5$ V

1. The input characteristics of the transistor for 25, 40 °C have similarity with semiconductor transistor for distance (D = 1.1.1.1 mm), flowrate = 40 drops/min
2. The output characteristics of the transistor for 25, 40 °C have similarity with semiconductor transistor for distance (D = 1.1.1.1 mm), flowrate = 40 drops/min

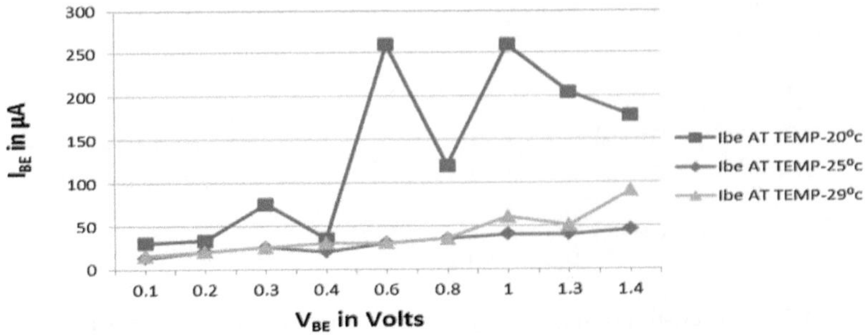

Graph 7 I/P characteristics of transistor spacing between probes D = 1.1.2.1, 60 drops/min, and $V_{\mathrm{CE}} = 3$ V

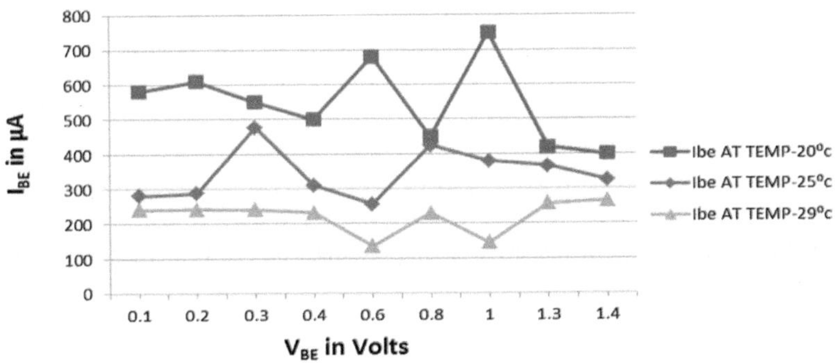

Graph 8 O/P characteristics of transistor spacing between probes D = 1.1.2.1, 60 drops/min, and $V_{\mathrm{BE}} = 3$ V

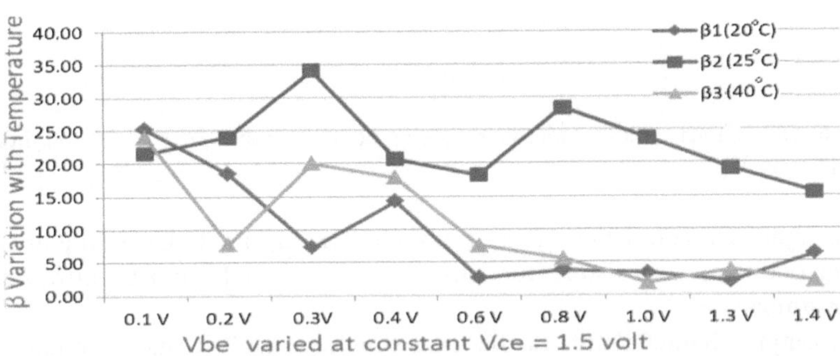

Graph 9 β-variation with blood temperature

Determination of Current Gain Factor

From the recorded tabular observations (Tables 9–11 not presented due to size limitations), the β was calculated ($\beta = I_{CE}/I_{BE}$) under various blood parameter variations and is depicted in a typical Graph 9.

Again, using the first order of approximation study of Graph 9 the following inference can be drawn: Typically, the variation of β for various blood variable conditions (nature wise) is similar to the conventional semiconductor transistor. Usually, β for semiconductor transistor ranges between 10 and 100.

Conclusions

Finally, it is philosophically concluded that under certain magnitudes of V_{BE}/V_{CE} bias conditions and appropriate pre-position of (1) distance between 1–2–3–4 probes, (2) temperature, and (3) flow rate, **the functioning of human blood transistor can be realized.** No attempts were made to optimize the transistor parameters as the study was **exploratory in nature.**

References

1. Google search on "Human blood liquid memristor" [1st week of April 2011]
2. Kosta SP, Bhatele M, Dubey YM, Gaur A, Kosta S et al (2011) Human blood liquid memristor. Int J Med Eng informatics 3:16–29
3. Kosta SP, Bhatele M, Dubey YM, Gaur A, Kosta S et al (2010) Novel Electronic device diode made from human blood. Int J Biomed Eng Consum Health Inf 2(1):7–13
4. Kosta SP, Kosta YP, Bhatele M, Dubey YM, Gaur A et al (2010) New applications of human blood electronic circuits for disease detection and healing ISSN: 2078-0273. J Med Biomed Sci 1(2):4–9
5. Kosta SP, Kosta YP, Bhatele M, Dubey YM, Gaur A, Kosta S et al (2011) Biological human tissue skin based memristor. Submitted to IEEE potential, New York

Endoscopic Treatment of Arachnoid Cyst

Y. R. Yadav, Vijay Parihar and Pushpraj Bhatele

Abstract *Introduction* The surgical options for symptomatic arachnoid cysts are shunting, endoscopic fenestration, and craniotomy with fenestration. The endoscopic procedure has been found to be minimally invasive, safe, and effective. Results of endoscopic treatment of 21 patients of arachnoid cyst in vicinity to cistern or ventricle are described. *Material and Methods* All except one of the symptomatic arachnoid cysts with raised intracranial pressure were operated by endoscopic procedure. One patient of convexity cyst without any adjoining cistern/ventricle was excluded from study. Gaab 6-degree rigid telescope was used. Burr hole was made keeping in mind the straight trajectory between the cyst and cistern/ventricle. A minimum of 1 cm hole was made in all the cases. Third ventriculostomy was also done for associated hydrocephalus in quadrigeminal arachnoid cyst. Both the procedures could be done by single burr hole placed about 3–4 cm anterior to coronal suture. *Results* This is a prospective study of 21 arachnoid cysts. There were 6, 8, 5, and 2 cases of vermian, quadrigeminal region, sylvian fissure region, and cerebello-pontine region arachnoid cyst respectively. Symptomatic improvement occurred in 20 cases, while one infant with quadrigeminal arachnoid cyst required a ventriculo-peritoneal (VP) shunt. There was no mortality or any other complication except 3 cases of CSF leak, which stopped in 7 days time in two cases. Third ventriculostomy was done in the same sitting in 8 cases of quadrigeminal region arachnoid cyst. Follow-up ranged from 6 to 54 months. *Conclusion* Endoscopic treatment of arachnoid cyst with an adjoining cistern or ventricle is safe and effective. Third ventriculostomy can be done in the same sitting.

Y. R. Yadav (✉) · V. Parihar
NSCB Medical College and MP MRI Centre, Jabalpur, Madhya Pradesh, India
e-mail: yadavyr@yahoo.co.in

P. Bhatele
Department of Neurosurgery and Radio diagnosis, NSCB Medical College and MP MRI Centre, Jabalpur, Madhya Pradesh, India

V. Kumar and M. Bhatele (eds.), *Proceedings of All India Seminar on Biomedical Engineering 2012 (AISOBE 2012)*, Lecture Notes in Bioengineering,
DOI: 10.1007/978-81-322-0970-6_4,

Keywords Arachnoid cyst · Neuro endoscopic · Endoscopic treatment

Introduction

The optimal surgical treatment for symptomatic arachnoid cysts is controversial. Therapeutic options include cyst shunting [1–5], endoscopic fenestration [6–11], and craniotomy for fenestration [12–14]. Endoscopy is having an increasingly prominent role in neurosurgery. The endoscopic procedure has been found to be minimally invasive, safe, and effective as compared to the traditional surgical craniotomy [15–20]. We are reporting our experience of endoscopic treatment of 21 arachnoid cysts.

Material and Methods

All the symptomatic patients of arachnoid cysts except one were operated by endoscopic procedure between Jan 2004 and Feb 2008. One patient of convexity cyst without any adjoining cistern/ventricle was managed by cystoperitoneal shunt was was excluded from study. There were a total of 21 patients. Detailed history and thorough physical examination was done. CT scans were done in all the cases. MRI scans were done in 19 cases. Gaab 6-degree rigid telescope (Karl Storz Germany) was used. Burr hole was placed at most superior point on the skull. This prevents entry of air in the cyst cavity. Presence of air in cyst cavity hampers proper visualization. Burr hole margins were drilled in such a way as to allow straight trajectory from the cyst to the cistern or the ventricle. Cruciate incision was made in the dura mater as small as possible but sufficient enough to pass a telescope. Hitch stitches taking dura mater and arachnoid cyst were applied to prevent separation of dura mater from bone. This also prevents separation of dura mater from cyst wall. Large-sized dural incision should be avoided as it allows entry of air which hampers proper endoscopic visualization. Cyst wall adjoining the cistern or the ventricle was coagulated and cut to make free communication taking care not to injure any vessel or cranial nerve. Communication between cyst and cistern is usually made parallel to the vessel or nerve. A minimum of 1 cm hole was made in all the patients.

Results

This was a prospective study of 21 arachnoid cysts. There were 14 male patients. There were 6 cases of inferior vermian region, 8 cases of quadrigeminal region, 5 of sylvian fissure region, and 2 of cerebello-pontine region cysts. Symptomatic improvement occurred in 20 cases after endoscopic treatment while one infant with quadrigeminal region arachnoid cyst required a ventriculo-peritoneal (VP) shunt. There was no mortality or any other complication except CSF leak in three patients. CSF leak stopped in two cases within 7 days' time. These patients required 2–3 ventricular taps. The third infant with quadrigeminal region arachnoid cyst required VP shunt. Hospital stay ranged from 4 to 12 days with an average of 5.4 days. Mean operating time was 50 min ranging from 40 to 90 min. The third ventriculostomy was done in the same sitting in 8 cases of quadrigeminal region arachnoid cysts; all these cases were associated with hydrocephalus. Both the procedures could be done by single burr hole placed about 3–4 cm anterior to coronal suture. There was gross ventriculomegaly in all these children. Minimum of 1 cm hole was made in all the cases taking care not to injure cranial nerve and vessel.

Discussion

The natural history and pathogenesis of arachnoid cyst remain poorly defined. Arachnoid cysts are commonly thought to arise from either congenital defects or trauma. There are reports of the spontaneous development of arachnoid cyst [6, 21]. Although most arachnoid cysts remain static fluid-filled compartments throughout life, some of them can be enlarged, exerting a mass effect on adjacent neural structures [22, 23]. There are reports of spontaneous disappearance of a suprasellar arachnoid cyst [24, 25]. These cysts may rupture producing subdural hygroma or chronic sub dura hematoma [26]. MR CSF flow imaging with a phase contrast cine sequence can be a reliable alternative to invasive CT cisternography for the functional evaluation of arachnoid cysts [27]. Optimal treatment guidelines are not yet established [24]. Alaani et al. [28] suggested a conservative management approach to the majority of these cysts as the cysts may not show change in size on repeated MRI scan and the patients' symptoms may not progress over the period of follow-up.

The preferred treatment for symptomatic arachnoid cysts is surgery. The indications for surgery are the presence of progressive hydrocephalus or intracranial hypertension [29]. The cystoperitoneal shunt was associated with clinical improvement in most cases [1]. Cysto ventricular shunting was also found to be simple as well as effective and reliable [2]. Shunt dependency and slit ventricle syndrome after cystoperitoneal shunting was found to be a real problem [5, 30, 31]. Insertion of an internal shunt from the cyst to the subdural compartment is also considered as a valuable alternative in the treatment of arachnoid cysts [3]. Arachnoid cysts can be successfully treated with a cystoperitoneal shunting with a programmable valve [4, 5]. Microsurgical keyhole fenestration was also found to be a safe and effective surgical procedure for the treatment of arachnoid cysts [12–14, 32]. Factors that influence outcome are the rate of volume reduction and cyst location [32]. Results are good if the cyst is in vicinity of the cistern/ventricle.

Endoscopic procedures were found to be safe and effective in our series also. Another advantage of this procedure is that third ventriculostomy can be done in the same sitting. In some cases hydrocephalus could be due to co-existing aqueductal stenosis, apart from the pressure due to cyst. Many researchers also advocated the endoscopic procedure as the primary procedure in arachnoid cysts in most cases because it is a minimally invasive procedure. The traditional surgical treatment can be performed without additional risk if endoscopic surgery fails [33–37]. Cerebro-spinal fluid leak was the only complication in this series. Results of endoscopic treatment of suprasellar arachnoid cysts were very good [38–45]. The outcome of endoscopic treatment of quadrigeminal cistern region arachnoid cyst was also good [46–48]. Similar good results in other location cysts like cerebello-pontine angle and posterior fossa cysts were also observed [28]. Abbott [49] and Strojnik [22] also predicted that most of the arachnoid cysts will be managed endoscopically in the future.

Endoscope-controlled microsurgery is a valid minimally invasive procedure for treating superficially located intracranial arachnoid cysts [50]. Arachnoid cyst can be successfully treated with the help of navigation. As the anatomical landmarks are not visible in some cases, navigated endoscopic procedures help in correct placement of communications between cyst and ventricle or cistern [38, 51].

Although endoscopic management of arachnoid cyst [6–11, 52], hydrocephalus [53–56], brain abscess [57, 58], intra ventricular hemorrhage [59], atlanto-axial dislocation [60], deep intra cerebral hematoma [61],and trigeminal neuralgia [62] is becoming the preferred and effective method because of its minimal invasive nature and safety, it also has some limitations. Normal anatomical landmarks are not visible, so the orientation may be a problem in some cases. Navigation is very helpful in such cases Follow-up is short in this study. This procedure may be possible if cyst is not in the vicinity to cistern or ventricle. Straight trajectory is needed for rigid scope, which may be difficult in some cases, to make communication between the cyst and cistern or the ventricle. This problem can be overcome by flexible endoscope. Air can enter inside the superficial cyst which may hamper proper visualization.

References

1. Gomez Escalonilla CI, Garcia Morales I, Galan Davila L, Gimenez-Torres MJ, Simon-Heras R, Valencia J, Mateos-Beato F (2001, 2002) Intracranial arachnoid cysts. A study of a series of 35 cases. Comment in: Rev Neurol 34(1):98, Rev Neurol 33(4):305–311
2. McBride LA, Winston KR, Freeman JE (2003) Cystoventricular shunting of intracranial arachnoid cysts. Pediatr Neurosurg 39(6):323–329
3. Helland CA, Wester K (2006) Arachnoid cysts in adults: long-term follow-up of patients treated with internal shunts to the subdural compartment. Surg Neurol. 66(1):56–61 (discussion 61)
4. Germano A, Caruso G, Caffo M, Baldari S, Calisto A, Meli F, Tomasello F (2003) The treatment of large supratentorial arachnoid cysts in infants with cyst-peritoneal shunting and Hakim programmable valve. Childs Nerv Syst 19(3):166–173 (Epub 2003 Feb 13)
5. Hamid NA, Sgouros S (2005) The use of an adjustable valve to treat over-drainage of a cyst-peritoneal shunt in a child with a large sylvian fissure arachnoid cyst. Childs Nerv Syst. 21(11):991–994 (Epub 2005 Jan 8)

6. Struck AF, Murphy MJ, Iskandar BJ (2006) Spontaneous development of a de novo suprasellar arachnoid cyst. Case report. J Neurosurg. 104(Suppl 6):426–428
7. Park SW, Yoon SH, Cho KH, Shin YS (2006) A large arachnoid cyst of the lateral ventricle extending from the supracerebellar cistern–case report. Surg Neurol 65(6):611–614
8. Mangano FT, Limbrick DD Jr, Leonard JR, Park TS, Smyth MD (2006) Simultaneous image-guided and endoscopic navigation without rigid cranial fixation: application in infants: technical case report. Neurosurgery 58(4 Suppl 2):ONS-E377 (discussion ONS-E377)
9. Nowoslawska E, Polis L, Kaniewska D, Mikolajczyk W, Krawczyk J, Szymanski W, Zakrzewski K, Podciechowska J, Polis B (2006) Neuroendoscopic techniques in the treatment of arachnoid cysts in children and comparison with other operative methods. Childs Nerv Syst 22(6):599–604 (Epub 2006 Mar 21)
10. Greenfield JP, Souweidane MM (2005) Endoscopic management of intracranial cysts. Neurosurg Focus 19(6):E7
11. Hagebeuk EE, Kloet A, Grotenhuis JA, Peeters EA (2005) Bobble-head doll syndrome successfully treated with an endoscopic ventriculocystocisternostomy. J Neurosurg 103(Suppl 3):253–259
12. Ozgur BM, Aryan HE, Levy ML (2005) Microsurgical keyhole middle fossa arachnoid cyst fenestration. J Clin Neurosci 12(7):804–806
13. Levy ML, Wang M, Aryan HE, Yoo K, Meltzer H (2003, 2005) Microsurgical keyhole approach for middle fossa arachnoid cyst fenestration. Comment in: Neurosurgery 53(5):1138–44 (discussion 1144–5), Neurosurgery 56(5):E1166 (author reply E1166)
14. Prat R, Galeano I, Conde FJ, Febles P (2003) Multiseptated arachnoid cyst treated with fenestration after valvular insufficiency in an adult. Neurocirugia (Astur) 14(2):149–151
15. Pulido-Rivas P, Villarejo-Ortega FJ, Cordobes-Tapia F, Pascual Martin-Gamero A, Perez-Diaz C (2005) Surgical treatment of symptomatic arachnoid cysts in children. Rev Neurol 41(7):385–390
16. Di Rocco F, Yoshino M, Oi S (2005) Neuroendoscopic transventricular ventriculocystostomy in treatment for intracranial cysts. J Neurosurg 103(Suppl 1):54–60
17. Dwarakanath S, Suri A, Mahapatra AK, Mehta VS, Gaikwad S, Sarkar C (2006) Endoscopic assisted excision of a retroclival arachnoid cyst presenting as hysterical breathlessness. Childs Nerv Syst 4:424–427 (Epub 2005 Jul 29)
18. Chernov MF, Kamikawa S, Yamane F, Hori T (2004) Double-endoscopic approach for management of convexity arachnoid cyst: case report. Surg Neurol. 61(5):483–486 (discussion 486–7)
19. Nomura S, Akimura T, Imoto H, Nishizaki T, Suzuki M (2002) Endoscopic fenestration of posterior fossa arachnoid cyst for the treatment of presyrinx myelopathy–case report. Neurol Med Chir (Tokyo) 42(10):452–454
20. Schonherr B, Wolf O, Meier U (2002) Endoscopy of intracranial cysts in the adult patient. Minim Invasive Neurosurg 45(3):181–184
21. Iglesias-Pais M, Gelabert-Gonzalez M, Lopez-Garcia E, Allut AG, Fernandez-Villa JM, Gonzalez-Garcia J, Rumbo RM (2003) De novo arachnoid cyst treated with a cystoperitoneal shunt. Rev Neurol 36(12):1149–1152
22. Strojnik T (2006) Different approaches to surgical treatment of arachnoid cysts. Wien Klin Wochenschr 118(Suppl 2):85–88
23. Rao G, Anderson RC, Feldstein NA, Brockmeyer DL (2005) Expansion of arachnoid cysts in children: report of two cases and review of the literature. J Neurosurg 102(Suppl 3):314–317
24. Moon KS, Lee JK, Kim JH, Kim SH (2006) Spontaneous disappearance of a suprasellar arachnoid cyst: case report and review of the literature. Childs Nerv Syst 23(1):99–104 (Epub 2006 Aug 30)
25. Pandey P, Tripathi M, Chandra PS, Singh VP, Mehta VS (2001) Spontaneous decompression of a posterior fossa arachnoid cyst: a case report. Pediatr Neurosurg 35(3):162–163
26. Mori K, Yamamoto T, Horinaka N, Maeda M (2002) Arachnoid cyst is a risk factor for chronic subdural hematoma in juveniles: twelve cases of chronic subdural hematoma associated with arachnoid cyst. J Neurotrauma 19(9):1017–1027

27. Yildiz H, Erdogan C, Yalcin R, Yazici Z, Hakyemez B, Parlak M, Tuncel E (2005) Evaluation of communication between intracranial arachnoid cysts and cisterns with phase-contrast cine MR imaging. AJNR Am J Neuroradiol 26(1):145–151
28. Alaani A, Hogg R, Siddiq MA, Chavda SV, Irving RM (2005) Cerebellopontine angle arachnoid cysts in adult patients: what is the appropriate management? J Laryngol Otol 119(5):337–341
29. Gelabert-Gonzalez M (2004) Intracranial arachnoid cysts. Rev Neurol 39(12):1161–1166
30. Kim SK, Cho BK, Chung YN, Kim HS, Wang KC (2002, 2003) Shunt dependency in shunted arachnoid cyst: a reason to avoid shunting. Comment in: Pediatr Neurosurg 37(4):178–85, Pediatr Neurosurg 38(3):164
31. Sunami K, Saeki N, Sunada S, Hoshi S, Murai H, Kubota M, Takanashi J, Yamaura A (2002) Slit ventricle syndrome after cyst-peritoneal shunting for temporal arachnoid cyst in children–a clinical entity difficult to detect on neuroimaging study. Brain Dev 24(8):776–779
32. Kandenwein JA, Richter HP, Borm W (2004) Surgical therapy of symptomatic arachnoid cysts—an outcome analysis. Acta Neurochir (Wien) 146(12):1317–1322 (discussion 1322. Epub 2004 Sep 13)
33. Kirollos RW, Javadpour M, May P, Mallucci C (2001) Endoscopic treatment of suprasellar and third ventricle-related arachnoid cysts. Childs Nerv Syst 17(12):713–718 (Epub 2001 Nov 1)
34. Hinojosa J, Esparza J, Munoz MJ, Valencia J (2001) Endoscopic treatment of suprasellar arachnoid cysts. Neurocirugia (Astur) 12(6):482–488 (discussion 489)
35. Utsunomiya A, Narita N, Jokura H (2001) [Treatment of symptomatic convexity arachnoid cyst in the elderly by neuroendoscope assisted-stereotactic surgery: a case report. No To Shinkei 53(11):1039–1042
36. Nakamura Y, Mizukawa K, Yamamoto K, Nagashima T (2001) Endoscopic treatment for a huge neonatal prepontine-suprasellar arachnoid cyst: a case report. Pediatr Neurosurg 35(4):220–224
37. Fitzpatrick MO, Barlow P (2001) Endoscopic treatment of prepontine arachnoid cysts. Br J Neurosurg 15(3):234–238
38. Van Beijnum J, Hanlo PW, Han KS, Ludo Van der Pol W, Verdaasdonk RM, Van Nieuwenhuizen O (2006) Navigated laser-assisted endoscopic fenestration of a suprasellar arachnoid cyst in a 2-year-old child with bobble-head doll syndrome. Case report. J Neurosurg 104(Suppl 5):348–351
39. Golash A, Mitchell G, Mallucci C, May P, Pilling D (2001) Prenatal diagnosis of suprasellar arachnoid cyst and postnatal endoscopic treatment. Childs Nerv Syst 17(12):739–742 (Epub 2001 May 17)
40. Fujimura J, Shima Y, Arai H, Ogawa R, Fukunaga Y (2006) Management of a suprasellar arachnoid cyst identified using prenatal sonography. J Clin Ultrasound 34(2):92–94
41. Charalampaki P, Filippi R, Welschehold S, Conrad J (2005) Endoscopic and endoscope-assisted neurosurgical treatment of suprasellar arachnoidal cysts (Mickey Mouse cysts). Minim Invasive Neurosurg 48(5):283–288
42. Sood S, Schuhmann MU, Cakan N, Ham SD (2005) Endoscopic fenestration and coagulation shrinkage of suprasellar arachnoid cysts: technical note. J Neurosurg 102(Suppl 1):127–133
43. Wang JC, Heier L, Souweidane MM (2004) Advances in the endoscopic management of suprasellar arachnoid cysts in children. Erratum in: J Neurosurg 100(Suppl 5 Pediatrics):418–26, J Neurosurg 101(Suppl 1):123
44. Fioravanti A, Godano U, Consales A, Mascari C, Calbucci F (2004) Bobble-head doll syndrome due to a suprasellar arachnoid cyst: endoscopic treatment in two cases. Childs Nerv Syst 20(10):770–773
45. Melikian G, Arutiunov NV, Melnikov AV (2003) Unusual intraventricular herniation of the suprasellar arachnoid cyst and its successful endoscopic management. Minim Invasive Neurosurg 46(2):113–116
46. Gangemi M, Maiuri F, Colella G, Magro F (2005) Endoscopic treatment of quadrigeminal cistern arachnoid cysts. Minim Invasive Neurosurg 48(5):289–292

47. Hayashi N, Hamada H, Umemura K, Kurosaki K, Kurimoto M, Endo S (2005) Selection of surgical approach for quadrigeminal cistern arachnoid cyst. No Shinkei Geka 33(5):457–465
48. Ohba S, Ichikizaki K (2003) Endoscopic ventriculo-cystomy for non-communicating hydrocephalus secondary to quadrigeminal cistern arachnoid cyst. Acta Neurol Scand 107(1):67–71
49. Abbott R (2004) The endoscopic management of arachnoidal cysts. Neurosurg Clin N Am 15(1):9–17
50. Godano U, Mascari C, Consales A, Calbucci F (2004) Endoscope-controlled micro neurosurgery for the treatment of intracranial fluid cysts. Childs Nerv Syst 20(11–12):839–841 (Epub 2004 Jun 5)
51. Selden NR, Durham SR, Anderson GJ, Braner DA (2005) Intracranial navigation using a novel device for endoscope fixation and targeting: technical innovation. Pediatr Neurosurg 41(5):233–236
52. Yadav YR, Parihar V, Sinha M, Jain N (2010) Endoscopic treatment of supra sellar arachnoid cyst. Neurol India 58:280–282
53. Yadav YR, Jaiswal S, Adam N, Basoor A, Jain G (2006) Endoscopic third ventriculostomy in infants. Neurol India 54(2):161–163
54. Yadav YR, Mukerji G, Parihar V, Sinha M, Pandey S (2009) Complex hydrocephalus (combination of communicating and obstructive type): an important cause of failed endoscopic third ventriculostomy. BMC Res Notes 2(1):137
55. Yadav YR, Parihar V, Agrawal M, Bhatele PR (2011) Endoscopic third ventriculostomy in tubercular meningitis with hydrocephalus. Neurol India 59:855–860
56. Yadav YR, Parihar V, Pande S, Namdev H, Agarwal M (2012) Endoscopic third ventriculostomy: review. J Neurosci Rural pract 3:163–173
57. Gajdhar M, Yadav YR (2005) A case of thalamic abscess treated by endoscopic surgery. Neurol India 53:345–346
58. Yadav YR, Sinha M, Neha, Parihar V (2008) Endoscopic management of brain abscesses. Neurol India 56(1):13–16
59. Yadav YR, Mukerji G, Shenoy R, Basoor A, Jain G, Nelson A (2007) Endoscopic management of hypertensive intraventricular haemorrhage with obstructive hydrocephalus. BMC Neurol 4(7):1
60. Yadav YR, Shenoy R, Mukerji G, Sherekar S, Parihar V (2010) Endoscopic transoral excision of odontoid process in irreducible atlanto-axial dislocation. In: Banerji APD (ed) Progress in clinical neurosciences, vol 24. Byword Books Private Limited, New Delhi, pp 118–128. ISBN ISBN 818193055X, ISBN13: 9788181930552
61. Yadav YR, Yadav S, Sherekar S, Parihar V (2011) A new minimally invasive tubular brain retractor system for microendoscopic removal of deep brain lesions. Neurol India 59:74–77
62. Yadav YR, Parihar V, Agarwal M, Sherekar S, Bhatele PR (2011) Endoscopic vascular decompression of the trigeminal nerve. Minim Invasive Neurosurg 54(3):110–114

Three-Dimensional Finite Element Analysis of Human Femur: A Comparative Study

Amrita Francis, Raji Nareliya and Veerendra Kumar

Abstract Three-dimensional finite element analysis (FEA) is widely used to generate reliable subject-specific finite element (FE) model using computed tomography (CT) data that accurately predicts information about bone morphology and tissue density. FEA provides detailed information regarding displacement, stress, and strain distributions along the entire bone. CT scan data is widely used to make realistic investigations on the mechanical behavior of bone structures. The purpose of this paper is to create anatomically accurate, three-dimensional finite element models of the right human femur of three male patients of different age groups of 17, 32, and 40 years, respectively, using CT scan data, loaded by physiologic forces, i.e., half-body weight. An average body weight of 70 kg (686.7 N) is assumed for this study, which is shared equally by the lower limbs according to the hip mechanism; hence, a load of 343.35 N (half-body weight analysis of this model will provide data unavailable at this time to orthopedic surgeons, engineers, and researchers) is applied on each right human proximal femur that affects femur during weight bearing action at different angles and to determine the total deformation, equivalent Von-Mises Stress distribution, maximum principal stress distribution, and fatigue tool throughout the whole femur and comparing the results of human orthopedics.

A. Francis (✉) · V. Kumar
Government Engineering College, Jabalpur, Madhya Pradesh, India
e-mail: amrita.francis21@gmail.com

V. Kumar
e-mail: prof.veerendra.kumar@gmail.com

R. Nareliya
Hitkarni College of Engineering and Technology, Jabalpur, Madhya Pradesh, India
e-mail: raji_nareliya@yahoo.co.in

V. Kumar and M. Bhatele (eds.), *Proceedings of All India Seminar on Biomedical Engineering 2012 (AISOBE 2012)*, Lecture Notes in Bioengineering,
DOI: 10.1007/978-81-322-0970-6_5, © Springer India 2013

Keywords Computed tomography · Finite element analysis · Human femur

Introduction

The femur is the thigh bone and the most important component of the lower limb, extending from the hip to the knee. It is the heaviest, longest, and strongest bone of the human body. Being an important structure, it serves two distinct functions: (1) acts as a supporting structure allowing the weight of the upper body to be transferred from the hip joint to the knee joint and (2) also acts as a stiff structure about which muscles act to facilitate movement at both the hip and knee joints. Koch was the first to give a complete and thorough description of the structure of the femur, and demonstrated the relations which exist between the structure and the function as well as between the external and internal architecture of the femur [1]. Macroscopically, the structure of the femur is of two types: (1) cortical or compact bone which is a dense outer layer mainly resisting bending and (2) cancellous or spongy or trabecular bone present in the interior of mature bones mainly resisting compression and bone elements placing or displacing themselves in the direction of functional pressure according to Wolff's Law [2]. The shape of the femur is asymmetric and curved in all three planes. Hence, a three-dimensional model is required for a quantitative stress analysis [3, 4]. With minor modifications, computed tomography (CT) scans of finite element (FE) models can be used to generate reliable subject-specific FE models that accurately predict strains in quasi-axial loading configurations [5–8]. A thorough understanding and behavior of the femur is essential to elucidate the femur fracture and provide better guidance to artificial femur replacement. Various works have been carried out to investigate the loading mode and stress distribution [9, 10]. For better understanding of femoral loading forces exerted by both the soft and hard tissues of the thigh, a 3D model is created taking into account all thigh muscles, body weight, contact forces at the hip, and patello-femoral and knee joints [11–14]. A mathematical model is developed to simulate 3D femur bone and femur bone with implant in the femoral canal, taking into account stress distribution and total displacement during horizontal walking [15]. Material properties of femur bones are evaluated to facilitate further study of total hip joint and replacement of joints in Indian subjects, as these properties are needed before finite element analysis (FEA) of indigenized hip joint to study its stability in the bone [16, 17]. The role of ante version in transferring the load from implant to bone and its influence on total hip arthroplasty (THA) is determined. In addition, loading of the proximal femur during daily activity, i.e., walking and stair climbing is determined. Experimental and analytical approaches are used to determine the in vivo loading of the hip joint. A numerical muscular skeleton model is validated against measured in vivo hip contact force [12, 18].

Materials and Methods

A quantitative assessment of femur stresses under physiologic conditions is essential for the understanding of failure mechanisms and providing guidance for the design and operation of femur replacement. Three-dimensional FE models are created using CT images in materialized interactive medical image control systems (MIMICS) and then its surface mesh is created in MIMICS after which this surface mesh is converted into volumetric mesh in ABAQUS and assigned material properties to these models in MIMICS, and finally transferred into ANSYS for FEA under physiological loading conditions where total deformation, stress distribution, and fatigue tools are obtained throughout the femur.

Image Acquisition

The CT data of total femur of normal individual male patients of 17, 32, and 40 years are collected. This geometrical data of real proximal human femur bone is in the form of digital imaging and communications in medicine (DICOM) file. The CT scanning of patient is obtained using GE Ultrafast High Resolution Multislice CT Scanner (16 Slice) containing a total number of 909, 667, and 1,714 images, respectively, pixel size of 0.7031, 0.8867, and 0.9766 mm, respectively, slice thickness of 0.4 mm, and resolution of 512 × 512. DICOM file is a standard for handling, storing, printing, and transmitting information in medical imaging and contains binary data elements. In MIMICS, distinctive CT images are a pixel map of the linear X-ray attenuation coefficient of tissue. The pixel values are scaled so that the linear X-ray attenuation coefficient of air equals −1,024 and that of water equals 0. This scale is called the Hounsfield scale after Godfrey Hounsfield, one of the pioneers in CT. Using this scale, fat is around −110, muscle is around 40, trabecular bone is in the range of 100–300, and cortical bone extends above trabecular bone to about 2,000. The pixel values are shown graphically by a set of gray levels that vary linearly from black to white. MIMICS displays CT images using up to 256 gray levels of the display setting.

Geometric Modeling/Image Segmentation

For this comparative study, we have created three models of right femur of male human patients: Model 1 of a 17-year-old male, Model 2 of a 32-year-old male, and Model 3 of a 40-year-old male. MIMICS is an interactive tool for the visualization and segmentation of CT images as well as MRI images and 3D rendering of objects. Therefore, in the medical field MIMICS is used for diagnostic, operation planning, or rehearsal purposes. Figure 1 shows the image of a normal individual total femur

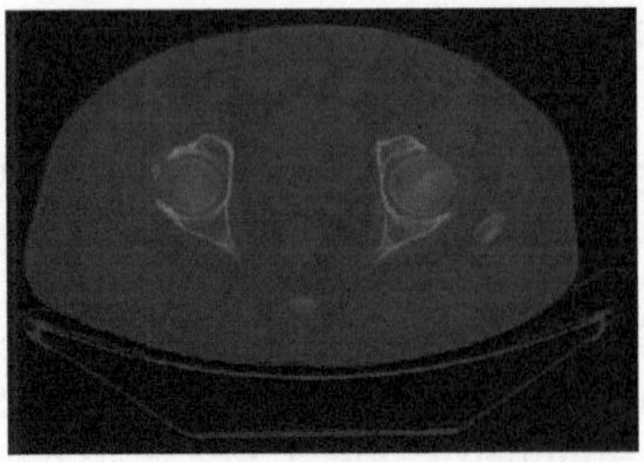

Fig. 1 The transverse section of total femur CT image

as acquired from the DICOM file images after conversion into MIMICS v10. Bone tissue is then extracted by means of thresholding using default values that range from 226 to 3,071 HU. The extracted bone tissue is put into a mask of volume 1,761,508.9874, 1,560,018.1976, and 1,841,722.1204 mm^3, respectively, and the number of pixels as 2,850,426, 1,984,073, and 3,089,900 pixels, respectively. These pixels in the masks are modified using various tools successively: edit masks, region growing, and calculation of 3D mask. Edit mask is used to separate the total femur from the adjoining hard tissues like pelvis, tibia, etc. The region growing tool provides the capacity to split the segmentation into separate masks with the following properties:

Model 1—minimum −238 to maximum 1,695 HU, number of pixels 143,227, and mask volume 88511.5585 mm^3,
Model 2—minimum −150 to maximum 1,630 HU, number of pixels 492,348, and mask volume 387118.7399 mm^3,
Model 3—minimum −118 to maximum 1,744 HU, number of pixels 445,600, and mask volume 265598.0377 mm^3, respectively.

Calculate 3D from mask tool converts the 2-Dimensional images into 3D models using an interpolation algorithm embedded in MIMICS as shown in Fig. 2, with the following properties of different models:

Model 1—mask volume 102228.88 mm^3, surface 26172.09 mm^2, triangles 42,360, and points 21,230,
Model 2—mask volume 471921.39 mm^3, surface 134009.90 mm^2, triangles 140,502, and points 69,989,
Model 3—mask volume 328208.31 mm^3, surface 115704.15 mm^2, triangles 146,142, and points 72,871.

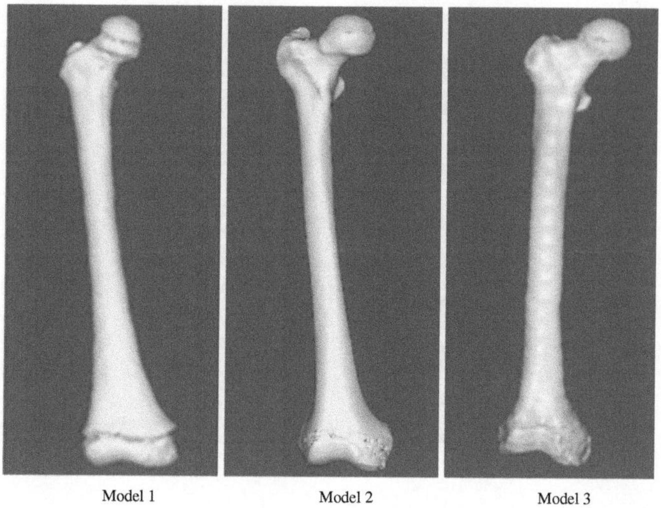

Fig. 2 Three-dimensional models of proximal femur

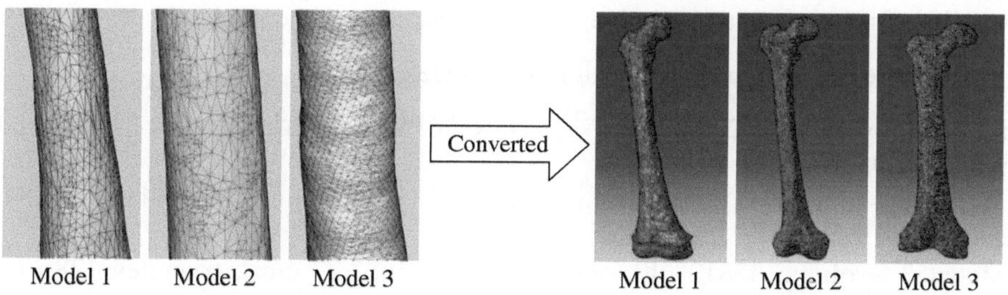

Fig. 3 Surface mesh in MIMICS converted into volumetric mesh in ABAQUS for all models of femur

Creation of FE Model

After creating 3D models in MIMICS, surface mesh is generated as shown in Fig. 3; for femur bone models for further FEA. FEA remeshing is a tool in MIMICS that allows us to create surface mesh of 3D models. In automatic remeshed operation, surface mesh of equilateral triangle is generated. All parameters are optimized here by optimize-based method using the ratio of the height of the triangle and the length of its base with quality parameter value above the maximum threshold of 0.3. The various other actions performed in FEA remeshing are:

- Triangle reduction of models normally.
- Improving qualities of the triangles.
- Triangle reduction of models preserving quality.

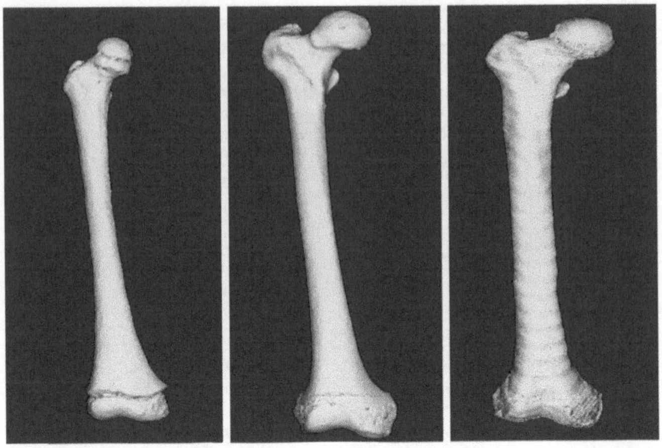

Model 1 Model 2 Model 3

Fig. 4 Volumetric meshed models in MIMICS

- Removal of extra shells.
- Self-intersection test to eliminate intersecting triangles completely.

Properties after remeshing of different models:

Model 1—volume 102094.20 mm^3, surface 26160.67 mm^2, triangles 23,816, and points 11,952,
Model 2—volume 471900.53 mm^3, surface 133994.83 mm^2, triangles 125,884, and points 62,644,
Model 3—volume 328123.40 mm^3, surface 115667.27 mm^2, triangles 128,374, and points 63,953.

These models are now imported in ABAQUS 6.10 to convert surface mesh into volumetric mesh. In mesh tool, choosing edit mesh category and then selecting convert tri to tetra generates volumetric meshed models. This volumetric meshing converts triangular elements of surface mesh into four-node linear tetrahedron elements (C3D4). The three models are meshed with the following number of 3D tetrahedron elements: 268,858, 959,083, and 809,524, respectively. Figure 3 shows volumetric meshed models of femur in ABAQUS. From ABAQUS, these volumetric meshed models are again imported into MIMICS for material assignment. Figure 4 shows volumetric meshed models after they are imported in MIMICS.

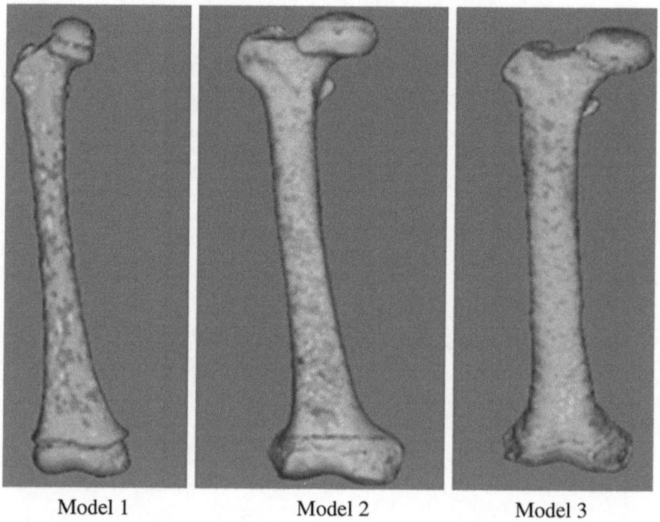

Fig. 5 The 3D model of proximal femurs after assigning material properties

Material Assignment

Femur is a complicated structured material composed of compact bone and cancellous bone. The compact bone is anisotropic material, while cancellous bone can be considered as isotropic material. Thus, it is difficult to assign material properties along each direction of bone model. In our study, material is assigned to all the models using MIMICS. In MIMICS, there are three ways to assign material properties: uniform, look-up file, and mask. We have considered the uniform method for realistic material assignment to each model using MIMICS. In this study, ten materials are assigned to each model and gray values are calculated for each material before realistic material assignment. Figure 5 shows all three models assigned with materials in MIMICS.

FE Analysis

The 3D FE Models of femur bone with volumetric mesh and realistic material assigned are imported into ANSYS v14. Since the femur bone models are nonlinear, asymmetric, and curved in all three planes, models are first imported in FE Modeler and then transferred to static structural module in ANSYS for FEA.

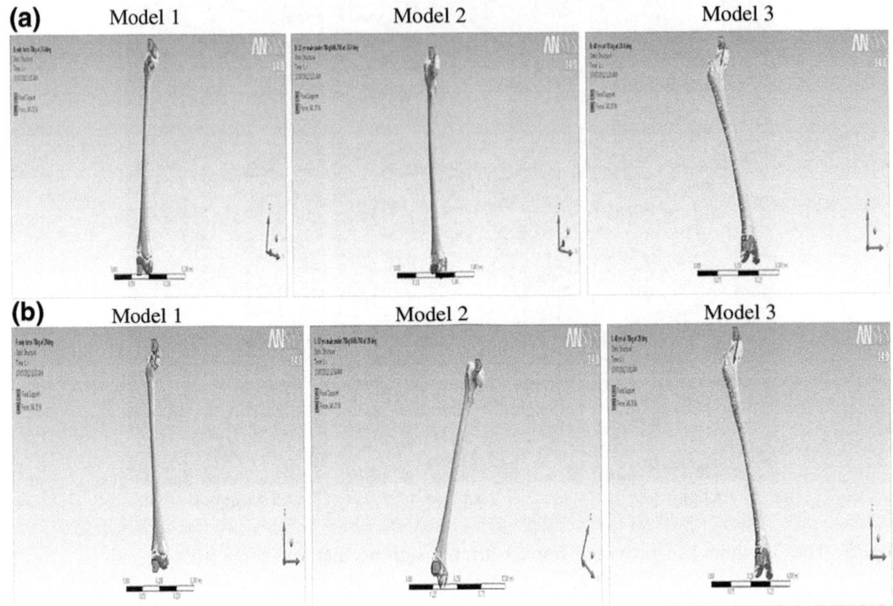

Fig. 6 **a** Load of 343.35 N acting at the head of right proximal femurs at 24.4°. **b** Load of 343.35 N acting at the head of right proximal femurs at 28°

Boundary Conditions

The femur is a thigh bone and both the left and right femurs in an individual human shares the whole body weight equally . Thus, in this study a constant body weight of 70 kg (686.7 N) is shared equally by both femurs [10]. Therefore, a load of 343.35 N is applied on the right femur head of every model at an angle of 24.4 and 28° for comparative study [10, 19, 20] and a fixed support is provided at lateral condyle, medial condyle, and patellar surface in every model. The boundary conditions are as shown in Fig. 6a, b.

Results

The total deformation, equivalent Von Mises stress, and maximum principal stress evaluated in the 3D FEA are shown Figs. 7, 8, and 9. A constant Fatigue life of 1e6 is obtained throughout the whole femur for all models of 17, 32, and 40-year-human male patients. The safety factor evaluated for each model is shown in Fig. 10. The comparative study shows the percentage variation in each model under study as shown in Table 1.

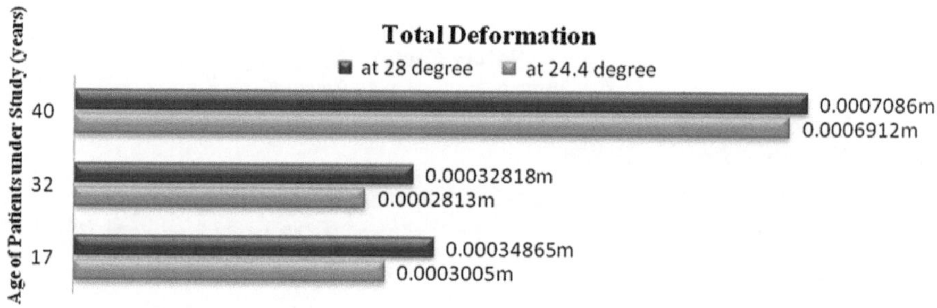

Fig. 7 Total deformation for 343.35 N acting at the head of right proximal femur of male patients at 24.4 and 28°

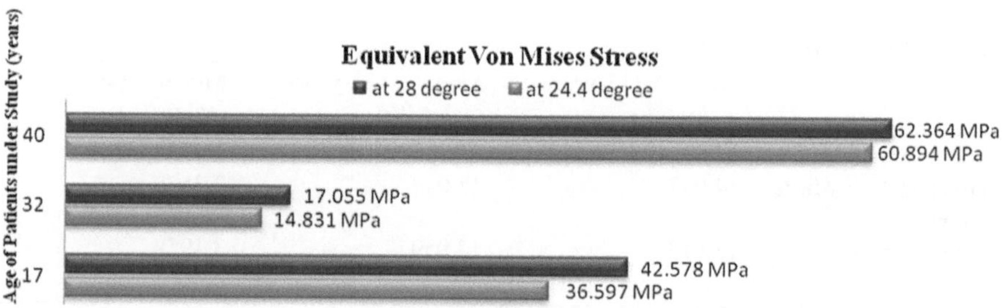

Fig. 8 Equivalent Von Mises stress for 343.35 N acting at the head of right proximal femur of male patients at 28 and 24°

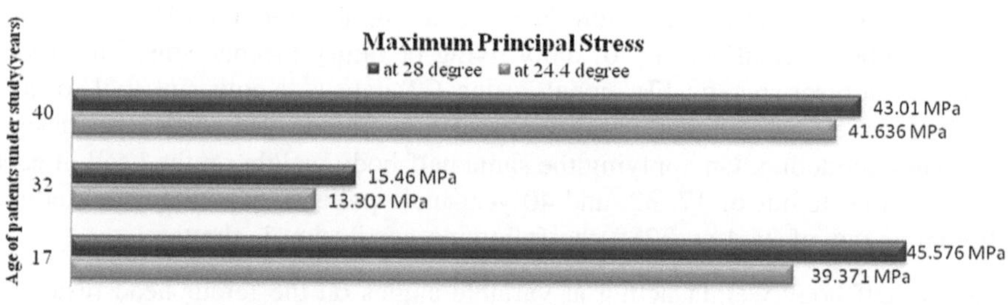

Fig. 9 Maximum principal stress for 343.35 N acting at the head of right proximal femur of male patients at 28 and 24°

Discussion and Conclusion

Patient-specific FE models generated from CT data have become of interest because of their high potential in clinical practice. Although automatic mesh generators may provide good and fast geometrical representation of bones, the determination of their cortical/trabecular subdomains and associated material properties is still one of the major difficulties in making these FE models reliable enough for clinical applications. Moreover, relatively fewer experimental and

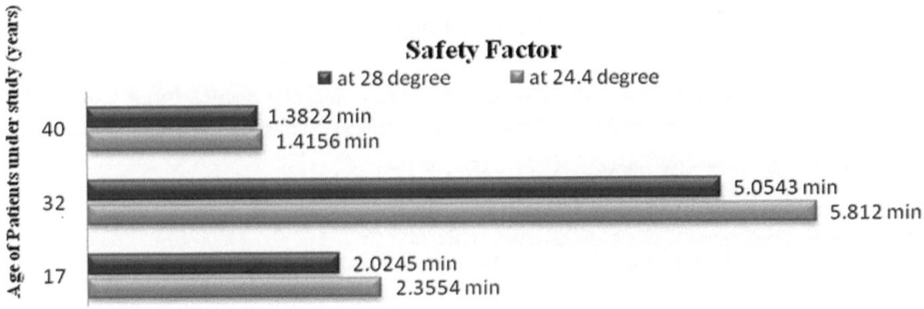

Fig. 10 Safety factor for 343.35 N acting at the head of right proximal femur of male patients at 28 and 24°

Table 1 Comparison of results

	Model 1 (17-year-male) (%)	Model 2 (32-year-male) (%)	Model 3 (40-year-male) (%)
Total deformation	13.81	14.285	2.455
Equivalent Von Mises stress	14.047	13.04	2.357
Maximum principal stress	13.615	13.959	3.195

computational studies have evaluated the intact whole femur's overall stiffness, strength, cyclic loading, and high-energy impact loading under various loading regimes, such as axial compression, lateral bending, and torsional loading, which simulate either normal activity of daily living or injury mechanisms. The development of subject-specific FE models using CT data is a powerful tool to non-invasively investigate clinical applications such as fracture risk, prosthesis design, and bone remodeling. On applying the same half-body weight on the head of each right proximal femur of 17, 32, and 40-year-male patients models under study at different angles of 24.4 and 28°, the following conclusion is drawn:

1. Same half-body weight acting at variable angles on the femur head results in increase in total deformation with increase in the inclination angle for all models of different age groups.
2. Same half-body weight acting at variable angles on the femur head results in increase in equivalent Von Mises stress and maximum principal stress with increase in the inclination angle for all models of different age groups.
3. The safety factor is the highest in the 32-year-male, then the 17-year-male, and least in the 40-year-male for the same half-body weight.
4. Safety factor is also decreasing with increase in inclination angle under physiologic loading.

5. The percentage variation in total deformation for different angles for different age group of male patients is found to be more in 32 years than in 17 years, and the least variation is found in 40 years.
6. For same body weight, maximum deformation is found to be at the age of 40 years, then 17 years, and least deformation at 32 years in male right femur for both the inclination angles.

Acknowledgments The authors would like to thank Dr. (Mrs.) Shobha Katheria, Principal Medical Officer, Ordnance Factory Hospital, Itarsi, M.P. India, Dr Rakesh Tirkey, Assistant Professor of Medical College, Jabalpur, M.P, India, and Dr. Pushpraj Bhatele, for providing medical imaging data and supporting our work.

Conflict of Interest Statement None of the authors have any conflict of interest to declare that could bias the presented work.

References

1. Gdoutos EE, Raftopoulos DD, Baril JD (1982) A critical review of the biomechanical stress analysis of the human femur. J Biomater 3:2–8
2. Nather A, Ong HJC, Aziz Z (2005) Bone grafts and bone substitutes: basic science and clinical applications, structure of bone. World Scientific Publishing Co. Pte. Ltd 5, Singapore
3. Rohlmann A, Mossner U, Bergmann G, Kolbel R (1982) Finite element analysis and experimental investigation of stresses in a femur. J Biomed Eng 4:242–246
4. Wille H, Rank E, Yosibash Z (2012) Prediction of the mechanical response of the femur with uncertain elastic properties. J Biomech. Accepted in Feb 2012
5. Grassi L, Schoileo E, Taddei F, Zani L, Juszczyk M, Cristofolini L, Viceconti M (2012) Accuracy of finite element predictions in sideways load configurations for the proximal human femur. J Biomech 45:394–399
6. Trabelsi N, Yosibash Z, Milgrom C (2009) Validation of subject-specific automated p-FE analysis of the proximal femur. J Biomech 42:234–241
7. Yosibash Z, Trabelsi N, Milgrom C (2007) Reliable simulations of the human proximal femur by high-order finite element analysis validated by experimental observations. J Biomech 40(16):3688–3699
8. Yosibash Z, Padan R, Joscowicz L, Milgrom C (2007) A CT-based high-order finite element analysis of the human proximal femur compared to in vitro experiments. ASME J Biomech Eng 129(3):297–309
9. Taylor ME, Tanner KE, Freeman MA, Yettram AL (1996) Stress and strain distribution within the intact femur: compression or bending? Med Eng Phys, Elsevier Science Ltd 18(2):122–131
10. Jun-hai Z, Shu-fang MA, Wue-ying WEI (2009) Finite element analysis of femur stress under bending moment and compression load. IEEE
11. Bitsakos C, Kerner J, Fisher I, Amis AA (2005) The effect of muscle loading on the simulation of bone remodelling in the proximal femur. J Biomech 38:133–139
12. Duda GN, Schneider E, Chao EYS (1997) Internal forces and moments in the femur during walking. J Biomech 30(9):933–941
13. Simoes JA, Vaz MA, Blatcher S, Taylor M (2000) Influence of head constraint and muscle forces on the strain distribution within the intact femur. Med Eng Phys 22:453–459
14. Brand RA, Crowninshield RD, Wittstock CE, Pederson DR, Clark CR, Van Krieken FM (1982) A model of lower extremity muscular anatomy. J Biomech 104:304–310

15. Amornsamankul S, Kaorapapong K, Wiwatanapataphee B (2010) Three-dimensional simulation of femur bone and implant in femoral canal using finite element method. Int J Math Comput Simul 4(4):171–178
16. Kulkarni MS, Sathe SR (2008) Experimental determination of material properties of cortical cadeveric femur bone. Trends Biomater Artif Organs 22(1):9–15
17. Burgers TA, Mason J, Niebur G, Ploeg HL (2008) Compressive properties of trabecular bone in the distal femur. J Biomech 4:1077–1085
18. Heller MO, Bergmann G, Deuretzbacher G, Claes L, Haas NP, Duda GN (2001) Influence of femoral anteversion on proximal femoral loading: measurement and simulation in four patients. Clin Biomech 16:644–649
19. Testi D, Viceconti M, Baruffaldi F, Cappello A (1999) Risk of fracture in elderly patients: a new predictive index based on bone mineral density and finite element analysis. Comput Methods Programs Biomed 60:23–33
20. Viceconti M, Bellingeri L, Cristofolini L, Toni A (1998) A comparative study on different methods of automatic mesh generation of human femurs. Med Eng Phys 20:1–10

A Novel Vital Sign Monitor Which Can Save Lives

Parimal Swamy

Abstract Few simple and easy to obtain physiological signs can predict the deteriorating status of pre-hospital and hospitalized patients. These signs together (after computation) generate a score known as Early Warning Score (EWS). Early Warning Score recognizes deteriorating status of patients objectively and quickly. Early recognition of deteriorating status in patients can save lives and prevent morbidity. But many studies have shown that though it is theoretically simple to compute EWS it is difficult to implement both at hospital and community levels. This is mainly due to multiple factors affecting the proper collection and analysis of clinical data (vital signs). We present the concept of a novel vital sign monitor which not only collects the clinical data but analyzes the data in such a manner that hospital staff can recognize patients at risk of deterioration and prevent unnecessary mortality and morbidity.

Keywords Early Warning Score · Clinical Data · Hospital Mortality Vital Sign Monitor

Introduction

Failure to recognize deteriorating status in hospitalized patients is common. This leads to unexpected deaths and unplanned ICU transfers which are associated with increased cost of treatment, dissatisfaction of clients (patients or relatives), and

P. Swamy (✉)
Jabalpur Hospital & Research Centre, Apollo Centre for Asthma & Diabetes Care, Jabalpur, Madhya Pradesh, India
e-mail: drparimals@rediffmail.com

V. Kumar and M. Bhatele (eds.), *Proceedings of All India Seminar on Biomedical Engineering 2012 (AISOBE 2012)*, Lecture Notes in Bioengineering,
DOI: 10.1007/978-81-322-0970-6_6,

The NHS Early Warning Score (NEWS) Scoring System and Weighting Chart							
Clinical Parameter	NEWS WEIGHTING SCORE						
	3	2	1	0	1	2	3
Pulse Rate (per minute)	≤40	41-50		51-100	101-110	111-130	>130
Systolic Blood Pressure (mmHg)	≤80	81-90	91-100	101-199		≥200	
Respiratory rate (per minute)	≤8			9-20	21-25	26-29	≥30
Oxygen Saturations (%)	<86	86-91	92-94	≥94			
Temperature (°C)	≤34	≤35	≤36	36.1–37.9	38.0–38.9	≥39	
Level of Consciousness (AVPU) Alert, Responds to; Voice, Pain, or U: Unresponsive				A	V	P	U
Age (years)				16-69	≥70		
Supplemental Oxygen required?				No	Yes		

Fig. 1 NHS early warning scoring system

disruption of hospital work flow. Even before hospitalization close family members of patients or even healthcare providers (general physician) may miss the warning signs of potentially lethal but treatable illnesses leading to delayed hospitalization, again leading to deaths or unplanned ICU admissions.

Common and potentially life-threatening conditions like severe asthma, impending heart attack, and serious infections (sepsis) are associated with delayed recognition.

Research has shown that a constellation of easily obtained clinical signs may predict future deterioration of clinical status in patients. This is applicable to both hospital and pre-hospital settings. These clinical signs are—respiratory rate, heart rate, blood pressure, body temperature, consciousness status, and percent oxygen saturation of blood (%SPO_2) which is obtained by a simple and cheap instrument.

NHS Early Warning Score

Manual recording of all these signs (except % SPO_2) is possible but multiple factors lead to suboptimal acquisition of these data. Once obtained these signs become variables for a simple calculation of a score commonly known as NHS Early Warning Score(NEWS) (Fig. 1). This score is a robust indicator of future

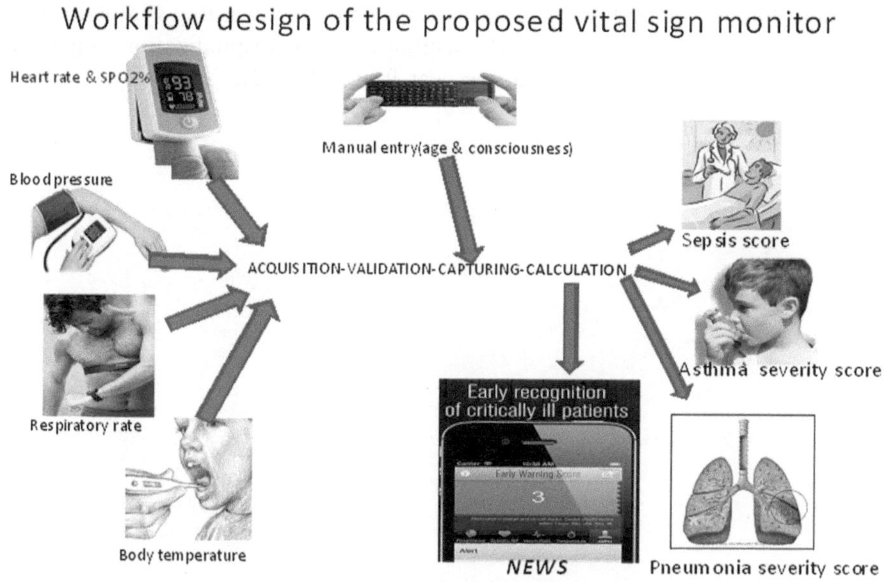

Fig. 2 Workflow design of the proposed vital sign monitor

deterioration. Not only this, NEWS guides the hospital staff regarding appropriate steps for patient care. As with recording of variables (clinical signs) calculation of NEWS is not done on regular basis due to multiple logistic factors.

From the above discussion, it appears that there are two road blocks in regular usage of NEWS:

1. Accurate acquisition of physical signs.
2. Calculation of NEWS.

To overcome these road blocks and to facilitate widespread implementation of NEWS, a unique vital sign monitor is proposed. This monitor will record the variables of NEWS, i.e., Heart Rate, Respiratory Rate, Blood Pressure, Body Temperature, and %SPO_2. Consciousness status can be entered manually. We do not foresee any technical or financial barrier as cheap and widely available technology already exists for recording of these clinical signs. After recording, clinical sign data will be calculated by a microcomputer which can generate—NEWS, sepsis score and pneumonia, and asthma severity. All these interpretations constitute important and frequent inputs for clinical decision making.

If we use existing technology then acquisition of data and interpretation will take 2–3 min per patient with the proposed monitor. This will greatly reduce the time required for patient assessment.

This monitor can play a life-saving role for the prehospital environment, i.e., hospital emergency room, general practice, and as a household health care device. Manual entry of variables like age, family history of heart problem, presence of conditions like high blood pressure or diabetes, and a few warning symptoms may make this monitor an important tool to facilitate timely hospitalization in patients who may deteriorate or even die in the near future (Fig. 2).

A Brief Review on Role of Nanotechnology in Medical Sciences

Kirti Vishwakarma, O. P. Vishwakarma and Mukta Bhatele

Abstract Medical nanotechnology or *nanomedicine* is the medical aspect or application of nanotechnology using different approaches such as nanoelectronic biosensors, nanomaterials, and a very futuristic but underdeveloped molecular nanotechnology that includes molecular manufacturing. Medical nanotechnology aims to provide cheaper yet quality health and medical equipment, facilities, and treatment strategies through continuous researches and studies. A number of pharmaceutical and medical companies all over the world have already adhered to medical nanotechnology because of its numerous benefits and practical uses. Current modalities of diagnosis and treatment of various diseases, especially cancer, have major limitations such as poor sensitivity or specificity and drug toxicities respectively. Newer and improved methods of cancer detection based on nanoparticles are being developed. They are used as contrast agents, fluorescent materials, molecular research tools, and drugs with targeting antibodies. Paramagnetic nanoparticles, quantum dots (qdots), nanoshells, and nanosomes are few of the nanoparticles used for diagnostic purposes. Drugs with high toxic potential like cancer chemotherapeutic drugs can be given with a better safety profile with the utility of nanotechnology. These can be made to act specifically at the target tissue by active as well as passive means. Other modalities of therapy such as heat-induced ablation of cancer cells by nanoshells and gene therapy are also being developed. This review discusses the various platforms of nanotechnology being used in different aspects of medicine. The safety of nanomedicine is not yet fully

K. Vishwakarma (✉)
Gyan Ganga Institute of Technology and Sciences, Jabalpur, India
e-mail: opkirti2007@gmail.com

O. P. Vishwakarma
Department of Nanotechnology, Gyan Ganga College of Technology, Jabalpur, India

M. Bhatele
Department of Computer Science, Gyan Ganga College of Technology, Jabalpur, India

V. Kumar and M. Bhatele (eds.), *Proceedings of All India Seminar on Biomedical Engineering 2012 (AISOBE 2012)*, Lecture Notes in Bioengineering,
DOI: 10.1007/978-81-322-0970-6_7,

defined. However, it is possible that nanomedicine in future would play a crucial role in the treatment of human diseases and also in enhancement of normal human physiology.

Keywords Diagnostics · Drugs · Nanomedicine · Nanotechnology · Therapeutics · Quantum dot

Introduction

"Nano" means very small, and it comes from the Greek word "nanos", meaning dwarf. It is also used as a prefix to indicate size in the series kilo-, milli-, micro-, nano-meter. A nanometer is one thousand millionth of a metre, 10^{-9} m.

Nanoscale is generally considered to be at a size below 0.1 μm or 100 nm. Nanoscience can be defined as the study of phenomena and manipulation of materials at atomic, molecular, and macromolecular scales where properties differ significantly from those at a larger particulate scale. Nanotechnology is then the design, characterization, production and application of structures, devices, and systems by controlling the shape and size at the nanometer scale.

Nanotechnology is considered an emerging technology with enormous potential in a range of applications. In addition to various industrial uses, great innovations are foreseen in metrology, electronics, biotechnology, medicine, and medical technology. It is anticipated that nanotechnology can have an enormous positive impact on human health. The potential medical applications are predominantly in diagnostics, monitoring, the availability of more durable and better prosthetics, and new drug delivery systems for potentially harmful drugs.

Nanoparticles and Nanostructures

Nanoparticles and nanostructures can be prepared either by the "top down" technique starting with large particles and making things smaller by grinding or pulverizing, or the "bottom up" technique making things larger by building atom by atom or molecule by molecule. The limit to making things smaller seems to be reached, while making nanostructures by synthesis has just started. In the latter case, avoiding random reactions and thus the control of the process is critical for the production of nanostructures. The development of enhanced microscopy techniques such as, Scanning Tunneling Microscopy and Atomic Force Microscopy, has facilitated the use of the bottom-up process. Some uses of nanotechnology include: Nanomaterials used in nanostructured materials, coatings, electronics, and active surfaces. Most of the time such nanoparticles will be fixed within or on the surface of materials.

Bionanotechnology and nanomedicine are rather promising areas for nanotechnology. Applications will probably include diagnostics, imaging techniques, materials for prosthetics, and drug delivery. Other applications may be as supporting structures in biomaterials and medical devices including the use in scaffolds for tissue engineering. Micro- and nano-grooves present on material surfaces may direct cellular growth; however, cell behavior is also influenced by chemical coating.

Private and public research efforts worldwide are developing nanoproducts aimed at improving health care and advancing medical research. Some of these products have entered the marketplace, more are on the verge of doing so, and others remain more a vision than a reality. The potential for these innovations is enormous, but questions remain about their long-term safety and the risk–benefit characteristics of their usage. Since 2000, when former President Bill Clinton announced the founding of the U.S. National Nanotechnology Initiative (NNI), governments in Europe, Japan, and other Asian nations have responded with competitive investments in national nano programs. The European Commission, a body of the European Union (EU) that funds about 24 % of the publicly financed research in the EU, and the Union's 15 member nations will spend about $180 million on nanotechnology in 2002. The NNI budget for fiscal year (FY) 2002 is $604 million, including $40.8 million for the National Institutes of Health (NIH). For FY 2003, proposed budgets amount to $710.2 million in the United States, and between $270 and $315 million in the EU.

Three applications of nanotechnology are particularly suited to biomedicine: diagnostic techniques, drugs, and prostheses and implants. Interest is booming in biomedical applications for use outside the body, such as diagnostic sensors and "labon- a-chip" techniques, which are suitable for analyzing blood and other samples, and for inclusion in analytical instruments for R&D on new drugs. For inside the body, many companies are developing nanotechnology applications for anticancer drugs, implanted insulin pumps, and gene therapy. Other researchers are working on prostheses and implants that include nanostructured materials.

Nanotechnology in Medicine: Application

The use of nanotechnology in medicine offers some exciting possibilities. Some techniques are only imagined, while others are at various stages of testing, or actually being used today. Nanotechnology in medicine involves applications of nanoparticles currently under development, as well as longer range researches that involve the use of manufactured nanorobots to make repairs at the cellular level.

Drug Delivery

One application of nanotechnology in medicine currently being developed involves employing nanoparticles to deliver drugs, heat, light, or other substances to specific types of cells (such as cancer cells). Particles are engineered so that they are attracted to diseased cells, which allows direct treatment of those cells. This technique reduces damage to healthy cells in the body and allows for earlier detection of disease. The basic point to use drug delivery is based upon three facts: (a) efficient encapsulation of the drugs, (b) successful delivery of the said drugs to the targeted region of the body, and (c) successful release of that drug there.

Nanomedical approaches to drug delivery enter on developing nanoscale particles or molecules to improve drug bioavailability. Bioavailability refers to the presence of drug molecules where they are needed in the body and where they will do the most good [1, 2]. Drug delivery focuses on maximizing bioavailability both at specific places in the body and over a period of time. This can potentially be achieved by molecular targeting by nanoengineered devices. It is all about targeting the molecules and delivering drugs with cell precision. More than $65 billion are wasted each year due to poor bioavailability. In vivo imaging is another area where tools and devices are being developed. Using nanoparticle contrast agents, images such as ultrasound and MRI have a favorable distribution and improved contrast. The new methods of nano-engineered materials that are being developed might be effective in treating illnesses and diseases such as cancer. What nano-scientists will be able to achieve in the future is beyond current imagination. This might be accomplished by self- assembled biocompatible nanodevices that will detect, evaluate, treat, and report to the clinical doctor automatically.

Drug delivery systems, lipid- or polymer-based nanoparticles can be designed to improve the pharmacological and therapeutic properties of drugs [3, 4]. The strength of drug delivery systems is their ability to alter the pharmacokinetics and biodistribution of the drug. When designed to avoid the body's defence mechanisms, nanoparticles have beneficial properties that can be used to improve drug delivery. Where larger particles would have been cleared from the body, cells take up these nanoparticles because of their size. Complex drug delivery mechanisms are being developed, including the ability to get drugs through cell membranes and into cell cytoplasm. Efficiency is important because many diseases depend upon processes within the cell and can only be impeded by drugs that make their way into the cell. Triggered response is one way for drug molecules to be used more efficiently. Drugs are placed in the body and only activate on encountering a particular signal. For example, a drug with poor solubility will be replaced by a drug delivery system where both hydrophilic and hydrophobic environments exist, improving the solubility. Also, a drug may cause tissue damage, but with drug delivery, regulated drug release can eliminate the problem. If a drug is cleared too quickly from the body, this could force a patient to use high doses, but with drug delivery systems clearance can be reduced by altering the pharmacokinetics of the drug. Poor biodistribution is a problem that can affect normal tissues through widespread distribution, but the particulates from drug delivery systems lower the volume of distribution and reduce the effect on non-target tissue. Potential nano drugs will work by very specific and well-understood mechanisms; one of the major impacts of nanotechnology and nanoscience will be in leading development of completely new drugs with more useful behavior and less side effects.

Diagnostic and Imaging Techniques

Carbon nanotubes and gold nanoparticles are being used in a sensor that detects proteins indicative of oral cancer. Tests have shown this sensor to be accurate in detecting oral cancer and provide results in less than an hour. Silver nanorods in a diagnostic system are being used to separate viruses, bacteria, and other microscopic components of blood samples, allowing clearer Raman spectroscopy signals of the components. This method has been demonstrated to allow identification of viruses and bacteria in less than an hour.

Iron oxide nanoparticles can be used to improve MRI images of cancer tumors. The nanoparticle is coated with a peptide that binds to a cancer tumor; once the nanoparticles are attached to the tumor the magnetic property of their oxide enhances the images from the Magnetic Resonance Imagining scan. Nanoparticles can attach to proteins or other molecules, allowing detection of disease indicators in a lab sample at a very early stage. There are several efforts to develop nanoparticle disease detection systems underway. One system being developed by Nanosphere, Inc. uses gold nanoparticles, nanosphere has clinical study results with their Verigene system involving its ability to detect four different nucleic acids, while another system being developed by T2 Biosystems uses magnetic nanoparticles to identify specimens, including proteins, nucleic acids, and other materials.

Gold nanoparticles that have antibodies attached can provide quick diagnosis of flu virus. When light is directed on a sample containing virus particles and nanoparticles the amount of light reflected back increases because the nanoparticles cluster around virus particles, allowing a much faster test than those currently used.

Quantum Dots (qdots) may be used in the future for locating cancer tumors in patients and in the near term for performing diagnostic tests in samples. Invitrogen's website provides information about qdots that are available for both uses, although at this time the use "in vivo" is limited to experiments with lab animals. Concerns about the toxicity of the material that qdots are made from are one of the reasons for restricting the use of qdots in human patients. However, work is being done with qdots composed of silicon, which is believed to be less toxic than the cadmium contained in many qdots.

Antimicrobial Techniques

One of the earliest nanomedicine applications was the use of nanocrystalline silver which is as an antimicrobial agent for the treatment of wounds. A nanoparticle cream has been shown to fight staph infections. The nanoparticles contain nitric oxide gas, which is known to kill bacteria. Studies on mice have shown that using the nanoparticle cream to release nitric oxide gas at the site of staph abscesses significantly reduced the infection.

Burn dressing that is coated with nanocapsules containing antibiotics. If an infection starts, the harmful bacteria in the wound causes the nanocapsules to break open, releasing the antibiotics. This allows much quicker treatment of an infection and reduces the number of times a dressing has to be changed.

Cell Repair

Nanorobots could actually be programmed to repair specific diseased cells, functioning in a similar way to antibodies in our natural healing processes [5].

Protein and Peptide Delivery

Protein and peptides exert multiple biological actions in the human body and they have been identified as showing great promise for treatment of various diseases and disorders. These macromolecules are called biopharmaceuticals. Targeted and/or controlled delivery of these biopharmaceuticals using nanomaterials like nanoparticles and Dendrimers is an emerging field called nano-biopharmaceutics, and these products are called nanobiopharmaceuticals.

Molecular Imaging and Therapy

The small size of nanoparticles endows them with properties that can be very useful in oncology, particularly in imaging. Qdots, when used in conjunction with MRI (magnetic resonance imaging), can produce exceptional images of tumor sites. These nanoparticles are brighter than organic dyes and only need one light source for excitation. This means that the use of fluorescent qdots could produce a higher contrast image and at a lower cost than today's organic dyes used as contrast media. The downside, however, is that qdots are usually made of quite toxic elements (Fig. 1).

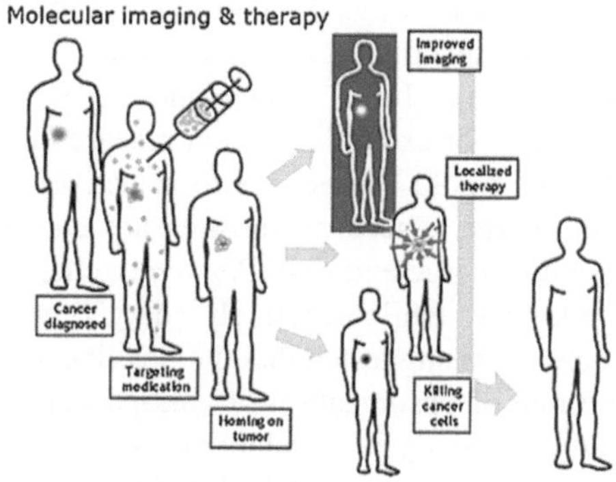

Fig. 1 A schematic illustration showing how nanoparticles or other cancer drugs might be used to treat cancer

Surgery

At Rice University, a flesh welder is used to fuse two pieces of chicken meat into a single piece. The two pieces of chicken are placed together touching each other. A greenish liquid containing gold-coated nanoshells is dribbled along the seam. An infrared laser is traced along the seam, causing the two sides to weld together. This could solve the difficulties and blood leaks caused when the surgeon tries to restitch the arteries that have been cut during a kidney or heart transplant. The flesh welder could weld the artery perfectly [6].

Visualization

Tracking movement can help to determine how well drugs are being distributed or how substances are metabolized. It is difficult to track a small group of cells throughout the body, so scientists dye the cells. These dyes need to be excited by light of a certain wavelength in order for them to light up. While different colored dyes absorb different frequencies of light, there is a need for as many light sources as cells. A way around this problem is with luminescent tags. These tags are qdots attached to proteins that penetrate cell membranes. The dots can be random in size, can be made of bio-inert material, and they demonstrate the nanoscale property that color is size-dependent. As a result, sizes are selected so that the frequency of light used to make a group of qdots fluoresce is an even multiple of the frequency required to make another group incandesce. Then both groups can be lit with a single light source.

Nanoparticle Targeting

It is increasingly observed that nanoparticles are promising tools for the advancement of drug delivery, medical imaging, and as diagnostic sensors. However, the biodistribution of these nanoparticles is still imperfect due to the complex host's reactions to nano- and micro-sized materials and the difficulty in targeting specific organs in the body. Nevertheless, a lot of work is still ongoing to optimize and better understand the potential and limitations of nanoparticulate systems. For example, current research in the excretory systems of mice shows the ability of gold composites to selectively target certain organs based on their size and charge. These composites are encapsulated by a dendrimer and assigned a specific charge and size. Positively charged gold nanoparticles were found to enter the kidneys while negatively charged gold nanoparticles remained in the liver and spleen. It is suggested that the positive surface charge of the nanoparticle decreases the rate of opsonization of nanoparticles in the liver, thus affecting the excretory pathway. Even at a relatively small size of 5 nm, though, these particles can become compartmentalized in the peripheral tissues, and will therefore accumulate in the body over time. While advancement of research proves that targeting and distribution can be augmented by nanoparticles, the dangers of nanotoxicity become an important next step in further understanding of their medical uses.

Neuro-Electronic Interfaces

Neuro-electronic interfacing is a visionary goal dealing with the construction of nanodevices that will permit computers to be joined and linked to the nervous system. This idea requires the building of a molecular structure that will permit control and detection of nerve impulses by an external computer. The computers will be able to interpret, register, and respond to signals the body gives off when it feels sensations. The demand for such structures is huge because many diseases involve the decay of the nervous system. Also, many injuries and accidents may impair the nervous system resulting in dysfunctional systems and paraplegia. If computers could control the nervous system through neuro-electronic interface, problems that impair the system could be controlled so that effects of diseases and injuries could be overcome. Two considerations must be made when selecting the power source for such applications. They are refuelable and non-refuelable strategies. A refuelable strategy implies energy is refilled continuously or periodically with external sonic, chemical, tethered, magnetic, or electrical sources. A non-refuelable strategy implies that all power is drawn from internal energy storage which would stop when all energy is drained.

Other Benefits of Medical Nanotechnology

Although some are still skeptical about the technology, scientists and researchers over continents have been practicing medicine using nanotechnology due to its numerous benefits. Some of these benefits to the medical field include the following:

- With nanotechnology, tools and equipment for surgery and diagnostic would be a lot cheaper yet remain to be effective and state of the art. Medical research and processes require highly advanced equipment that could be very expensive but once the equipment is fully developed, its manufacturing would be a lot easier and faster with the use of nanotechnology. The creation of complex tools that can diagnose serious diseases with a single laboratory test would minimize diagnostic costs and treatment. Using tiny nano-built sensors inserted into the human body for direct contact with the source of ailment would definitely make medical treatments easier and cheaper.
- With medical nanotechnology, treatment would be more efficient and precise. Instead of opening the whole body area for surgical purposes, a microscopic nanotool would spare the patient from bloody and risky surgical processes. With nanotechnology in the medical field, treatment would be precise, eliminating trial-and-error drug prescription. With a single laboratory test and highly technical computers, a detailed image of the body's system and processes can be automatically spotted including the cause of the disease and its possible treatment. With nanotechnology in the fields of medicine, medical malpractice would be eliminated and the side effects of taking medicines out of sheer guessing from the physicians would be avoided.
- With highly advanced medical equipment, potential diseases can easily be detected and prevented.
- Since diseases can be prevented, the quality of life for mankind would be improved and lifespan would be increased.
- With the application of nanotechnology in medicine, replacement of body organs using machines smaller than body cells can be possible. Because of advanced nanotechnology, candidates for organ replacement and augmentation will receive far better body organs enhanced by tiny machines introduced to the body for better organ performance and functions.
- Medical nanotechnology can largely contribute to genetic therapy and improvement. Diseases can be easily treated if approached at the genetic level. So instead of treating diseases based on the symptoms, nanotechnology will help medical practitioners treat the problem by looking at the root cause.

Nanotechnology and Nanomedicine in the Future

Medical diagnosis, proper and efficient delivery of pharmaceuticals, and development of artificial cells are the medical fields where nanosized materials have found practical implementations. As *suggested* by Freitas, the application of nanotechnology to medicine, nanomedicine, subsumes three mutually overlapping and progressively more powerful molecular technologies. First, nanoscale-structured materials and devices that can be fabricated today hold great promise for advanced diagnostics and biosensors, targeted drug delivery and smart drugs, and immunoisolation therapies. Second, biotechnology offers the benefits of molecular medicine via genomics, proteomics, and artificial engineered microbes. Third, in the longer term, molecular machine systems and medical nanorobots will allow instant pathogen diagnosis and extermination, chromosome replacement and individual cell surgery in vivo, and the efficient augmentation and improvement of natural physiological function. There are several other intriguing, still theoretical, proposals for practical applications of nanomechanical tools into the fields of medical research and clinical practice. One function of nanodevices in medical sciences could be the replacement of defective or incorrectly functioning cells, such as the respirocyte proposed by Freitas. It has also been postulated that nanomachines could distribute drugs within the patient's body. Such nanoconstructions could deliver medicines to particular sites, making more adequate and precise treatment possible. Such devices would have a small computer, several binding sites to determine the concentration of specific molecules, and a supply of some 'poison' that could be released selectively. Similar machines equipped with specific 'weapons' could be used to remove obstructions in the circulatory system or identify and kill cancer cells. It has been also proposed that nanorobots may be modified bacteria and viruses that already have most of the motorization and target delivery of genetic information. Moreover, nanorobots, operating in the human body could monitor levels of different compounds and store that information in internal memory. They could be used to rapidly examine a given tissue location, surveying its biochemistry, biomechanics, and histometric characteristics in greater detail. This would help in better disease diagnosing. The use of nanodevices would give the additional benefits of reduced intrusiveness, increased patient comfort, and greater fidelity of results, since the target tissue can be examined in its active state in the actual host environment.

Over the next couple of years it is widely anticipated that nanotechnology will continue to evolve and expand in many areas of life and science, and the achievements of nanotechnology will be applied in medical sciences, including diagnostics, drug delivery systems, and patient treatment. According to Dr Brazil from the Royal Society of Medicine (July 2003) opinion: "Nanotechnology provides the potential for significant advances over the next 50 years" with potential applications of:

1. biological nanosensors for diagnostics in the next 1–5 years,
2. generation of artificial muscles, development lab-on-a chip technology for more efficient drug discovery and targeted drug and gene delivery within the next 6–10 year, and
3. later on (after 10–50 years) introduction of nanomachines for in vivo treatment and nanopumps/vales for tissue engineering and generation of artificial organs, in health care and medicine.

Conclusion

Although the expectations from nanotechnology in medicine are high and the potential benefits are endlessly enlisted, the safety of nanomedicine is not yet fully defined. Use of nanotechnology in medical therapeutics needs adequate evaluation of its risk and safety factors. However, it is possible that nanomedicine in the future will play a crucial role in treatment of human diseases and also in enhancement of normal human physiology. With concurrent application of nanotechnology in other fields, its utility is likely to extend further into diagnostics, molecular research techniques, and tools.

References

1. Lavan DA, McGuire T, Langer R (2003) Small-scale systems for in vivo drug delivery. Nat Biotechnol 21(10):1184–1191
2. Cavalcanti A, Shirinzadeh B, Freitas RA Jr, Hogg T (2008) Nanorobot architecture for medical target identification. Nanotechnology 19(1):015103(15pp)
3. University of Waterloo, Nanotechnology in Targeted Cancer Therapy, 15 January 2010
4. Allen TM, Cullis PR (2004) Drug delivery systems: entering the mainstream. Science 303(5665):1818–1822
5. Loo C, Lin A, Hirsch L, Lee MH, Barton J, Halas N, West J, Drezek R (2004) Nanoshell-enabled photonics-based imaging and therapy of cancer. Technol Cancer Res Treat 3(1):33–40
6. Gobin AM, O'Neal DP, Watkins DM, Halas NJ, Drezek RA, West JL (2005) Near infrared laser-tissue welding using nanoshells as an exogenous absorber. Lasers Surg Med 37(2): 123–129

Finite Element Modeling of Human Femur Using CT Data: A Biomechanical Analysis

Amrita Francis, Ashwani Shrivastava, Chetna Masih, Nidhi Dwivedi, Priyanka Tiwari, Raji Nareliya and Veerendra Kumar

Abstract Biomechanics is the development, extension, and application of mechanics for the purpose of understanding better the influence of mechanical loads on the structure, properties, and function of living things. Biomechanics focuses on design and analysis, each of which is the foundation of engineering. CT scan data is widely used to make realistic investigations on the mechanical behavior of bone structures using Finite Element Analysis (FEA). The purpose of this paper is to create anatomically accurate, 3D finite element models of the right human proximal femur for 17, 32, and 40-year-old-male patients using individual CT scan data. Thus, allowing the biomechanical analysis of the male right human proximal femur of different age groups loaded under physiologic forces at constant angle of 28°, i.e., at varying body weights of 70 and 75 kg, respectively which is shared equally by the lower limbs, that affect femur during weight bearing acting at different conditions and to determine the total deformation, equivalent Von-Mises stress distribution, maximum principal stress distribution, and fatigue tool throughout the whole femur, and comparing the results. Analysis of this model will provide data unavailable at this time to orthopedic surgeons, engineers, and researchers of human orthopedics.

A. Francis (✉) · A. Shrivastava · N. Dwivedi · P. Tiwari
Government Engineering College, Jabarlpu, MP, India
e-mail: amrita.francis21@gmail.com

V. Kumar
Government Engineering College, Jabalpur, MP, India
e-mail: prof.veerendra.kumar@gmail.com

R. Nareliya
Hitkarni College of Engineering and Technology, Jabalpur, MP, India
e-mail: raji_nareliya@yahoo.co.in

C. Masih
Government Engineering College, Gokhalpur, Jabarlpur, MP 482 011, India
e-mail: chetnamasih@gmail.com

V. Kumar and M. Bhatele (eds.), *Proceedings of All India Seminar on Biomedical Engineering 2012 (AISOBE 2012)*, Lecture Notes in Bioengineering,
DOI: 10.1007/978-81-322-0970-6_8,

Keywords Biomechanics computed tomography · Finite element modeling · Human femur

Introduction

Femur, the longest and strongest bone in the skeleton is almost perfectly cylindrical in the greater part of its extent. In the erect posture it is not vertical, being separated above from its fellow by a considerable interval, which corresponds to the breadth of the pelvis, but inclining gradually downward and medial ward, so as to approach its fellow toward its lower part, for the purpose of bringing the knee joint near the line of gravity of the body. The degree of this inclination varies in different persons, and is greater in the female than in the male, on account of the greater breadth of the pelvis [1]. Being an important structure, femur serves two distinct functions: it acts as a supporting structure allowing the weight of the upper body to be transferred from the hip joint to the knee joint and it also acts as a stiff structure about which muscles act to facilitate movement at both the hip and knee joints. The neck of the femur is a point of structural weakness and a common fracture site in elderly people, especially in women suffering from osteoporosis and is usually associated with a fall and at age of 65 or above. Fracture of the shaft of the femur occurs when subjected to extreme force such as in a road traffic accident. Thus, this complete study of human femur is addressed under biomechanics. As biomechanics is the study of motions experienced by living things in response to applied loads. Koch was the first who gave a complete and thorough description of the structure of the femur and demonstrated the relations which exist between the structure and the function as well as between the external and internal architecture of the femur [2]. Macroscopically, the structure of femur consists of two types: (1) cortical or compact bone which is a dense outer layer mainly resisting bending and (2) cancellous or spongy or trabecular bone present in the interior of mature bones; this structure mainly resists compression and bone elements placing or displacing themselves in the direction of functional pressure according to Wolff's Law [3]. The shape of the femur is asymmetric and curved in all three planes. Hence, a 3D model is required for a quantitative stress analysis [4, 5]. With minor modifications CT scans of FE models can be used to generate reliable subject-specific FE models that accurately predicts strains in quasi-axial loading configurations [6–9]. A thorough understanding and behavior of femur is essential to elucidate the femur fracture and provide better guidance to the artificial femur replacement. Various works have been carried out to investigate the loading mode and stress distribution [10, 11]. For better understanding of femoral loading forces exerted by the soft and hard tissues of the thigh together are considered, a 3D model is created taking into account all thigh muscles, body weight, contact forces at the hip, patellofemoral, and knee joints [12–15]. A mathematical model is developed to simulate 3D femur bone and femur bone with implant in the femoral canal, taking into account stress distribution and total displacement during horizontal walking [16]. Material properties of femur bones are evaluated to facilitate further study of total hip joint and

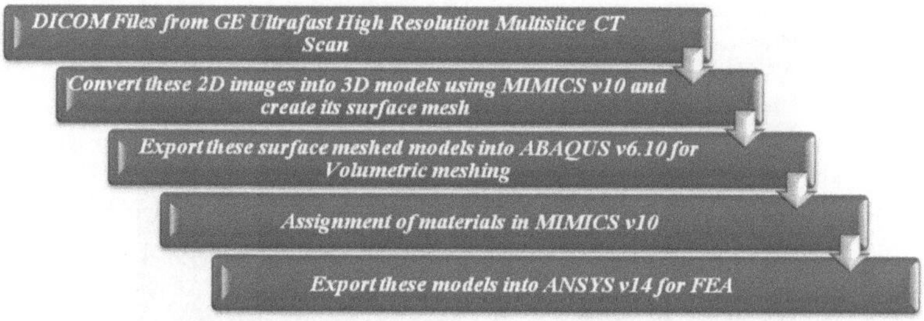

Fig. 1 Steps involved in finite element modeling

replacement of joint in Indian subjects, as these properties are needed before finite element analysis of indigenized hip joint to study its stability in the bone [17, 18]. The role of ante version in transferring the load from implant to bone and its influence on total hip arthroplasty (THA) is determined. Also, loading of the proximal femur during daily activity, i.e., walking and stair climbing is determined. Experimental and analytical approaches are used to determine the in vivo loading of the hip joint. A numerical muscular skeleton model is validated against measured in vivo hip contact force [13, 19].

Materials and Methods

A biomechanical analysis of human femur under half the body weight which varies with the shift of the vertical axis of body center where center of gravity of the body lies as one leg is lifted in air while the other leg is on the ground. This condition of instability is essential for the understanding of failure mechanisms during day-to-day life conditions or any accidental cases, as with every half-centimeter shift of this vertical axis of body center 5 kg weight is added to the body weight acting on the leg touching the ground, for providing guidance for the design and operation of human femur replacement. 3D FE models are created using CT images in materialized interactive medical image control system (MIMICS) and the various steps involved are described in Fig. 1. For biomechanical investigation of total deformation, stress distribution, and fatigue tools throughout the right proximal human femur of all male patients, under physiological loading conditions, FEA is performed.

Image Acquisition

The CT data of total femur of normal individual male patients of 17, 32, and 40 years are collected. This geometrical data of real proximal human femur bone are in the form of digital imaging and communications in medicine (DICOM) files. The CT

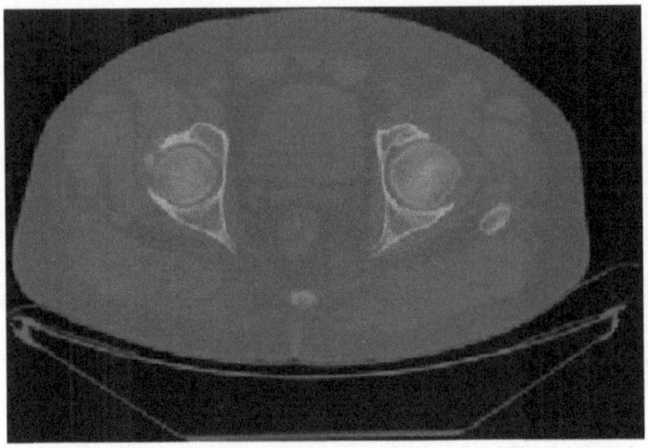

Fig. 2 The transverse section of total femur CT image

scanning of patients are obtained using GE Ultrafast High-resolution Multislice CT Scanner (16 Slice) containing a total number of 909, 667, and 1,714 images, respectively, pixel size of 0.7031, 0.8867, and 0.9766 mm, respectively, slice thickness of 0.4 mm, and resolution of 512 × 512. DICOM file is a standard for handling, storing, printing, and transmitting information in medical imaging and contains binary data elements. In MIMICS, distinctive CT images are a pixel map of the linear X-ray attenuation coefficient of tissue. The pixel values are scaled so that the linear X-ray attenuation coefficient of air equals −1024 and that of water equals 0. This scale is called the Hounsfield scale after Godfrey Hounsfield, one of the pioneers in computerized tomography. Using this scale, fat is around −110, muscle is around 40, trabecular bone is in the range of 100–300, and cortical bone extends above trabecular bone to about 2,000. The pixel values are shown graphically by a set of gray levels that vary linearly from black to white [20].

Image Segmentation

Three models of right proximal human femur of three individual male human patients are created: Model 1 of 17-year-old male, Model 2 of 32-year-old male, and Model 3 of 40-year-old male. MIMICS is an interactive tool for the visualization and segmentation of CT images as well as MRI images and 3D rendering of objects. Therefore, in the medical field MIMICS is used for diagnostic, operation planning, or rehearsal purposes. Figure 2 shows the image of normal individual total femur as acquired from the DICOM file images after conversion in MIMICS v10. Bone tissue is then extracted by means of thresholding using default values range. The extracted bone tissue is put into a mask. Mask is a collection of pixels which can be modified using various tools successively: edit masks, region growing, and calculate of 3D mask. Edit mask is used to separate the whole total femur from the adjoining hard tissues like pelvis, tibia, etc. The region growing

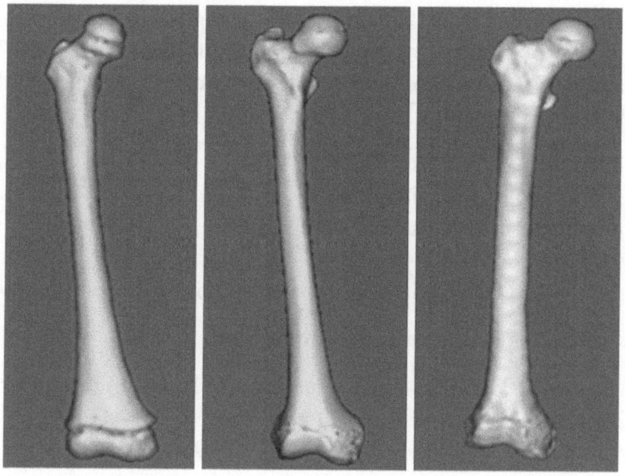

Fig. 3 Three-dimensional models of proximal femur

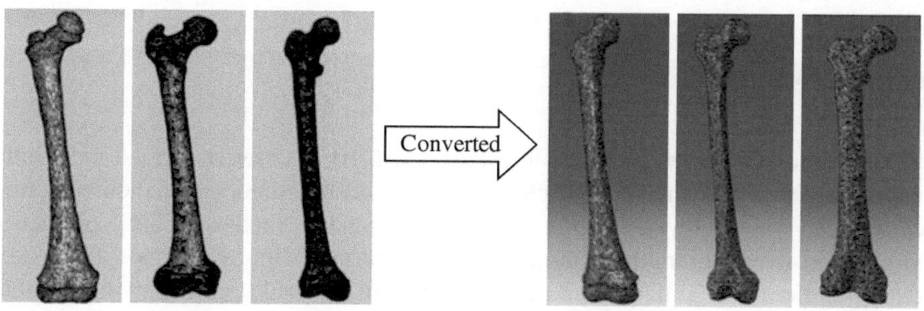

Fig. 4 Surface mesh in MIMICS converted into volumetric mesh in ABAQUS for all models of femur

tool provides the capacity to split the segmentation into separate masks. Calculate 3D from mask tool converts the 2D images into 3D models using an interpolation algorithm embedded in MIMICS as shown in Fig. 3.

Creation of FE Model

After creating 3D models in MIMICS, surface mesh is generated as shown in Fig. 4, for femur bone models and for further finite element analysis (FEA). FEA remeshing is a tool in MIMICS that allows us to create surface mesh of 3D models. In automatic remeshed operation surface mesh of equilateral triangle is generated. All parameters are optimized here by optimize-based method using the ratio of the height of the triangle and the length of its base with quality parameter value above the maximum threshold 0.3. The various other actions performed in FEA remeshing are:

- Triangle reduction of models normally.
- Improving qualities of the triangles.
- Triangle reduction of models preserving quality.
- Removal of extra shells.
- Self-intersection test to eliminate intersecting triangles completely.

Properties after remeshing of different models:

Model 1—volume 102094.20 mm^3, surface 26160.67 mm^2, triangles 23816, points 11952,
Model 2—volume 471900.53 mm^3, surface 133994.83 mm^2, triangles 125884, points 62644,
Model 3—volume 328123.40 mm^3, surface 115667.27 mm^2, triangles 128374, points 63953.

Converted

These models are now imported in ABAQUS 6.10 to convert surface mesh into volumetric mesh. In mesh tool, choosing edit mesh category and then selecting convert tri into tetra generates volumetric meshed models. This volumetric meshing converts triangular elements of surface mesh into four node linear tetrahedron elements (C3D4). The three models are meshed with following number of 3D tetrahedron elements: 268858, 959083, and 809524, respectively. Figure 4 shows volumetric meshed models of femur in ABAQUS. From ABAQUS these volumetric meshed models are again imported into MIMICS for material assignment. Figure 5 shows volumetric meshed models after they are imported in MIMICS.

Material Assignment

Once an FE mesh has been generated, the next step is to assign material properties to the elements. Bone is a biological substance and has complicated mechanical properties. Femur is a complicated structured material composed of compact bone and cancellous bone. The compact bone is anisotropic material while cancellous bone can be considered as isotropic material. Thus, it is difficult to assign material properties along each direction of bone model. In our study, ten materials are assigned to all the models using MIMICS. In MIMICS, there are three ways to

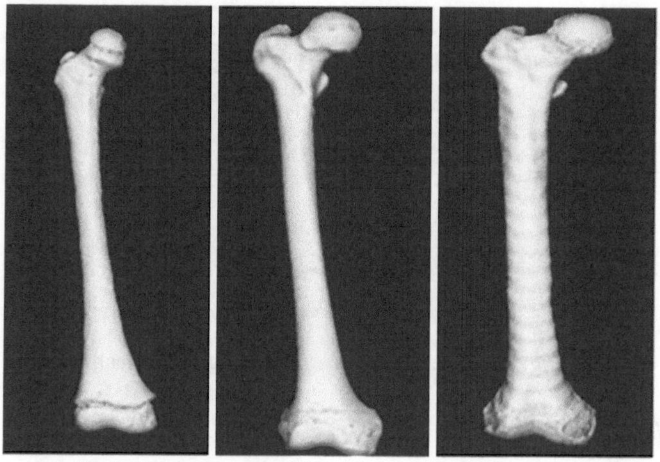

Fig. 5 Volumetric meshed models in MIMICS

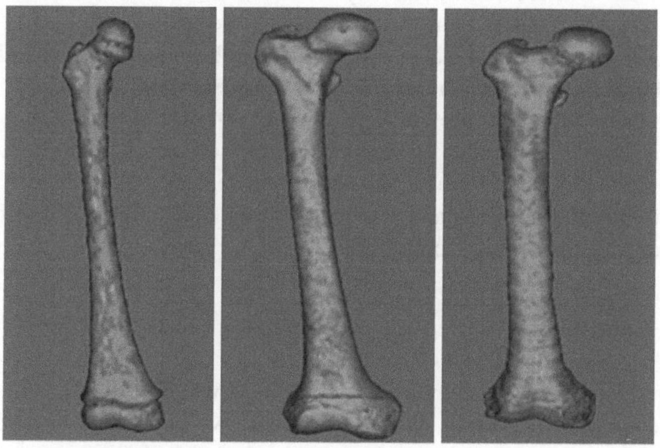

Fig. 6 The 3D model of proximal femurs after assigning material properties

assign material properties: uniform, look-up file, and mask. We have considered a uniform method for realistic material assignment to each model using MIMICS. In this study, ten materials are assigned to each model by default and gray values are calculated for each model before realistic material assignment. Figure 6 shows all three models assigned with materials in MIMICS.

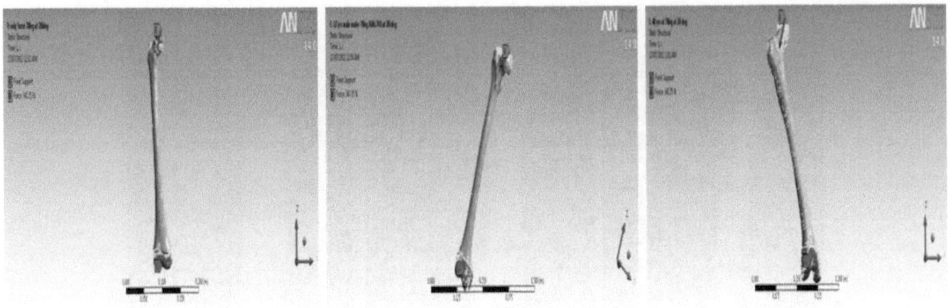

Model 1 Model 2 Model 3

Fig. 7 Half of 70 and 75 kg loads acting on the head of right proximal femurs at 28°

Finite Element Analysis

The 3D Finite Element Models of femur bone of all male patients with volumetric mesh and realistic material assigned are imported into ANSYS v14. Since the femur bone models are nonlinear, asymmetric, and curved in all three planes, the models are first imported in Finite Element Modeler and initial geometry are created for each model, then transferred individually to static structural module in ANSYS 14 for FEA. Three-dimensional FE models of human femur bone with realistic material properties are analyzed in static structural workbench of ANSYS 14 capabilities. The boundary conditions discussed below are applied to each model for the investigation of total deformation, equivalent Von-Mises stress distribution, maximum principal stress distribution, and fatigue tool throughout the whole femur and the results compared.

Boundary Conditions

Femur being a thigh bone shares the whole body weight equally by both the left and right femurs. In our study, the varying body weights of 70 kg (686.7 N) and 75 kg (735.75 N) are considered to be equally shared by both femurs according to the hip mechanism. Thus, load of 343.35 N and 367.875 N which is half the whole body weight is applied on the right femur head of every model at a constant angle of 28° [11, 21–23] without consideration of muscle forces to resist the bending stress produced in all the models during load application and a fixed support is provided at lateral condyle, medial condyle, and patellar surface in every model; thus, the femur is assumed to be a cantilever beam with one end fixed and the other end subjected to load. The boundary conditions are shown in Fig. 7.

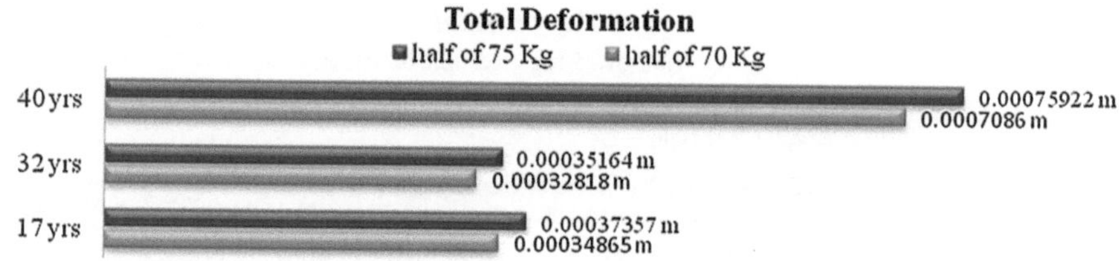

Fig. 8 Total deformation for loads acting on the head of right proximal femur of male patients at 28°

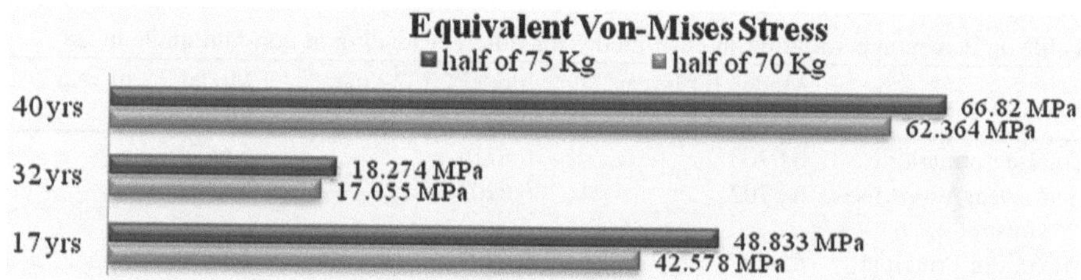

Fig. 9 Equivalent Von-Mises stress for loads acting on the head of right proximal femur of male patients at 28°

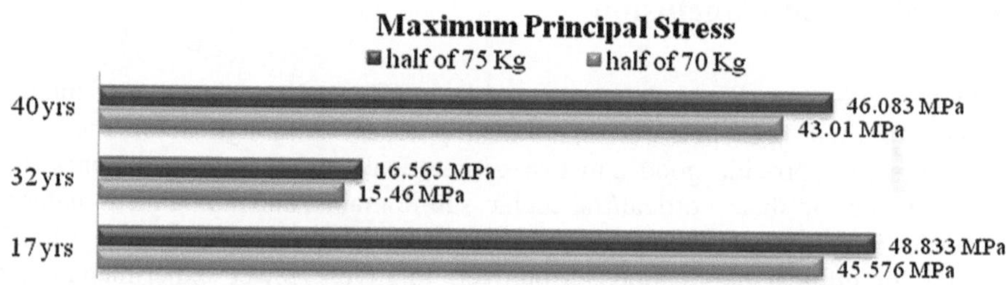

Fig. 10 Maximum principal stress for load acting on the head of right proximal femur of male patients at 28°

Results

The total deformation, equivalent Von-Mises stress, and maximum principal stress evaluated in the 3D Finite Element Analysis is shown in Figs. 8, 9, and 10. A constant fatigue life of 1e6 is obtained throughout the whole femur for all models of 17, 32, and 40-year human male patients. The safety factor evaluated for each model is shown in Fig. 11. This biomechanical study also shows the percentage variation in each model due to increase in curvature or bend in human femur with age which results in the increase in inclination angle of load application as shown in Table 1.

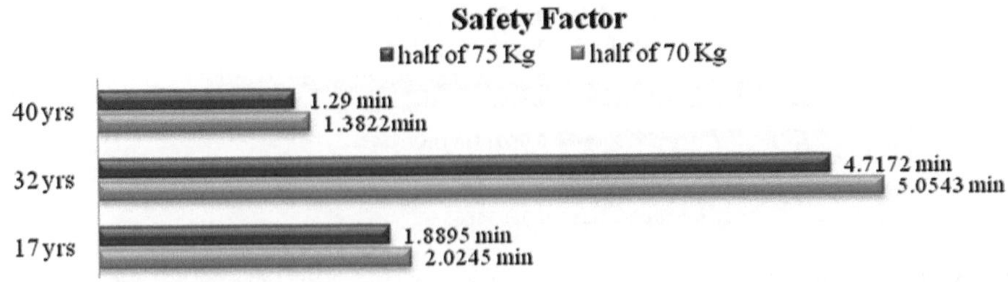

Fig. 11 Safety factor for loads acting on the head of right proximal femur of male patients at 28°

Table 1 Percentage variation in each model for different loading at constant angle of 28°

	Model 1(17-year male) (%)	Model 2 (32-year male) (%)	Model 3 (40-year male) (%)
Total deformation	6.6708	6.6716	6.6674
Equivalent Von-Mises stress	6.6702	6.6707	6.6687
Maximum Principal stress	6.6697	6.6707	6.6684

Discussion and Conclusion

Patient-specific bone FE models generated from CT data have become of interest because of their high potential in clinical practice. Although automatic mesh generators may provide good and fast geometrical representation of bones, the determination of their cortical/trabecular sub-domains and associated material properties is still one of the major difficulties in making these FE models reliable enough for clinical applications. Moreover, relatively fewer experimental and computational studies have evaluated the intact whole femur's overall stiffness, strength, cyclic loading, and high-energy impact loading under various loading regimes, such as axial compression, lateral bending, and torsional loading, which simulate either normal activity of daily living or injury mechanisms. The development of subject-specific finite element (FE) models using computed tomography (CT) data is a powerful tool to noninvasively investigate clinical applications, such as fracture risk, prosthesis design, and bone remodeling. On applying half of the body weight on the head of the right proximal femur of 17-, 32-, and 40-year male patients 3D models under study at constant inclination angle, the following conclusion is drawn:

1. Total deformation increases with increase in body weight.
2. Equivalent Von-Mises stress and maximum principal stress increases with increase in body weight.

3. The total deformation is found to be highest in 40-year-old male, then in 17-year-old male, and least in 32-year-old male.
4. The safety factor is highest in 32-year-old male, then in 17-year-old male, and least in 40-year-old male for variable body weight at constant angle.
5. Safety factor is also decreasing with increase in body weight in all cases under study.
6. The percentage variation is highest in 40-year-old male, then in 32-year–old male, and least in 17-year-old male for all investigation done.

Acknowledgments The authors would like to thank Dr. (Mrs.) Shobha Katheria, Principal Medical Officer, Ordnance Factory Hospital, Itarsi, M.P. India, Dr Rakesh Tirkey, Assistant Professor of Medical College, Jabalpur, M.P, India and Dr. Pushpraj Bhatele, for providing medical imaging data and supporting our work.

Conflict of Interest Statement None of the authors have any conflict of interest to declare that could bias the presented work.

References

1. Hanumantharaju HG, Shivanand HK (2010) Strength analysis and comparison of SS316L, Ti-6AI-4 V and Ti-35Nb-7Zr-5Ta used as orthopaedic implant materials by FEA, 2nd international conference on chemical, biological and environmental engineering (ICBEE 2010): 101–105
2. Gdoutos EE, Raftopoulos DD, Baril JD (1982) A critical review of the biomechanical stress analysis of the human femur. J Biomater 3:2–8
3. Nather A, Ong HJC, Aziz Z (2005) Bone grafts and bone substitutes—basic science and clinical applications. World Scientific Publishing Co. Pte. Ltd, Structure of bone; 5
4. Rohlmann A, Mossner U, Bergmann G, Kolbel R (1982) Finite element analysis and experimental investigation of stresses in a femur. J Biomed Eng 4:242–246
5. Wille H, Rank E, Yosibash Z (2012) Prediction of the mechanical response of the femur with uncertain elastic properties. J Biomech 45(7):1140–1148
6. Grassi L, Schoileo E, Taddei F, Zani L, Juszczyk M, Cristofolini L, Viceconti M (2012) Accuracy of finite element predictions in sideways load configurations for the proximal human femur. J Biomech 45:394–399
7. Trabelsi N, Yosibash Z, Milgrom C (2009) Validation of subject-specific automated p-FE analysis of the proximal femur. J Biomech 42: 234–241
8. Yosibash Z, Trabelsi N, Milgrom C (2007a) Reliable simulations of the human proximal femur by high-order finite element analysis validated by experimental observations. J Biomech 40: 3688–3699
9. Yosibash Z, Padan R, Joscowicz L, Milgrom C (2007b) A CT-based high-order finite element analysis of the human proximal femur compared to in vitro experiments. ASME J Biomech Eng 129(3): 297–309
10. Taylor ME, Tanner KE, Freeman MAR, Yettram AL (1996) Stress and strain distribution within the intact femur: compression or bending? Medical Eng Phy, Elsevier Science Ltd 18(2):122–131
11. Jun-hai Z, Shu-fang MA, Wue-ying W (2009) Finite element analysis of femur stress under bending moment and compression load, 2nd international conference on biomedical engineering and informatics (BMEI 2009): 1–4

12. Bitsakos JK, Fisher I, Amis AA (2005) The effect of muscle loading on the simulation of bone remodelling in the proximal femur. J Biomech 38: 133–139
13. Duda GN, Schneider E, Chao EYS (1997) Internal forces and moments in the femur during walking. J Biomech 30(9): 933–941
14. Simoes JA, Vaz MA, Blatcher S, Taylor M (2000) Influence of head constraint and muscle forces on the strain distribution within the intact femur. Med Eng Phys 22:453–459
15. Brand RA, Crowninshield RD, Wittstock CE, Pederson DR, Clark CR, Van Krieken FM (1982) A model of lower extremity muscular anatomy. J Biomech 104: 304–310
16. Amornsamankul S, Kaorapapong K, Wiwatanapataphee B (2010) Three-dimensional simulation of femur bone and implant in femoral canal using finite element method. Int J Math Comput Simulation 4(4): 171–178
17. Kulkarni MS, Sathe SR (2008) Experimental determination of material properties of cortical cadeveric femur bone. Trends Biomater Artif Organs 22(1):9–15
18. Burgers TA, Mason J, Niebur G, Ploeg HL (2008) Compressive properties of trabecular bone in the distal femur. J Biomech 4: 1077–1085
19. Heller MO, Bergmann G, Deuretzbacher G, Claes L, Haas NP, Duda GN (2001) Influence of femoral anteversion on proximal femoral loading: measurement and simulation in four patients. Clinical Biomech 16: 644–649
20. Materialise's Interactive Medical Image Control System (MIMICS) 10.01: User Manual: Materialise, http://www.materialise.com/mimics/
21. Testi D, Viceconti M, Baruffaldi F, Cappello A (1999) Risk of fracture in elderly patients: a new predictive index based on bone mineral density and finite element analysis. Comput Methods Programs Biomed 60:23–33
22. Viceconti M, Bellingeri L, Cristofolini L, Toni A (1998) A comparative study on different methods of automatic mesh generation of human femurs. Medical Eng Phy 20: 1–10
23. Nareliya R, Kumar V (2011) Biomechanical analysis of human femur bone. Int J Eng Sci Technol 3(4): 3090–3094

Chondroitin Sulfate Surface Engineered Docetaxel-Loaded Liposomes for Tumor Targeting: Design, Development, and Characterization

Aditya Ganeshpurkar, Ankit Ganeshpurkar, Abhishek Agnihotri, Vikas Pandey, Nikhar Vishwakarma, Divya Bansal and Nazneen Dubey

Abstract Cancer is amongst the most devastating uncontrolled cellular growth that hampers the growth of normal cells leading to their malfunctioning and organ failure. Anticancer agents are widely used to limit the progression of cancer; however, it suffers from severe side effects. Development of novel modes of drug delivery has minimized the side effects and has increased the therapeutic index of drugs. In the current work, chondroitin sulfate-coupled liposomes of docetaxel were prepared and characterized. The formulation was also studied for in vivo efficacy and biodistribution. The formulation effectively enhanced the life period of experimental animals, which reflects the success of formulation. Thus, use of chondroitin sulfate-coupled docetaxel-loaded liposomes could be advocated to treat cancer. However, systemic in vivo studies are required to extrapolate its effects on humans.

Keywords Surface engineered liposomes · Chondroitin sulfate · Docetaxel · Tumor targeting

Introduction

Cancer is characterized by the rapid growth of abnormal cells. Various external and internal factors predispose to progression of cancer [1]. Currently, along with new drug discovery, development of a suitable carrier system becomes essential to

A. Ganeshpurkar (✉) · A. Ganeshpurkar · A. Agnihotri · N. Vishwakarma · N. Dubey
Drug Discovery Laboratory, Shri Ram Institute of Technology-Pharmacy, Jabalpur, Madhya Pradesh, India

V. Pandey · D. Bansal
Pharmaceutics Research Laboratory, Shri Ram Institute of Technology-Pharmacy, Jabalpur, Madhya Pradesh, India

V. Kumar and M. Bhatele (eds.), *Proceedings of All India Seminar on Biomedical Engineering 2012 (AISOBE 2012)*, Lecture Notes in Bioengineering,
DOI: 10.1007/978-81-322-0970-6_9,

deliver drug safely at the target site. Some of the anticancer agents are believed to suppress the progression of cancer cells while others modulate the proliferation or differentiation. Use of anticancer agents is associated with the risk of sustained damage to DNA. Thus, it proves to be of no satisfactory treatment for cancer. The traditional mode of drug administration generally is unable to provide target specificity. A sharp increase in drug release is also observed in such systems and drug toxicity is observed, while, sometimes, less therapeutic effect is also observed. Thus it becomes a need to deliver target molecule at target tissue with high degree of specificity [2].

Lipid-based drug carrier systems viz., solid lipid nanoparticles and solid lipid microspheres emerge as one of the promising carrier systems for the delivery of water-insoluble drugs [3]. Docetaxel is clinically well-established anti-mitotic chemotherapy medicament used mainly used for the treatment of breast, ovarian, and non-small cell lung cancer [3]. Its short biological half-life necessitates the need to be administered in two or three doses of 20–80 mg per day [4]. The development of chondroitin sulfate-coupled liposomes would be beneficial.

Materials and Method

Chemicals

Docetaxel was obtained as a generous gift sample from Dabur, India. Phosphatidyl choline was obtained as a gift sample from Lipoid, GmbH, Germany. Stearylamine, cholesterol, chondroitin sulfate, Triton-X100, 1-ethyl-3-(3-dimethylaminopropyl) carbodiimide Sephadex G-50, Calcein, RPMI-1640, 3-(4,5-dimethylthiazol- 2-2-yl)-2,5-diphenyl) tetrazolium bromide (MTT) were procured from Sigma Chemicals (St Louis, MO). Dialysis membrane (MWCO 12–14 kDa) were procured from Himedia (Mumbai, India). Chloroform, methanol was purchased from Loba, India. All other reagents and solvents used were of analytical grade and were used as received. MiliQ water was used throughout the study.

Animals

Swiss albino mice of either sex were used for the studies. The animals were maintained under standard conditions (27 ± 2 °C; relative humidity 60 ± 5 %, light–dark cycle of 12 h) and fed with standard pellet diet and water *ad libidum* were used for the present study. The research protocol was approved by the Institutional Animal Ethical Committee.

Preparation

Liposomes were prepared by film cast method as reported elsewhere; phosphatidylcholine, cholesterol, stearylamine, and drug (7:3:1.5:1.0 molar ratio) were dissolved in minimum quantity of chloroform and methanol (2:1) in a round-bottomed flask, and a thin film was casted by evaporating the solvent under reduced pressure using rotatory flash. Finally, traces of solvent were removed under vacuum. The dried lipid film was hydrated with phosphate buffer saline (PBS) (pH 7.4, 0.1 mL/mg lipid) [5]. To 5 ml suspension of liposomes, 5 mg chondroitin sulfate was dissolved in PBS (pH 7.4). To it 10 mg of EDC per ml was added. The mixture was incubated at room temperature (25 ± 2 °C) for 3 h, and coupling was confirmed by IR spectroscopy [6].

Characterization

Surface Morphology

The morphological examination of liposomes was performed using a transmission electron microscope (TEM) following negative staining with sodium phosphotungstate solution (0.2 %, w/v), at various magnifications.

Zeta Potential Measurements

Suitably diluted aqueous suspension of liposomes at concentration of 1.0 ± 0.3 mg/mL was taken for zeta potential measurements using Malvern Zetasizer (DTS Ver, 4.10, Malvern Instruments).

Entrapment Efficiency

Entrapment efficiency was determined by separating the unentrapped drug by minicolumn centrifugation and disrupting the liposomes with 0.1 % Triton X-100. Drug content was determined spectrophotometrically using UV-Vis spectrophotometer.

In Vitro Drug Release

Liposomal suspension was held in dialysis membrane (mol. wt. cut off 3,500) and hung in a beaker with PBS (pH 7.4); the system was shaken with a magnetic stirrer. Samples were withdrawn periodically and analyzed for drug content.

Table 1 Formulation characteristics for the liposome formulations

Diameter (nm) (mean ± SD)	20.17 ± 5.8
Zeta potential (ZP) (mV) (mean ± SD)	−19.45 ± 0.27
Encapsulation efficiency (EE) (%) (mean ± SD)	62.39 ± 2.54

Each value is the mean of three independent determinations

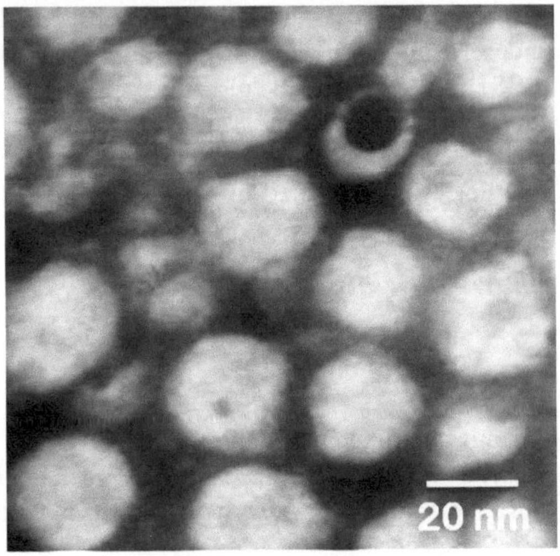

Fig. 1 TEM image of liposomes

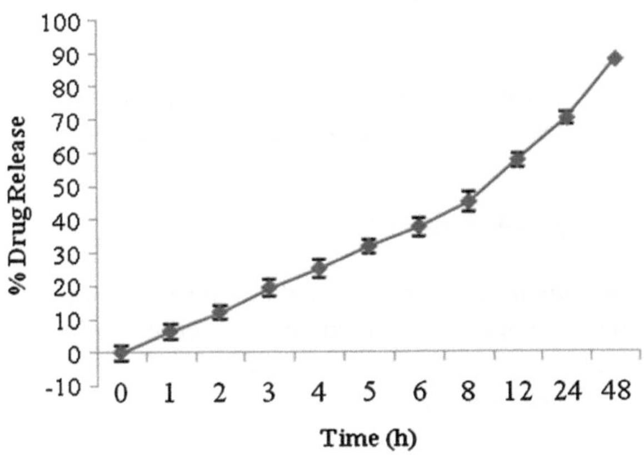

Fig. 2 In vitro drug release from liposomes

In Vivo Studies

Swiss albino mice of weight group below 25 g were selected for the study. 1×10^5 EAC cells cultured in MEM, 10 % FCS, were injected i.p. Treatment was started when mice weight reached above 30 g (Day 1). Mice weight is proportional to the development of ascetic fluid in peritoneal cavity and observed for longevity.

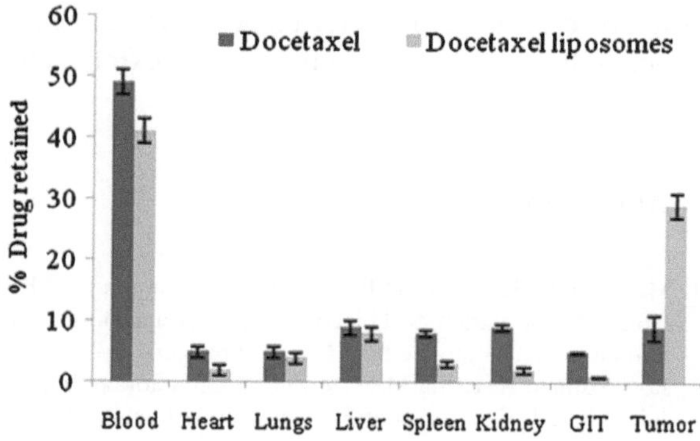

Fig. 3 Organ distribution studies

Biodistribution Studies

To determine the distribution of liposomal formulation in EAC bearing mice, the animals were divided into three groups ($n = 5$); administration of drug was done through the tail vein. The mice of first group served as control. The second group was injected with Docetaxel (10 mg/kg), and the third group was treated with Docetaxed-loaded liposomes (eq 10 mg/kg). After 12 h of administration the animals were sacrificed and the organs were subjected to estimation of docetaxel spectrophotometrically.

Results and Discussion

The evaluated characters of liposomal formulation are summarized in Table 1. In general, the liposomes were spherical in shape and average particle was in the range of 15–25 nm (Fig. 1). As shown in Fig. 2, after initial burst within 3 h, the liposomes effectively released drug which sustained for a period of 48 h. Biodistribution studies revealed that liposomal docetaxel concentrated more in tumor as compared to free drug (Fig. 3). Animals treated with liposomal docetaxel survived 29 % more ($p < 0.01$) as compared to docetaxel alone. Thus, chondritin linked docetaxel liposomes demonstrated efficacy in terms of improvement in quality of life of experimental animals.

Conclusion

The ultimate goal of anticancer chemotherapy is either to destroy or to limit the growth of cancer cells. Use of chondroitin sulfate-coupled liposomes for effective delivery of docetaxel is an innovative approach. This concept is advantageous in terms of drug targeting with reduced side effects. However, for such a system, systemic in vivo studies are required to extrapolate its effects on humans.

References

1. Madhumitha RY, Chakaraborty S, Roy M, Taraphdar AK, Bhattacharya RK (2004) Cytotoxic effect of root extract of Tiliacora racemosa and oil of Semecarpus anacardium nut in human tumour cells. Asian Pacific J Cancer Prev 3:61–67
2. Jayakrishnan A, Latha MS (1997) Biodegradable polymeric microspheres as drug carriers. In: Jain NK (ed) Controlled and novel drug delivery. CBS publishers, New Delhi, pp 55–236
3. Bunjes H, Koch MHJ (2005) Saturated phospholipids promote crystallization but slow down polymorphic transitions in triglyceride nanoparticles. J Control Release 107:229–243
4. Williamson KA, Fenton C (2005) Docetaxel: a review of its use in metastatic breast cancer. Drugs 65:2513–2531
5. Bangham AD, Standish MM, Watkins JC (1965) Diffusion of univalent ions across the lamellae of swollen phospholipids. J Mol Biol 13:238–252
6. Hoare DG, Koshland DE (1966) A procedure for the selective modification of carboxyl group in proteins. J Amer Chem Soc 88:2057–2058

Photoluminescence Studies of CdS Nanoparticles

Kirti Vishwakarma, O. P. Vishwakarma and S. K. Pandey

Abstract II–VI semiconductor nanoparticles are presently of great interest for their practical applications such as zero-dimensional quantum confined materials and for their applications in optoelectronics and photonics. The optical properties get modified dramatically due to the confinement of charge carriers within the nanoparticles. Similar to the effects of charge carriers on optical properties, confinement of optical and acoustic phonon leads to interesting changes in the phonon spectra. In the present work, we have synthesized nanoparticles of cadmium sulfide (CdS) using chemical precipitation technique. A detailed study on CdS sample is done by characterizing photoluminescence (PL) spectra. Photoluminescence studies of CdS nanoparticle samples show a red shift. The intensity of red luminescence decreases and its peak position shifts to the lower energy with increasing size of the particles.

Keywords Cadmium sulfide · Nanoparticles · Photoluminescence spectra · Optical properties

Introduction

There is presently widespread interest in the physical and optical properties of nanometer-sized semiconductor particles, the so-called nanoparticles or quantum dots. It is known that the optical properties of such particles depend on their size

K. Vishwakarma (✉) · O. P. Vishwakarma
Department of Engineering Physics, Gyan Ganga College of Technology, Jabalpur, India
e-mail: opkirti2007@gmail.com

S. K. Pandey
Rani Durgawati Vishwavidalaya, Jabalpur, India

V. Kumar and M. Bhatele (eds.), *Proceedings of All India Seminar on Biomedical Engineering 2012 (AISOBE 2012)*, Lecture Notes in Bioengineering,
DOI: 10.1007/978-81-322-0970-6_10,

[1–6]. Such particles display optical and physical properties which are intermediate between those of the bulk materials and those of the isolated molecules. For example, the optical absorption of bulk cadmium sulfide (CdS) typically extends to 690 nm. When CdS is made into 40 Å nanoparticles the longest absorption band shifts to 530 nm. In nanoparticles a large percentage of the atoms are on the surface, rather than in the bulk phase. Consequently, the chemical and physical properties of the material, such as the melting point or phase transition temperature, depend on the particle size. Nanoparticles can be made from a wide variety of materials, including CdS, ZnS, Cd_3P_2, and PbS, to name a few. The nanoparticles frequently display photoluminescence and sometimes display electroluminescence [7–12]. Additionally, some nanoparticles can form self-assembled arrays. Because of such favorable properties, nanoparticles are being extensively studied for use in optoelectronic displays. The CdS nanocrystalline has become a subject of both scientific and industrial importance in the past one decade.

Nanomaterials can be characterized using different techniques like X-ray diffraction, Ultra-violets spectroscopy, Scanning electron microscopy, Atomic force microscopy, and Tunneling electron microscopy. Many features of nanocrystals differ from those of their bulk counterparts and are dependent on their individual sizes. It has always been a prime goal, since the beginning of research in this field, to prepare samples of nanocrystals as identical as possible.

As the crystalline size decreases the band gap values increase. In principle, the band gap can be varied by changing the crystalline size. Thus, for low band gap material, one has to control the crystalline size to obtain the required band gap. Light emission from these nanocrystals is possible through a radiative recombination process of charge carriers generated by higher energy photon absorption. The color of the emission can be layered by changing the crystalline size and appropriate doping. The efficiency changes from 3 % in bulk to 18 % in nanocrystallites, leading to a tremendous improvement in the brightness of emitted light; because of the small size, the intensity of emitted light increases [13].

Experimental Support

It is a great challenge to synthesize particles of nanometer dimension with narrow size distribution without any impurity. Various methods have been attempted for the synthesis. Nanoparticles of CdS are synthesized in aqueous medium through chemical precipitation technique starting from cadmium salt and sodium sulfide, and using tri-ethanolamine as capping agent. These compounds are weighted in a microbalance. The stoichiometric solution was taken in a burette and was added in drops with continuous sitting to precipitate of CdS was formed. After complete precipitation, the solution in conical flask was constantly stirred for about 20 h. Then the precipitates were filtered out. The nanoparticles are separated from the reaction medium by centrifugation, washing, and drying. Photoluminescence

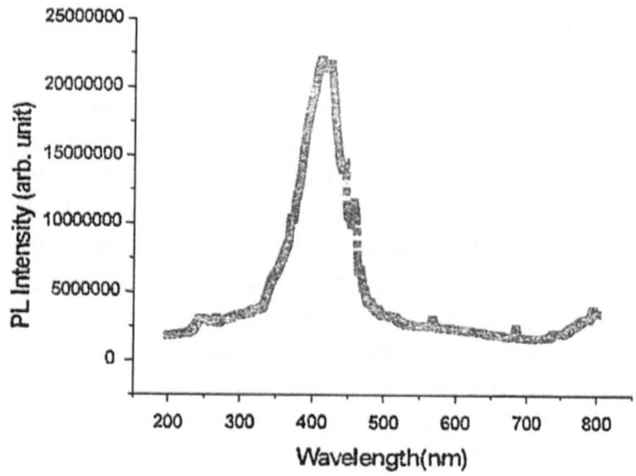

Fig. 1 Photoluminescence spectra of Cds

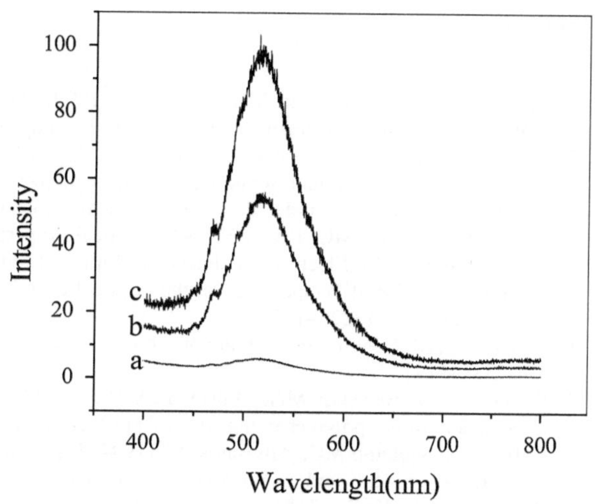

Fig. 2 Photoluminescence spectra of nanoparticles of CdS for different excitation wavelengths: **a** 300 nm, **b** 240 nm, and **c** 230 nm

of the sample is recorded using spectrofluorometer or different excitation wavelengths.

For the measurement of photoluminescence (PL) intensity, the particle was placed on a bare glass slide by using toluene and the glass slide was fixed onto the entrance slit of the monochromator. A filter was used between the sodium mercury lamp and the nanoparticles so that photoluminescence excitation can take place. By rotating the drum of the monochromator, the wavelength can be varied and thus relative PL intensity can be measured, and subsequently the PL spectra can be recorded.

Results and Discussions

Figure 1 shows the photoluminescence spectra of nanoparticles of CdS for different excitation wavelengths of 328 nm and the PL peak is about 410 nm. The luminescence from the surface states has also been observed. The peak of eigen-transition is strong and steep; the emission peak of surface states is flat and weak. The PL full-width half-maximum is only about 30 nm, it reveals the narrow size distribution of nanoparticles. Photoluminescence analysis in 400–650 nm emission wavelengths shows the well-known green emission band in CdS nanoparticles.

We have seen that the intensity peaks and its full-width half-maximum increases with increasing the crystalline size. Our result is similar to the work done [14] in 2005 by Prabhu et al. Figure 2 shows the PL spectra of CdS nanocrystal obtained [14].

References

1. Bawendi MG, Steigerwald ML, Brus LE (1990) The quantum mechanics of larger semiconductors clusters (quantum dots). Annu Rev Phys Chem 41:477–496
2. Martin CR, Mitchell DT (1998) Nanomaterials. Anal Chem News Features 322A–327A
3. Weller H (1993) Colloidal semiconductor Q-particles: chemistry in the transition region between solid state and molecules. Angew Chem Int Ed Engl 32:41–53
4. Norris DJ, Bawendi MG, Brus LE (1997) Optical properties of semiconductor nanocrystals (quantum dots). Mol Electron. In: Jortner J, Ratner M (eds) Blackwell, Oxford, pp 281–323
5. Alivisatos AP (1996) Perspectives on the physical chemistry of semiconductor nanocrystals. J Phys Chem 100:13226–13239
6. Alivisatos AP (1996) Semiconductor clusters, nanocrystals and quantum dots. Science 271:933–937
7. Dabbousi BO, Bawendi MG, Onitsuka O, Rubner MF (1995) Electroluminescence from CdSe quantum-dot/polymer composites. Appl Phys Lett 66(11):1316–1318
8. Colvin VL, Schlamp MC, Alivisatos AP (1994) Light-emitting diodes made from cadmium selenide nanocrystals and a semiconducting polymer. Nature 370:354–357
9. Zhang L, Coffer JL (1997) Electrochemiluminescence from calixarenecoated porous Si liquid junction cells. J Phys Chem B 101(35):6874–6878
10. Artemyev MV, Sperling V, Woggon U (1997) Electroluminescence in thin solid films of closely packed CdS nanocrystals. J Appl Phys 81(10):6975–6977
11. Huang J, Yang Y, Xue S, Yang B, Liu S, Shen J (1997) Photoluminescence and electroluminescence of ZnS: Cu nanocrystals in polymeric networks. Appl Phys Lett 70(18):2335–2337
12. Artemyev MV, Sperling V, Woggon U (1998) Electroluminescence in thin solid films of closely packed CdS nanocrystals. J Cryst Growth 184/185:374–376
13. Seigel RW (1996) Sci Am 275:74–79
14. Prabhu Rajiv R (2005) Characterization of chemically synthesized CdS nanoparticles. J Phys 65(5):801–807

Biomechanical Analysis of the RP Model of Human Humerus Bone and its Comparison with the Real Proximal Humeral Bone

Chetna Masih, Raji Nareliya and Veerendra Kumar

Abstract The goal of this study is to biomechanically evaluate the rapid prototype (RP) model of the human humeral bone and to compare it with the real proximal humeral bone under the similar loading and boundary conditions. Composite bones provide a reliable source of consistent geometry for finite element (FE) models, as they allow for repeatable experimental validation of the FE model, and avoid handling and preservation issues associated with post-mortem specimens. The altered model of the bone can be considered as patient-specific bone geometry and the loading and boundary conditions are applied accordingly.

Keywords Biomechanically · Finite element · Proximal humeral bone · Rapid prototype

Introduction

Biomechanics is the application of mechanical principles on living organisms. By applying the laws and concepts of physics, biomechanical mechanisms and structures can be simulated and studied [1]. This work illustrates the potential that a combination of knowledge from biology and engineering can help for

C. Masih (✉)
Government Engineering College, Gokhalpur, Jabarlpur, MP 482 011, India
e-mail: chetnamasih@gmail.com

R. Nareliya
Hitkarni College of Engineering and Technology, Jabalpur, India
e-mail: raji_nareliya@yahoo.co.in

V. Kumar
Government Engineering College, Jabalpur, India
e-mail: prof.veerendra.kumar@gmail.com

V. Kumar and M. Bhatele (eds.), *Proceedings of All India Seminar on Biomedical Engineering 2012 (AISOBE 2012)*, Lecture Notes in Bioengineering,
DOI: 10.1007/978-81-322-0970-6_11,

understanding the behaviour of human bones. Here, our focus is on the upper arm bone, the humerus, which is a long bone, composed of a head, neck and body, or shaft [2].

The study of the model has been done by creating its Rapid Prototype (RP). RP Technology is a group of manufacturing processes that enable the direct physical realisation of 3D computer models. This technology converts the 3D computer data provided by a dedicated file format directly into a physical model, layer-by-layer with a high degree of accuracy. With the advancements in medical-based modeling technologies like Medical device prototyping, biomodeling, anatomical modeling, and Reverse Engineering it is possible to construct three-dimensional (3D) models of anatomical structures of the human body. This is possible by collating scan data attained from CT and MRI scans. These 3D models of anatomical structures can be used for preoperative planning, diagnosis of diseases, surgical simulation, and medical device prototyping [3].

Objectives

1. To obtain a 3D model of human humerus CT image using MIMICS and ABAQUS.
2. Application of FEA on the 3D model and obtaining its results using ANSYS.
3. Conversion of the data into STL file format for the creation of the RP model.
4. RP model of human humerus bone created at DRDO, Bangalore.
5. 3D model obtained from the CT images of the RP model.
6. Again applying the FEA for the results of the RP model using ANSYS 14.
7. Comparison of the results of Real Proximal Human Humerus Bone with the RP model.

The first three objectives have been fulfilled in our previous work and the rest of it has been explained below including some of the crucial steps of the previous work.

Materials and Methods

(a) Data Collection:

The geometrical data of real proximal human humerus bone in the format of Digital Imaging and Communications in Medicine (DICOM) images of a 17-year-old male, whose weight is 75 kg, is obtained from CT scan data. This DICOM data set is obtained from GE Signa HDXt 2008 Multi Channel 1.5 Tesla Superconducting Helium Cooled whole-body MR module machine and contains a total of 909 slices. This machine can perform with highest precision the humongous task of MR spectroscopy. The slice thickness is 0.4 mm and the resolutions $1,024 \times 1,024$.

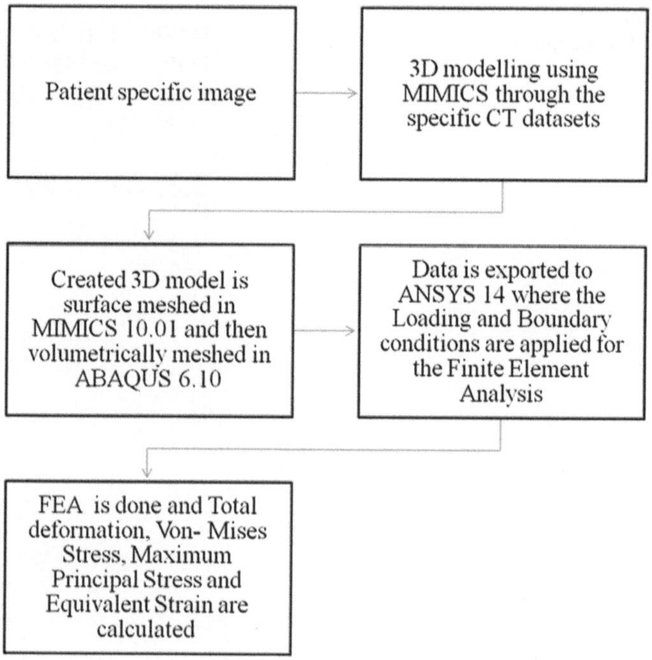

Fig. 1 Steps followed for the required resultants

(b) Methodology:

(Figure 1).

(c) Software's Used:

MIMICS 10.01software is used to view the collected CT scan data of the patient and importing these images for the generation of the 3D model of the patient's humerus bone. When the model has been created it is meshed, but the limitation is that it only has a shell. So to give it a solid form ABAQUS 6.10 software is used and volumetric meshes are created. ANSYS 14 software is used for the FEA.

(d) Segmentation:

Medical images from the CT or MRI consist of the grayscale information. The required part is obtained by segmenting the image. Various tools are used for segmentation. They are: thresholding, region growing, and calculate 3D [4].

(e) Thresholding:

Thresholding is performed to create a segmentation mask. It classifies all pixels within a Hounsfield as a same color or a mask. A lower threshold is used for the segmentation of soft tissue and a higher one is used for the segmentation of bone. The grey values were defined for selecting a region of interest. The specific area was selected by delineating the grey values.

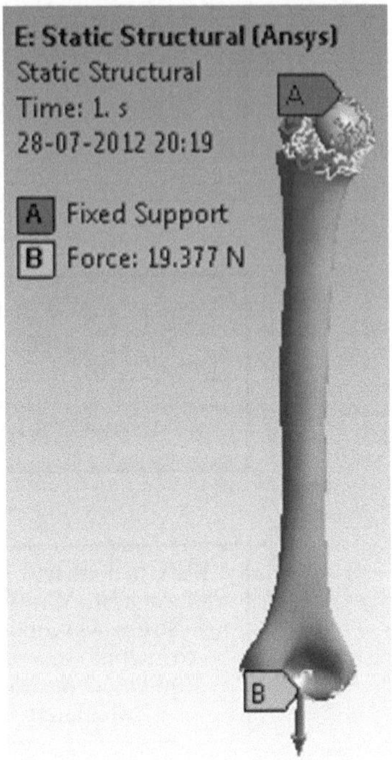

Fig. 2 Loading and boundary condition applied in ANSYS 14

(f) Region growing:

Region growing provides the capacity to split the segmentation into separate objects. The separation of masks into different parts is obtained by region growing method. The floating pixels can also be eliminated.

(g) Calculate 3D:

Calculate 3D is used for transformation of the data from 2D images into 3D model [5].

(h) Meshing:

Meshing is needed in order to raise the quality of the triangles so that the pre-processor of an FEA package can build a tetrahedron mesh from them. In other words meshing provides a better geometric quality.

(i) Material assignment:

When the volumetric mesh is created in ABAQUS 6.10 from the remeshed object, this volume mesh is loaded in MIMICS for material assignment.

(j) Converting to STL files:

3D solid model can be directly converted into STL format for use in subsequent rapid prototyping process. The STL files provide interface options via triangulated formats: Binary STL, ASCII STL. By using this, a triangle mesh will be generated

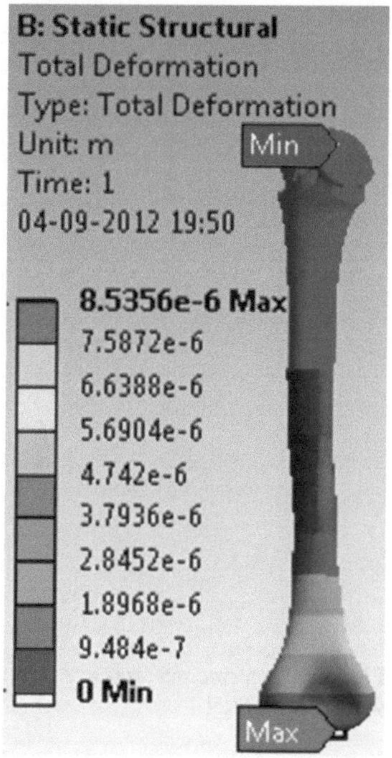

Fig. 3 Total deformation with F = 9.689N

around the selected volume. The number of triangles determines the quality of the reconstruction: the more the triangles, the higher the quality [6].

(k) Importing the geometry to ANSYS:

ANSYS is an engineering simulation software developer. The humeral head is fixed and the elbow is considered a motor rotation couple having some angular variation. The load is applied according to the force values calculated with respect to the angular variation (Fig. 2). The parameters like total deformation (Fig. 3), Von-Mises Stress (Fig. 4), maximum principal stress (Fig. 5) and equivalent strain (Fig. 6) are calculated.

Steps Involved in RP Process

- The STL files are checked for flaws within the file.
- The data have been sent to the machine for the Stereo lithography (SLA) process to take place which is the most widely distributed process of RP.
- A photosensitive liquid, i.e., a photopolymer resin that solidifies when exposed to light, is in a vat.
- A laser, emitting ultraviolet light, is placed on top of this vat.
- The movement of the laser light on the surface of the resin is controlled by a movable mirror, using the data from the STL files.

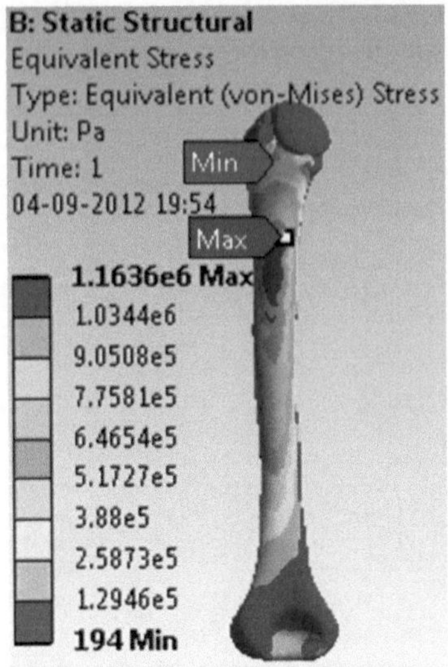

Fig. 4 Equivalent von-mises stress with F = 9.689N

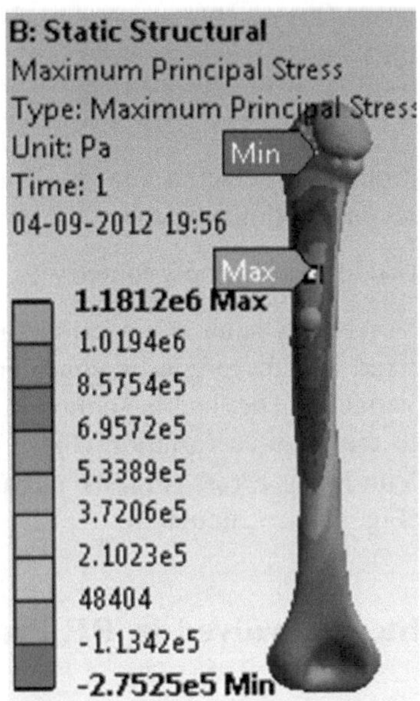

Fig. 5 Max principal stress with F = 9.689N

- A building platform within the vat is moved down one layer thickness after the surface layer is solidified.
- The final 3D physical model is obtained (Fig. 7) [7].

After the RP model is created the same process as above is followed using the CT images of the RP model. CT data was obtained from the same machine specified above with the slice thickness of 0.5 mm. Similar parameters: Total deformation

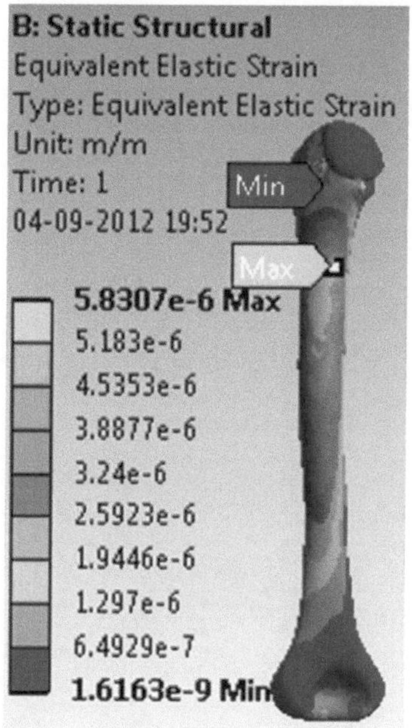

Fig. 6 Equivalent elastic strain with F = 9.689N

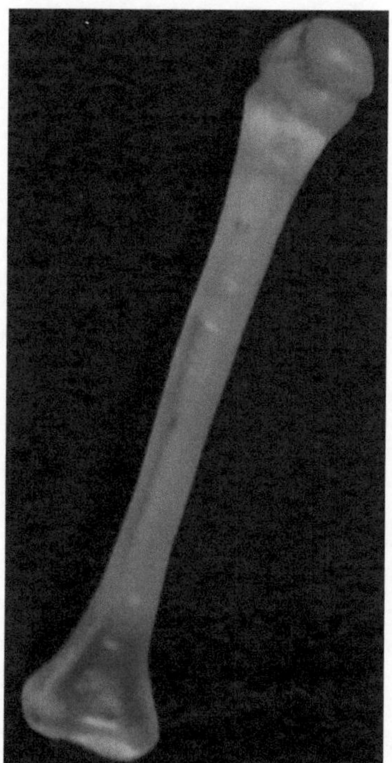

Fig. 7 RP model of human humerus bone

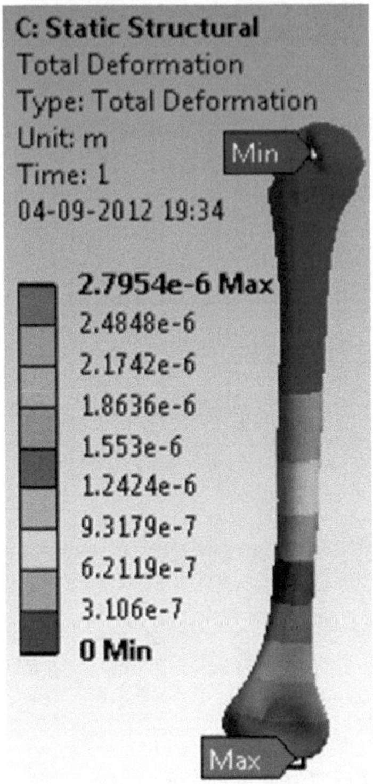

Fig. 8 Total deformation with F = 9.689N

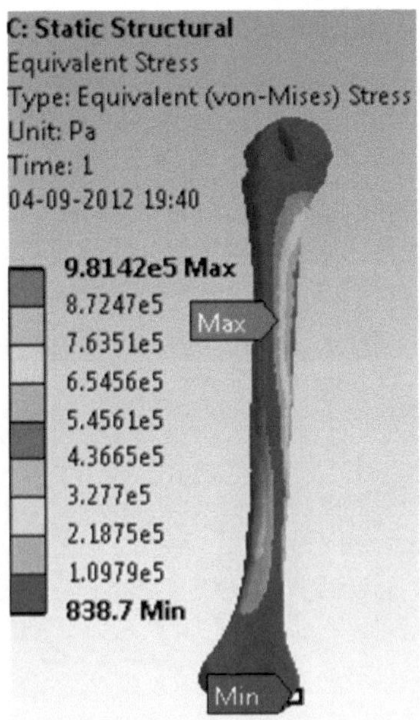

Fig. 9 Equivalent von-mises stress with F = 9.689N

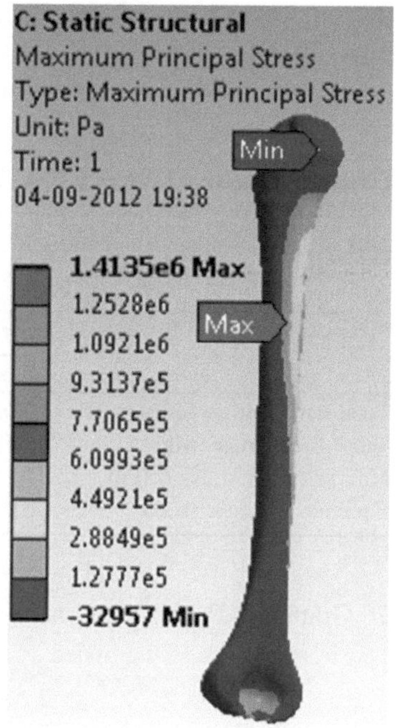

Fig. 10 Max principal stress with F = 9.689N

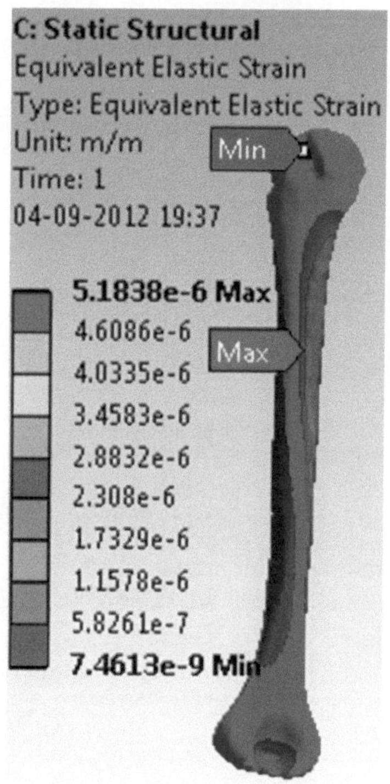

Fig. 11 Equivalent elastic strain with F = 9.689N

(Fig. 8), Von-Mises Stress (Fig. 9), Maximum Principal Stress (Fig. 10) and Equivalent Strain (Fig. 11) are calculated for the RP model and graphically compared with the Real Proximal Humerus bone.

Comparison of the FEA Results

1. Tabular representation

Parameters	For $F = 9.689$		For $F = 19.377$	
Model type	Real	RP	Real	RP
Total deformation (mm)	0.0085356	0.002754	0.014691	0.005702
Von-Mises stress (MPa)	1.1636	0.98142	2.3172	1.9627
Max principal stress (MPa)	1.1812	1.4135	2.1997	2.8269
Equivalent elastic strain	5.8307e-6	5.1838e-6	1.3775 e-5	1.0367e-5

2. Graphical Representation

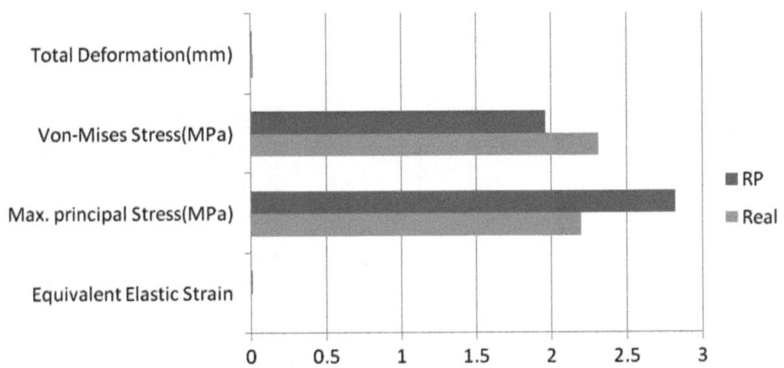

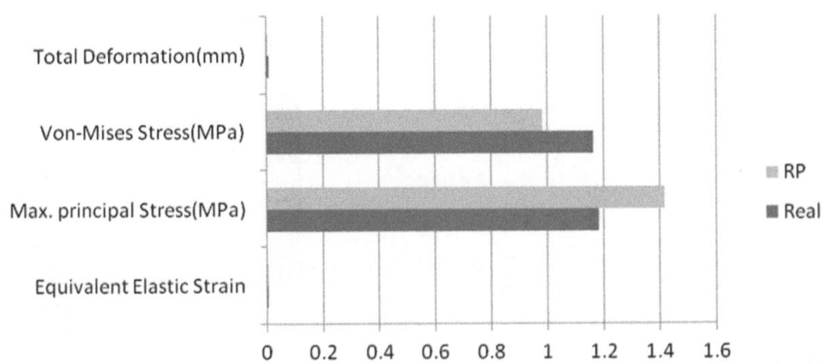

Results and Discussions

This paper focuses on a new method of using data obtained from CT images combined with digital CAD and rapid prototyping model for surgical planning and this new application enables the surgeon to choose the proper configuration and location of internal fixation of plate on humerus bone during orthopaedic surgery. The method gives rise to various advantages and disadvantages. Oka et al. [8] found that the process can be used in various studies of biomechanics, computational stress analysis. Design of optimal training regimens to minimize the risk of injury can also be performed. The verification required from the biological experiments for the structure analysis makes the process slightly difficult. The study of parameters and loads of the bone makes the process a time-consuming one.

The limitations of this study are that the soft tissue considerations were not employed. The strengths of this work are that the resultants are very close to the previous works performed using RP. In conclusion, the virtual bone that we studied can be used as prototype model for the studies regarding humerus fracture with application in medical researches.

Acknowledgments The authors thank the Additional Director, Dr. Chandra Sekhar (Scientist 'G'), R. Anbazhagan (Scientist 'D'), G.T.R.E, R&D, DRDO, Bangalore, who helped us for the creation of the RP model and Dr. Pushpraj Bhatele for providing the medical imaging data. We also thank Dr. (Mrs.) Shobha Katheria, Principal Medical Officer, Ordnance Factory Hospital, Itarsi, M.P. India, for a back support, making us aware of the doctoral issues and practices. We are also thankful to all the faculty members of the Department of Mechanical Engineering, Government Engineering College, Jabalpur, M.P, India.

Conflict of Interest Statement The authors disclose that they have no financial or personal relationships with organisations or people that could inappropriately influence this work.

References

1. Houston RL (2009) Principles of biomechanics. Taylor & Francis Group, LLC, ISBN 13:978-0-8493-3494-8
2. "Kinesiology of the Upper Extremity" Part II, Unit 2, Oatis_CH08-117-149.qxd 4/18/07 2:29 PM, pp 117–121
3. Brennan J (2010–2011) Production of anatomical models from CT scan data. Masters Dissertation, De Montfort University, Leicester, 2010–2011
4. Materialise Interactive Medical Image Control System (MIMICS) 10.01: User Guide
5. Truscott M, Prof. de Beer DJ, Booysen GJ, Barnard LJ (2004) Bone development through CT/CAD/CAM/RP. Central University of Technology, Bloemfontein
6. Chandramohan D, Dr Marimuthu K (2011) Humerus bone development through CT/CAD/RPT. Int J Eng Res Appl 1(4):1256–1261. ISSN: 2248-9622
7. Chandramohan D, Marimuthu K (2011) Natural fiber bone plates as substitutes for orthopaedic alloy plates. Biotechnol Bioinf Bioeng 1(4):405–413. ISSN 2249-9075 (Society for applied biotechnology)
8. Oka K, Murase T, Moritomo H, Goto A, Sugamoto K, Yoshikawa H (2009) Accuracy analysis of three-dimensional bone surface models of the forearm constructed from multidetector computed tomography data. Int J Med Rob Comp Assist Surg 5:452–457

Finite Element Application to Human Humerus Bone: A Biomechanical Study

Chetna Masih, Raji Nareliya and Veerendra Kumar

Abstract The purpose of this retrospective study is to evaluate the biomechanical behavior of the human humerus bone under specific boundary and loading conditions. The shape and material properties of the bones are based on the computed tomography (CT) data set, which was obtained from the Medical College, Jabalpur. Here, the Finite Element Analysis (FEA) which has an important significance in the biomechanical research has been used and its purpose in the field of biomechanics is to predict the mechanical behavior of bones; it is also a powerful computational tool that permits accurate structural analysis. Here, an analytical model of human humerus bone is developed to predict the stress and strain distribution developed. In the model, stress values increased with the increase of the axial load. The results of this analysis are helpful for orthopedic surgeons for clinical interest and bone prosthesis.

Keywords Biomechanical · Computed tomography · Finite element analysis · Humerus bone and prosthesis

V. Kumar
Government Engineering College, Jabalpur, India
e-mail: prof.veerendra.kumar@gmail.com

R. Nareliya
Hitkarni College of Engineering and Technology, Jabalpur, India
e-mail: raji_nareliya@yahoo.co.in

C. Masih (✉)
Government Engineering College, Gokhalpur, Jabarlpur, MP 482 011, India
e-mail: chetnamasih@gmail.com

V. Kumar and M. Bhatele (eds.), *Proceedings of All India Seminar on Biomedical Engineering 2012 (AISOBE 2012)*, Lecture Notes in Bioengineering,
DOI: 10.1007/978-81-322-0970-6_12, © Springer India 2013

Introduction

Anatomy of Humerus Bone

Humerus is the longest and the largest bone of the upper limb. It comprises a rounded head at the upper end, the shaft, and the expanded lower end. This bone pivots in three rotational degrees of freedom from its proximal end at the shoulder joint [1]. The head of the humerus forms less than half of the sphere and its smooth surface is covered by hyaline cartilage which articulates with the glenoid cavity with the scapula forming a ball and socket joint. It lies at an angle to the shaft and fits into a shallow socket of the scapula also known as shoulder blade to form the shoulder joint [2]. The anatomical neck is a slight constriction separating the head from the rest of the upper end of the humerus. The shaft is almost cylindrical in the upper half of its extent, prismatic and is flattened below [3]. It is not a weight bearing bone and therefore weight bearing is not a factor and shortening does not significantly worsen the end results. Humeral shaft fractures result from direct and indirect trauma. Pure compressive forces result in proximal and distal humerus fractures; bending forces, however, typically result in transverse fractures of the humerus shaft [4]. Humerus connects the shoulder by articulating the humeral head with the glenoid of the scapula, to the elbow by articulating the testal humerus with the ulna and radius, as shown in Fig. 1 [5]. The elbow is one of the few places in the body where two bones articulate with one bone [6].

Biomechanics of Bones

FE models of long bones constructed from CT data are an invaluable tool in the field of bone biomechanics. The structural properties of bone consist of the size, shape, and architecture of bones in addition to mechanical properties of bone tissue [7]. Bone tissue is a type of dense connective hard tissue. Bones are composed of inorganic salts impregnated in a matrix of collagen fibers, proteins, and minerals. They maintain the shape of the body and assist in force transmission during movement [8]. The mechanical properties of bone vary between species and individuals or due to age and disease [9]. Bone mass is increased by mechanical loading through the application of resistance or increased weight bearing activity [10]. One method to analyze the loading of the bone is by biomechanical modeling [11].

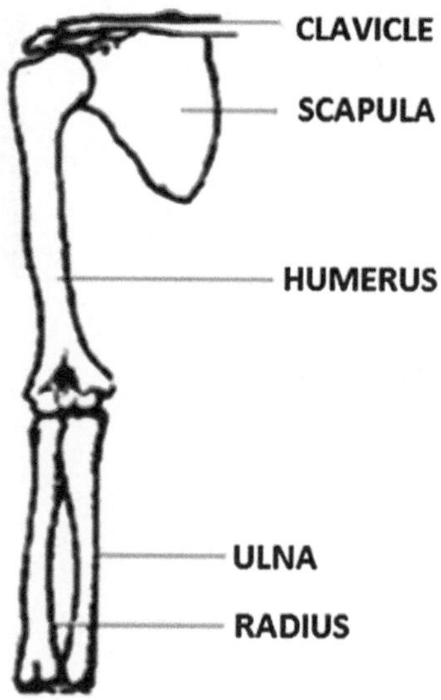

Fig. 1 Humerus bone in human arm

Adaption of Bone to Mechanical Loading

In loading, pure longitudinal, axial force such as compression slightly shortens and widens the bone while tension lengthens and narrows the bone. Bending mainly compresses the other side of the long bone and elongates the other. Bone is at its weakest at coping with the shear forces, better at coping with tension, and at its best for coping with compression [12]. Forces in habitual loading are most likely a combination of more than one, however, [13]. The anisotropic nature of bone reflects its function since bone structure is strongest in the primary loading condition [14].

Research Methodology

1. Obtain the sample data

The geometrical data of real proximal human humerus bone in the format of Digital Imaging and Communications in Medicine (DICOM) images of a 17-year-old male, whose weight is 75 kg, is obtained from CT scan data. A single DICOM file contains a header that stores information about the patient's names, the type of scan, image dimensions, and the image data, which contains information in three dimensions [15]. This DICOM data set is obtained from GE Signa HDXt 2008 Multi Channel 1.5 Tesla Superconducting Helium Cooled whole-body MR module machine and contains a total of 909 slices. This machine can perform with highest

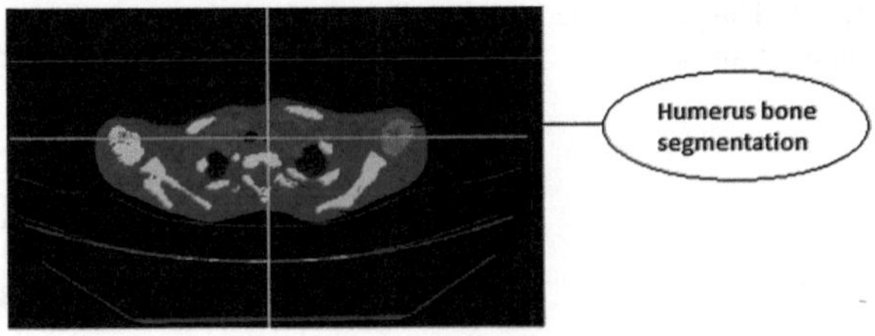

Fig. 2 *Yellow*-colored mask of Humerus bone

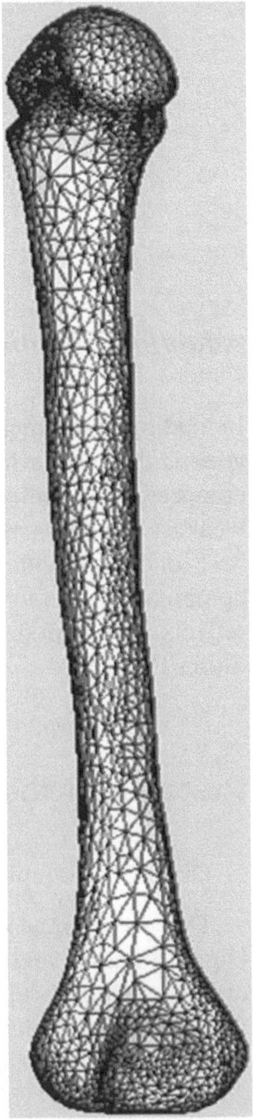

Fig. 3 Surface mesh

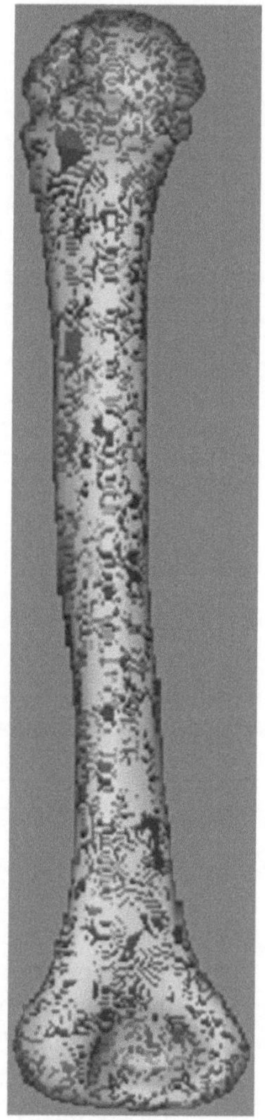

Fig. 4 Volumetric Mesh with material assignment

precision, the humongous task of MR spectroscopy. The slice thickness is 0.4 mm and resolutions are 1,024 × 1,024.

2. Procedure of establishing the model
   (a) *Import the DICOM into MIMICS* 10.01-
   All DICOM images are loaded and displayed and then by assigning a proper threshold value, based on Hounsfield Unit, the segmentation object is obtained, which is visualized by a colored mask containing only those pixels of images that we are interested in [16]. MIMICS 10.01 predefined a threshold of bone (CT), so we could easily select all bone tissue, the green

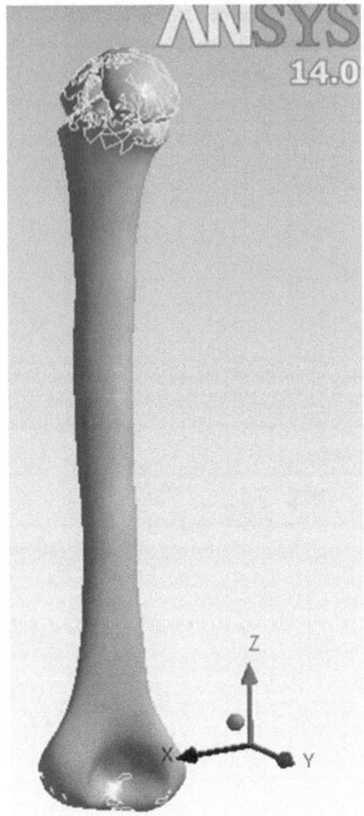

Fig. 5 3D Model for analysis

area was bone tissue pixels, we defined this as a mask. Based on the mask the humerus was selected, as in Fig. 2. This mask is modified until we get the satisfactory mask.

(b) *Establishing FE model and generate surface mesh with MIMICS* 10.01-
The generated region mask was used to develop 3D model for the bone. Based on 3D Grayvalue interpolation techniques 2D images are transformed into 3D model. It is a real 3D interpolation technique that takes into account the Partial Volume effect and therefore it is more accurate [16]. To obtain surface mesh, the option remeshing is used in order to raise the quality of the triangles so that the preprocessor of an FEA package can build a tetrahedron meshes from them (Fig. 3).

(c) *Convert surface mesh into volumetric mesh with ABAQUS* 6.10-
This mesh is exported to ABAQUS 6.10 and is converted from tri into tetra by using the mesh edit option. This is done because the denser the mesh the more realistic and more accurate will be the solution.

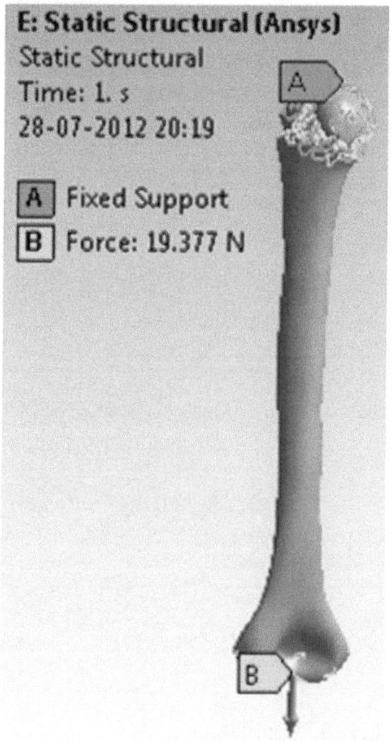

Fig. 6 Loading and boundary condition applied in ANSYS 14

(d) *Assign material properties in MIMICS* 10.01-
Materials are assigned to FEA meshes via the FEA menu or the FEA mesh tab. Before assigning materials to the elements of the volumetric mesh, Mimics will first calculate grayvalue for each element. After the calculation of the gray values of the elements of the volumetric mesh, the material assignment window will appear. We consider the default material properties of the CT data set. Using MIMICS STL+ module, humerus bone was converted into stereo lithography files for FE Analysis (Fig. 4).

3. Finite Element Analysis (FEA) using ANSYS 14
Elbow is one of the most complex joint in the human body and they are studied statically in a system [17]. Thus, the FEA mesh files are added in the FE modeler and then the model is transferred to static structural and further analysis is done under specific boundary and loading conditions (Fig. 5).
4. Loading and boundary condition
This biomechanical study was done based on some values calculated from some simulation studies done previously. The load was applied axially at the lower end of the humerus, in tension, keeping the humeral head fixed (Fig. 6).

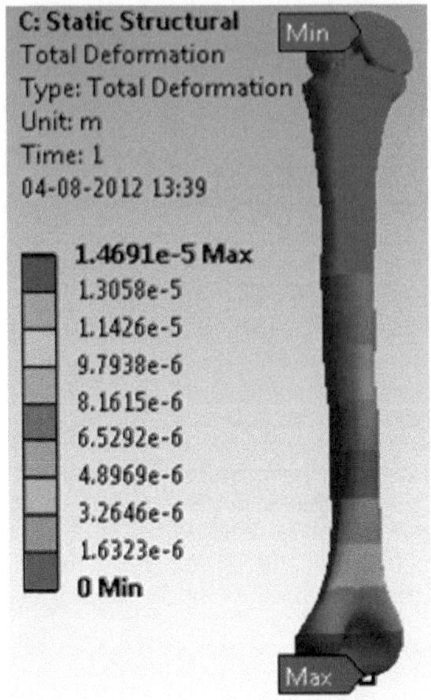

Fig. 7 Maximum total deformation

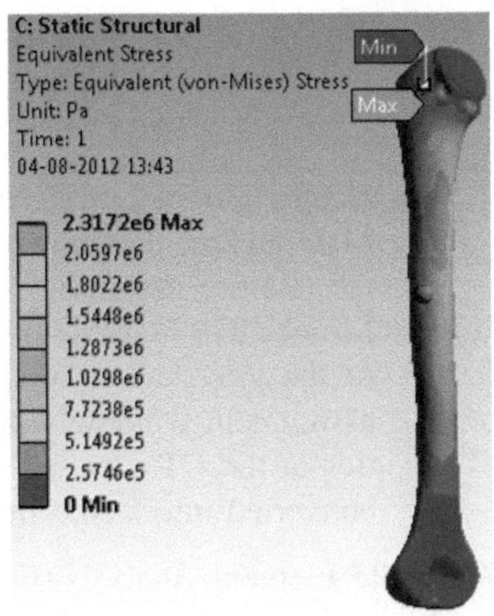

Fig. 8 Equivalent Von-Mises stress

Results and Discussions

Based on the analysis of the FE model, it was seen that the total deformation, equivalent stress, and strain increase with the increased load values. The fatigue safety factor for the bone is found to be appropriate considering the daily activities performed [18].

The purpose of our study was to establish a 3D FE model of humerus bones from volumetric CT data that will accurately capture the varying bone geometry and material properties. Arm bones are usually subjected to tensile forces during

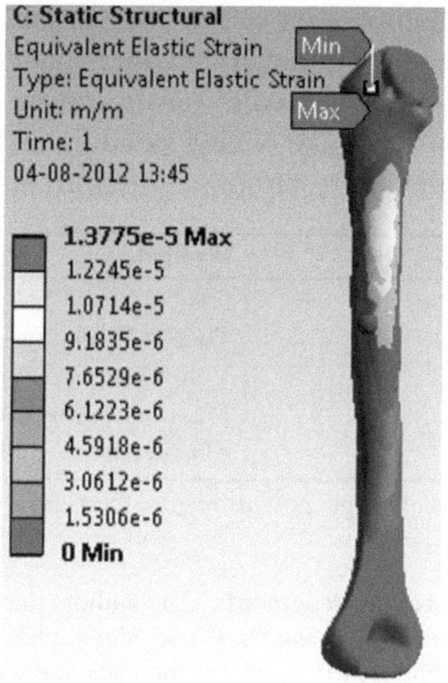

Fig. 9 Elastic strain

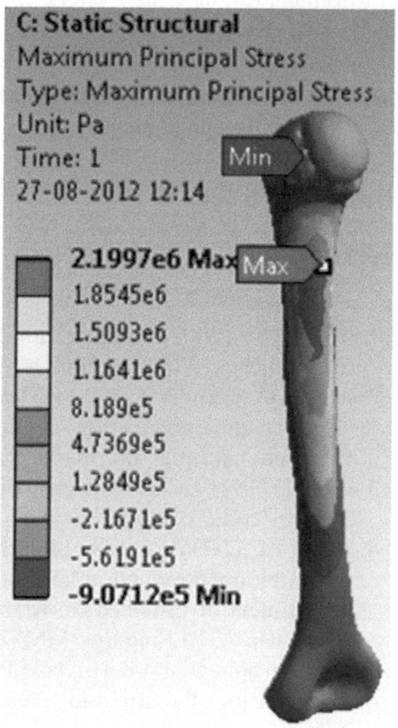

Fig. 10 Maximum principal stress

everyday weight lifting-related activities. In bending there is a combination of tensile and compressive force, tensile stress and strains on one side of the neutral axis and compressive stresses and strains on the other side [19]. By testing under tension, we cover the basic loading conditions to which the humerus bone can be subjected. The data collected from FEA showed the pattern of stress, strain, and deformation of the bone at the interface that can be used to predict the failure of the bone material under load as shown in Figs. 7, 8, 9 and 10. This can help surgeons predict postoperative failures and analyze the cause of fractures taking place in the bone depending on the regions or zones where the maximum values of the stress, strain, and deformation exist.

S. No.	Parameters	$F = 707 \cdot \sin(7.8525 \cdot t)$	
	Case	t = 0.1	t = 0.2
1.	Total deformation (mm)	0.0085356	0.014691
2.	Von-mises stress (MPa)	1.1636	2.3172
3.	Maximum principal stress (MPa)	1.1812	2.1997
4.	Elastic strain	5.8307e−6	1.3775e−5

Note Figures with results for Case t = 0.2 are shown in Figs. 7, 8, 9 and 10

Acknowledgments The authors thank Dr. Pushpraj Bhatele for providing medical imaging data. We also thank Dr. (Mrs.) Shobha Katheria, Principal Medical Officer, Ordnance Factory Hospital, Itarsi, M.P. India, for the back support, making us aware of the doctoral issues and practices. We are also thankful to all the faculty members of the Department of Mechanical Engineering, Government Engineering College, Jabalpur, M.P, India. Also, thanks to all study participants for their great effort and cooperation.

Conflict of Interest Statement None of the authors have any conflict of interest with the work described in this manuscript.

References

1. Toddes SP (2007) Optimization for commercialization of a two degree of freedom powered arm orthosis, Worcester Polytechnic Institute
2. Masih C, Francis A, Shriwastava A, Diwedi N, Tiwari P, Nareliya R, Kumar V (2012) Biomechanical evaluation of human humerus and scapula bone: a review. vol 3(1) Bioinfo Publications, India, pp 63–66, ISSN: 0976-8084 & E-ISSN: 0976-8092
3. Gray H (1821–1865) Anatomy of the human body-osteology-the humerus, 1918, http://www.bartleby.com/107/51.html
4. Kiran KC (2006) A study of surgical management of diaphyseal fractures of the humerus in adults by open reduction and internal fixation with dynamic compression plate and screws. Department of orthopedics. Kempegowda Institute of Medical Sciences, Banglore
5. Alsamhan A, ELSingergy MM, Zamzam MM, Darwish SM (2011) Engineering judgment of children bone fracture. Hindawi Publishing Corporation, Cairo, Vol 2011, Article ID 737054: 7
6. The skeleton: the arm and forearm. http://home.comcast.net/~barbbranham/arm.htm
7. Nikander R (2009) Exercise loading and bone structure,studies in sports, physical education and health, University of Jyvaskyla, ISBN 978-95131-3597-9
8. Nareliya R, Kumar V Biomechanical analysis of human femur bone. Int J Eng Sci Technol 3(4). ISSN: 0975-5462
9. Fung YC (1993) Biomechanics: mechanical properties of living tissues, 2nd edn. Springer, New York, p 511
10. Greene DA, Naughton GA (2006) Adaptive skeletal responses to mechanical loading during adolescence. Sports Med 36(9):723–732

11. Nieminen H, Niemi J, Takala EP, Juntura EV (1995) Load-sharing patterns in the shoulder during isometric flexion tasks. J Biomech 28:555–566
12. Einhorn TA (1992) Bone strength: the bottom line. Calcif Tissue Int 51:333–339
13. Turner CH, Burr DB (1993) Basic biomechanical measurements of bone: a tutorial. Bone 14:595–608
14. Bouxsein ML (2008) Technology inside: non invasive assessment of bone strength in osteoporosis. Nat Clin Pract Rheumatol 4:310–318
15. Gupta S, Dan P (2004) Trends biomaterial artificial organs, bone geometry and mechanical properties of the human scapula using computed tomography data 17(2):61–70
16. Materialise Interactive Medical Image Control System (MIMICS) (2011) 10.01: user guide
17. Lungu R, Borgazi E, Lungu M, Popa D, Tutunea D, Calbureanu MX (2010) New methods for the simulation with finite element of the human elbow.In: Proceedings of the international conference on circuits, systems, signals, pp 45–50
18. Westerhoff P, Graichen F, Bender A, Halder A, Beier A, Rohlmann A, Bergmann G (2009) In vivo measurement of shoulder joint loads during activities of daily living. J Biomech 42:1840–1849
19. Varghese BA (2011) Quantitative computed-tomography based bone-strength indicators for the identification of low bone-strength individuals in a clinical environment. Dissertation, Doctor of Philosophy, Wright State University

Digital Watermarking of Medical Images

Siddharth Bhalerao, Manas Mehta, Neelu Dubey and Mukta Bhatele

Abstract Security is one of the major aspects of medical imagery. Various methods have been evolved which ensure the integrity and confidentiality of medical images stored as electronic patient record (EPR). In this paper, digital watermarking is proposed as a method to enhance medical data security. Watermarking also ensures that the image presented for insurance claims and before law is the authentic image. The proposed scheme is a software-dependent watermarking technique. The software used for watermarking can only reconstruct the image.

Keywords Medical image security · Digital watermarking · EPR

Introduction

This chapter deals with the security aspect of digital imaging and communications in medicine (DICOM) images, using digital watermarking techniques. Although these techniques could be applied to any image, they are a must in case of medical images. Similarly, digital watermarking techniques are not limited to images but could also be applied on audio as well as video media. Medical images include all scan images like CT scans, Ultrasounds, MRIs, etc. In today's environment medical images are parts of electronic patient record (EPR) and are not only stored

S. Bhalerao (✉) · M. Mehta
Department of Digital Communication, Gyan Ganga College of Technology, Jabalpur, India
e-mail: siddharth.b2010@gmail.com

N. Dubey
CTA, Gyan Ganga College of Technology, Jabalpur, India

M. Bhatele
Department of Computer Science, Gyan Ganga College of Technology, Jabalpur, India

V. Kumar and M. Bhatele (eds.), *Proceedings of All India Seminar on Biomedical Engineering 2012 (AISOBE 2012)*, Lecture Notes in Bioengineering,
DOI: 10.1007/978-81-322-0970-6_13, © Springer India 2013

in computers, but also transferred across networks and with advent of cloud computing sometimes stored on network clouds. In such a scenario, there is a chance of images getting distorted on the way. Even stored images can be distorted due to activities of hackers and malicious software like malwares and viruses. The distortion may not severely affect the image, but will make its user skeptic toward originality of image. Therefore, the distorted images are of no use to medical professionals and also cannot be used as a proof in legal matters before the law. The digital watermarking techniques discussed here would reinstantiate the originality of images after transmission over a network or if the images are stored for very long. Reference [1] provides a detailed description of medical security.

Classification of different watermarking techniques is provided first and then we cover the details of the watermarking method that we have used.

Classification

Digitally watermarked images can be classified on various grounds depending on the different aspects of watermarking. One classification is made on the robustness of watermarking; a watermark is said to be fragile if it gets changed, if any change is made to image. On the other hand, a watermark is said to be robust if it can survive attacks like compression, cropping, etc.

Another classification can be made on the basis of the technique used in watermarking. If image pixel information is changed to create a watermark, it is known as the spatial domain technique. Sometimes, image is transformed into frequency domain using transforms, of which are the well-known Fast Fourier Transform (FFT), Discrete Cosine Transform (DCT) and Discrete Wavelet Transform (DWT). Such techniques are called frequency domain techniques.

Watermarking techniques can also be classified as reversible and non-reversible. When it is possible to get the original image from the watermarked one, the method is said to be reversible or else it is non-reversible watermarking. Other classifications can be made on the basis of whether watermark is included in the region of interest (ROI). If watermark is embedded in ROI it should not affect the medical detection, hence some of the techniques decide an ROI and embed watermarking in the non-ROI region.

Spatial Domain Techniques

Spatial domain techniques of watermark embedding which modify the pixel information of image and thus provide watermarking are fragile techniques. The watermark is sometimes embedded in LSB of every image pixel, thus creating digital watermark but keeping the image usable. These techniques could be both reversible as well as non-reversible.

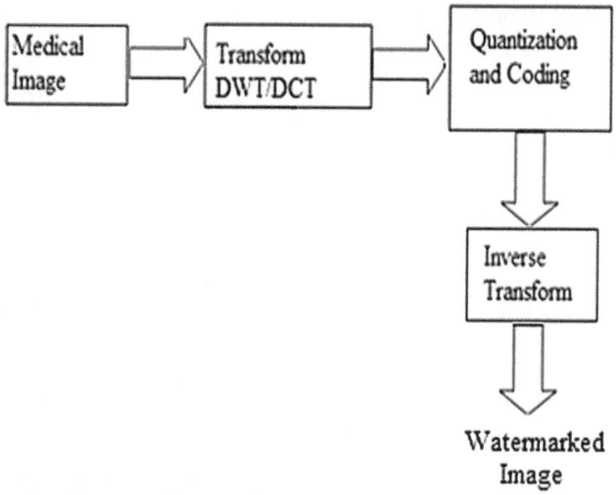

Fig. 1 Frequency domain techniques

Frequency Domain Techniques

As discussed above in these techniques, image data is transformed using some well-known transforms like FFT, DCT, DWT etc. The coefficients of transformed images are then coded and again inverse transformed to get a watermarked image. Quantisation of coefficients is done prior to coding (Fig. 1).

More on these techniques is presented in Ref. [2, 3].

Proposed Method

The method presented here is a digital watermarking technique which extracts some crucial information from the image, and maps that information in the non-ROI region of the image. The parameters required to extract the data from the non-ROI region is embedded into the ROI of the image. The whole process is software dependent and can be reversed by using the same piece of software used to watermark the image. Figure 2 depicts the watermarking process.

In our method, ROI is first determined from the image and separated from the complete image. The remaining, i.e., non-ROI region includes patient data and other medical information. This information is then extracted from the non-ROI region. This data are extracted on the basis of font color, which is mostly white in DICOM images although OCR can also be used. The row and column information is obtained from white pixels, which is scrambled and then embedded in the non ROI region surrounding the ROI. The start and end information of these data are then randomly mapped to the ROI region. Other than start and end, information about where row and column is present with the information about extant of ROI area which is also embedded in ROI region in a way that it does not deform the image.

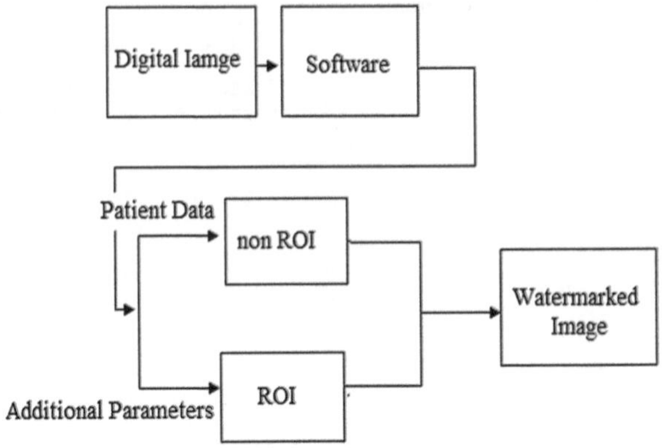

Fig. 2 Proposed method

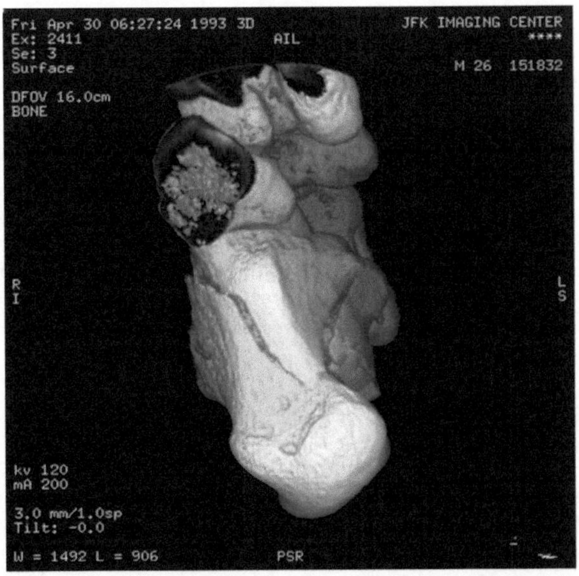

Fig. 3 Original image

The coding for software is done in MATLAB™ and the test image used is also the default image provided in MATLAB™. Figure 3 shows the original image which is digitally watermarked

Figure 3 shows the watermarked image in which patient information is hidden in the area surrounding ROI, the figure also shows the clear difference between ROI and the rest of the image.

Figure 4 is the reconstructed image by the same software; if the information is preserved in watermarked image then only software can reconstruct the image. In case of any information loss in non-ROI region software will create a deformed image. Similarly, loss of additional parameters present in ROI region will give an error on reconstruction.

Figure 5 shows the reconstructed image.

Fig. 4 Watermarked image

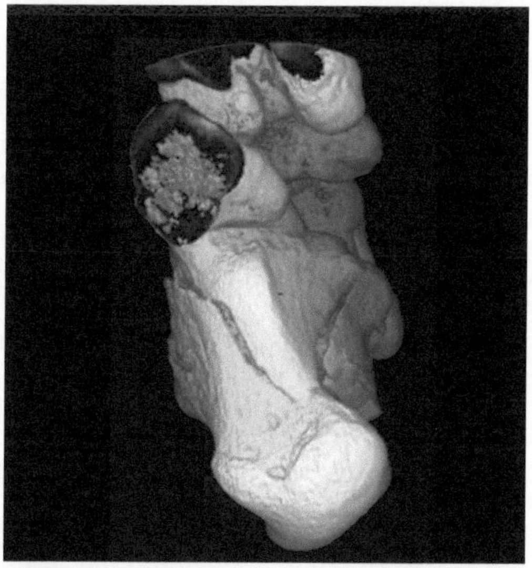

Fig. 5 Recovered image

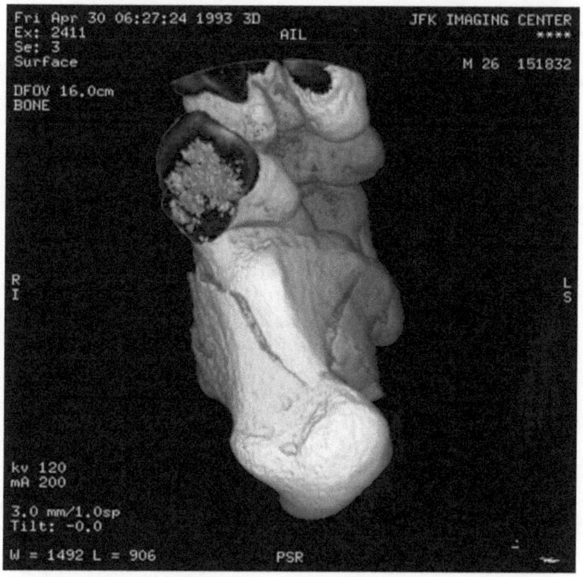

Conclusion

The watermarking method present here is a software-dependent reversible watermarking method; unlike other methods it does not use any algorithm to validate the watermarked image. If the image is recovered without deformation by the software, it guarantees that the image is authentic.

References

1. Coatrieux G, Maître H, Sankur B, Rolland Y, Collorec R (2000) Relevance of watermarking in medical imaging. In: IEEE International conference on information technology applications in biomedicine, EMBS, November 2000, pp 250–255
2. Zain JM, Baldwin LP, Clarke M (2009) Reversible watermarking for authentication of DICOM images. In: Proceedings of 26th annual international conference on engineering medical biological society (EMBC 2004), vol 2, pp 3237–3240
3. Umaamaheshvari A, Thanushkodi K (2012) High PERFORMANCE AND EFFECTIVE WATERMARKING SCHEME FOR MEDICAL IMAGES. European Journal of Scientific Research 2012:283–293
4. Tian J (2003) High capacity reversible data embedding and content authentication. IEEE Int Conf Acoust Speech Sign Process 2003:517–520

Applications of Wavelet Transform in Registration, Segmentation, Denoising, and Compression of Medical Images

Neelu Dubey, Meghna Jain and Mukta Bhatele

Abstract Wavelet transforms and other multiscale analysis functions have been used for compact signal and image representations in denoising, compression, and feature detection processing problems. The wavelet transform itself offers great design flexibility. Basis selection, spatial-frequency tiling, and various wavelet threshold strategies can be optimized for best adaptation to a processing application, data characteristics, and feature of interest. Fast implementation of wavelet transforms using a filter-bank framework enables real-time processing capability. Instead of trying to replace standard image processing techniques, wavelet transforms offer an efficient representation of the signal, finely tuned to its intrinsic properties. By combining such representations with simple processing techniques in the transform domain, multiscale analysis can accomplish remarkable performance and efficiency for many image processing problems.

Keywords Wavelet transform using Matlab · Image edge detection · Segmentation · Registration · De-noising · Lossless image compression · Digital imaging and communications in medicine (DICOM) · Security issue in transmission · Transmission of medical images · Measuring lossless compression effectiveness parameters · Compression algorithm

N. Dubey
CTA, Gyan Ganga College of Technology, Jabalpur, India

M. Jain (✉)
Digital Communication, Gyan Ganga College of Technology, Jabalpur, India
e-mail: jain.meghna@yahoo.com

M. Bhatele
Department of Computer Science, Gyan Ganga College of Technology, Jabalpur, India
e-mail: mukta_bhatele@rediffmail.com

V. Kumar and M. Bhatele (eds.), *Proceedings of All India Seminar on Biomedical Engineering 2012 (AISOBE 2012)*, Lecture Notes in Bioengineering,
DOI: 10.1007/978-81-322-0970-6_14,

Introduction

The increasing adoption of information systems in health care has led to a scenario where patient information security is more and more being regarded as a critical issue. Allowing patient information to be in jeopardy may lead to irreparable damage, physically, morally, and socially to the patient, potentially shaking the credibility of the health care institution. This demands adoption of security mechanisms to assure information integrity and authenticity. Structured descriptions attached to medical image series conforming to the digital imaging and communications in medicine (DICOM) standard make possible to fit the collections of existing digitized images into an educational and research framework.

Our aim is to design an application of Wavelet transform in Edge detection, segmentation, image registration, denoising, providing lossless compression of DICOM images by applying Daubechie's wavelet, and run length encoding. This helps in better bandwidth utilization of the networks and at the same time, also aims at providing the security mechanism for DICOM images by removing the texual elements of the medical image.

Wavelet Edge Detection and Segmentation

Edge detection plays an important role in image segmentation. In many cases, boundary delineation is the ultimate goal for an image segmentation and a good edge detector itself can then fulfill the requirement of segmentation [1]. On the other hand, many segmentation techniques require an estimation of object edges for their initialization.

Most multiscale edge detectors smooth the input signal at various scales and detect sharp variation locations (edges) from their first or second derivatives. Edge locations are related to the extrema of the first derivative of the signal and the zero crossings of the second derivative of the signal.

It was also pointed out that first-derivative wavelet functions are more appropriate for edge detection since the magnitude of wavelet modulus represents the relative "strength" of the edges, and therefore enables to differentiate meaningful edges from small fluctuations caused by noise (Fig. 1).

Wavelet Image Registration

Another very important application of wavelets in image processing: image registration. Image registration is required for many image processing applications. In medical imaging, co-registration problems are important for many clinical tasks:

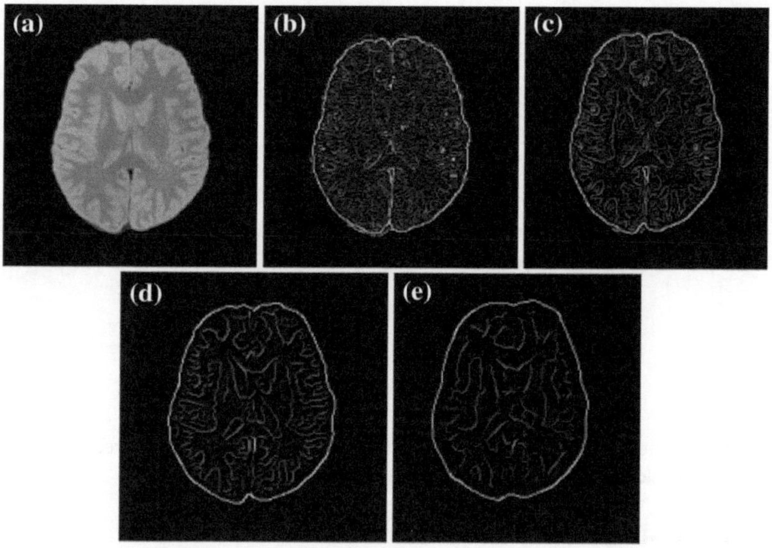

Fig. 1 Example of a multiscale edge detection method finding local maxima of wavelet modulus, with a first-derivative wavelet function. **a** Input image. **b–e** Multiscale edge map at expansion scale 1–4

- Multimodalities study.
- Cross-subject normalization and template/atlas analysis.
- Patient monitoring over time with tracking of the pathological evolution for the same patient and the same modality.

Many registration methods follow a feature matching procedure. Feature points (often referred to as "control points", or CP) are first identified in both the reference image and the input image. An optimal spatial transformation (rigid or non-rigid) is then computed that can connect and correlate the two sets of control points with minimal error. Registration has always been considered as very costly in terms of computational load. Besides, when the input image is highly deviated from the reference image, the optimization process can be easily trapped into local minima before reaching the correct transformation mapping. Both issues can be alleviated by embedding the registration into a "coarse to fine" procedure.

Registration at higher resolution is initialized with the result from the lower resolution, and only need to refine the mapping between the two images with local deformations for updating the transformation parameters.

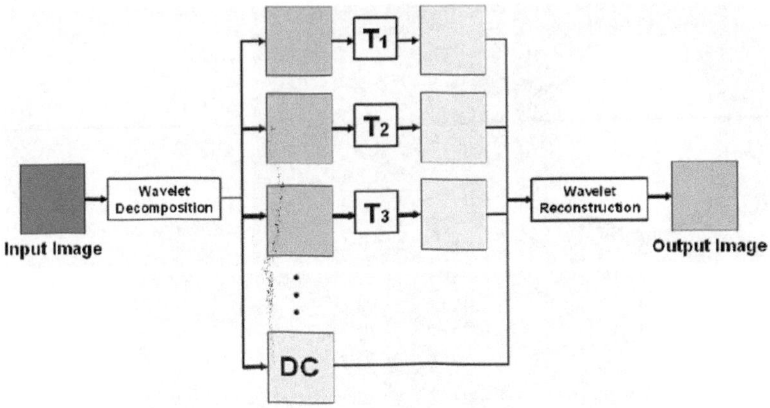

Fig. 2 A Multiscale framework of denoising and enhancement using discrete dyadic wavelet transform. A three-level decomposition was shown

Denoising Using Wavelet Transform

Denoising can be viewed as an estimation problem trying to recover a true signal component X from an observation Y where the signal component has been degraded by a noise component N:

$$Y = X + N$$

The estimation is computed with a thresholding estimator in an orthonormal basis $B = \{\text{gm}\}0<m<N$

$$X = \sum \rho_m(X, g_m)\, g_m$$

where ρ_m is a thresholding function that aims at eliminating noise components (via attenuating of decreasing some coefficient sets) in the transform domain while preserving the true signal coefficients. If the function ρ_m is modified to rather preserve or increase coefficient values in the transform domain, it is possible to enhance some features of interest in the true signal component with the framework of equation (Fig. 2).

Figure 3 illustrates a multiscale enhancement and denoising framework using wavelet transforms. An over-complete dyadic wavelet transform using bi-orthogonal basis is used. Notice that since the DC-cap contains the overall energy distribution, it is usually kept untouched during the procedure. As shown in this figure, thresholding and enhancement functions can be implemented independently from the wavelet filters and easily incorporated into the filter bank framework.

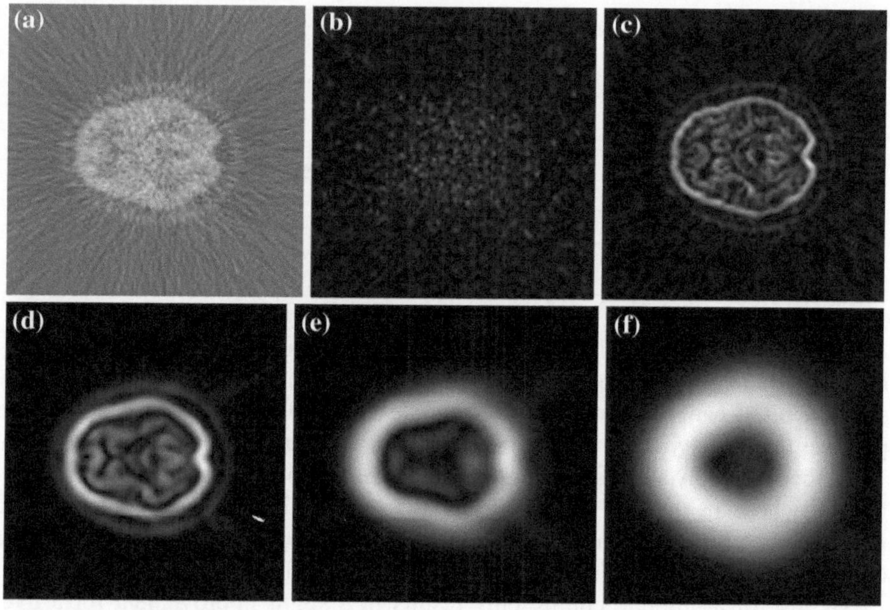

Fig. 3 **a** A brain PET image from a 3D data set with high level of noise, **b–f** modulus of wavelet coefficients at expansion scale 1–5

Wavelet Image Compression

Existing Systems

- Keynotes on JPEG2000

The JPEG2000 standard provides a set of features that are of importance to many high-end and emerging applications by taking advantage of new technologies. It addresses areas where current standards fail to produce the best quality or performance and provides capabilities to markets that currently do not use compression. The markets and applications better served by the JPEG2000 standard are internet, color facsimile, printing, scanning, digital photography, remote sensing, mobile, and medical image. Each application area imposes some requirements that the standard should fulfill. Some of the most important features that this standard should possess are as follows [2]:

- Improved compression efficiency
- Lossy to lossless compression
- Multiple resolution representation
- Region of interest (ROI) coding
- Random code-stream access and processing
- Keynotes on CSPIHT

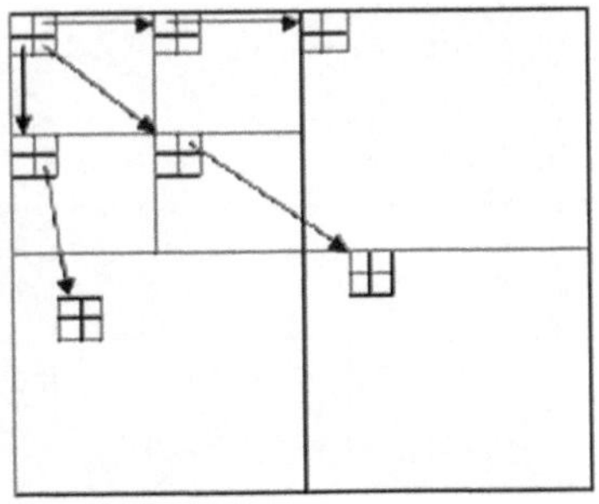

Fig. 4 Level wavelet decomposition with spacial orientation tree

In a wavelet-based still image, coding algorithm known as contexual set partitioning in hierarchical trees (CSPIHT) is developed that generates a continuously scalable bit stream. This means that a single encoded bit stream can be used to produce images at various bit-rates and quality, without any drop in compression. The decoder simply stops decoding when a target rate or reconstruction quality has been reached. In the CSPIHT algorithm, the image is first decomposed into a number of subbands using hierarchical wavelet decomposition. The subbands obtained for a two-level decomposition are shown in Fig. 4.

The use of arithmetic coding only results in a slight improvement for a five-level decomposition. The information that we know about the image file that is produced from wavelet transformation is that it can be represented in a binary tree format with the root of the tree having a much larger probably of containing a greater pixel magnitude level than that of the branches of the root. The algorithm that takes advantage of this information is the CSPIHT algorithm. The architecture of CSPIHT is shown in Figs. 5 and 6.

Proposed System

With the DICOM standard, it is easy to eliminate textual information such as patient name and ID. The problem of text identification arises in many applications other than medical security. However, the algorithms used in such systems are not designed to handle superimposed text because it is difficult to differentiate the edges of text from the edges of the medical objects in the image. We use Daubechies' wavelets and analysis techniques to detect the high frequency variation in the diagonal direction that is indicative of text. With some basic knowledge of the machine used to create the image, we are able to eliminate only sensitive patient identification information while retaining the medical information in the image. Excellent results have been obtained in experiments using a large set of real-world medical images many with superimposed text (Fig. 7).

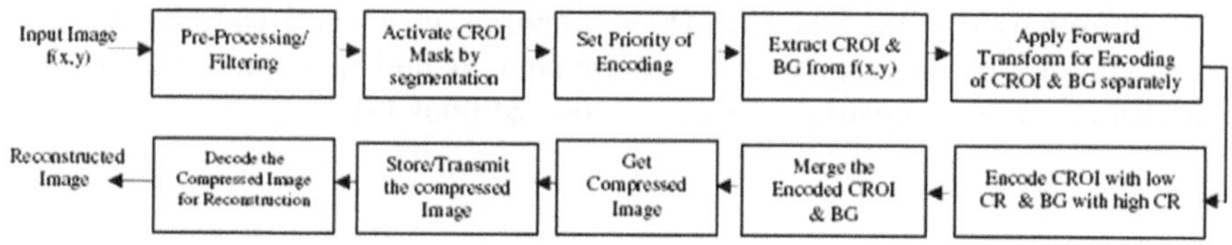

Fig. 5 Architecture of contexual (CSPIHT) compression system

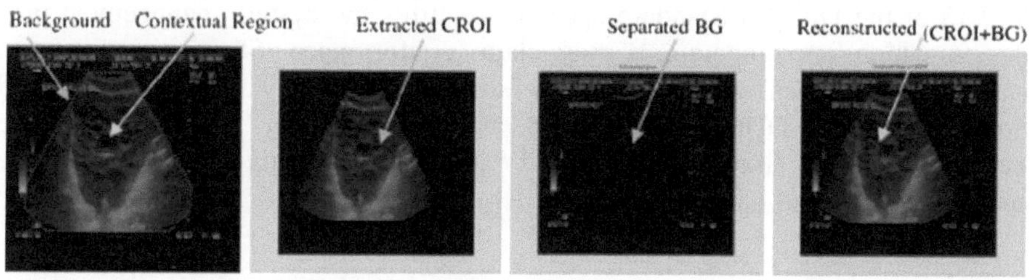

Fig. 6 Separation of CROI and BG from the ultrasound (*US*) image and its reconstructed image

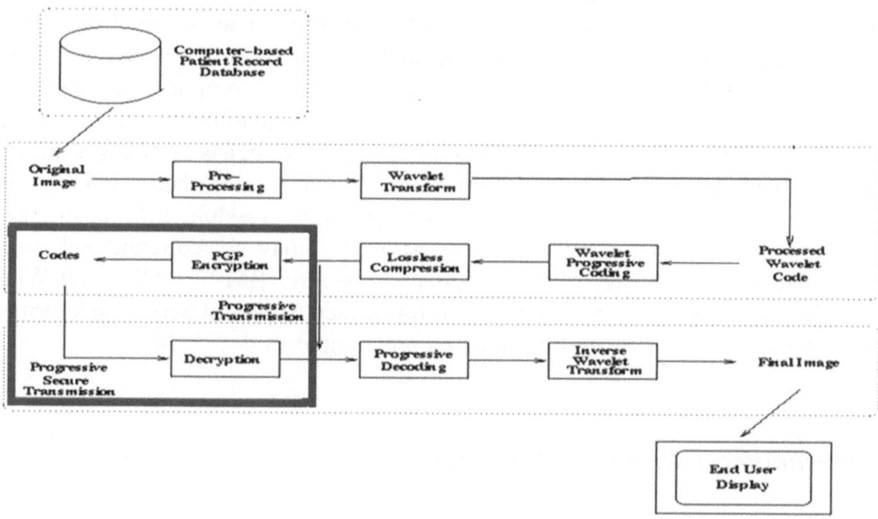

Fig. 7 Architecture of the proposed system

Transmission of Medical Images

The DICOM Standard is an evolving standard and it is maintained in accordance with the Procedures of the DICOM Standards Committee. Proposals for enhancements are forthcoming from the DICOM Committee member organizations based on input from users of the Standard. These proposals are considered for inclusion in future editions of the Standard. A requirement in updating the Standard is to maintain effective compatibility with previous editions [3].

Security Issue in Transmission

PS 3.15 of the DICOM Standard specifies security and system management profiles to which implementations may claim conformance. Security and system management profiles are defined by referencing externally developed standard protocols, such as DHCP, LDAP, TLS, and ISCL. Security protocols may use security techniques like public keys and “smart cards”. Data encryption can use various standardized data encryption schemes.

Choosing Lossless Compression Technique for Medical Images

Medical images are compressed due to their large size and repeated usage for diagnosing purposes. Certified radiologists and doctors assess the degree of image degradation resulting from various types and amounts of compression associated with several different digital image file formats. A qualitative, rather than a quantitative approach is normally chosen because radiologists typically evaluate images qualitatively in their day-to-day practice and, also, because common metrics used for comparing images pre- and post-compression, e.g., mean pixel error, root mean square error, maximum error, etc., may not correlate well with visual assessment of image quality. Bitmapped picture (BMP) is Microsoft Windows device-independent bitmap standard for lossless format. Users of this format can depend on images being displayed on any Windows device [4, 5].

Performance Evaluation Parameters

The effectiveness of lossless compression schemes can be described using the following parameters:

- Compression Ratio: it is defined as the ratio of original file size to that of compressed file size.
- Bit Rate: the bit rate is the average number of bits (fractional) required to encode a pixel and is computed from the total number of bits encoded divided by the number of pixels.
- Mean Square Error: the cumulative squared error between the original and the compressed image is shown by MSE

$$\mathrm{MSE} = \frac{1}{MN}\sum_{y=1}^{N}\sum_{x=1}^{M}[I(x,y) - I'(x,y)]^2$$

- Peak Signal to Noise Ratio: the peak error between the original and the compressed image is shown by PSNR

$$\mathrm{PSNR} = 10\log_{10}\left(\frac{\mathrm{MAX}_i^2}{\mathrm{MSE}}\right) = 20\log_{10}\left(\frac{\mathrm{MAX}_I}{\sqrt{\mathrm{MSE}}}\right)$$

System Implementation

Matlab Software Version 7.0.1 consists of various modules:

1. The input module to retrieve the medical image as input.
2. Provide security feature by changing the DICOM unique identifier (UID).
3. Wavelet decomposition module to provide wavelet compression using Daubechies wavelet of order 2.
4. Compression module to compress the input image by applying run length encoding.
5. Reconstruct original image from compressed image data applying run length decoding.
6. Wavelet reconstruction to decompress the image and extract the original image.

Compression Algorithm

General flow of the various modules of Matlab Software is shown by the algorithm below. Source code of this program is given in Appendix-A.

- Read an image from a DICOM file into the MATLAB workspace.
- Read the metadata from the same DICOM file.
- Remove all the text from the image.
- Generate a new DICOM UID using the dicomuid function.
- Set the value of the SeriesInstanceUID field in the metadata associated with the original DICOM file to the generated value.
- Write the modified image to a new DICOM file, specifying the modified metadata structure, info, as an argument.
- Apply wavelet decomposition and run length encoding to provide lossless compression of image.
- To verify this operation, view the SeriesInstanceUID metadata field in the new file.
- Apply run length decoding and wavelet reconstruction to decompress the Image.

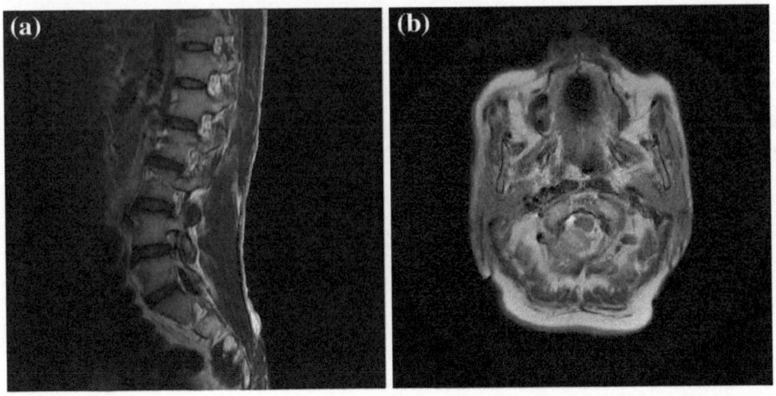

Fig. 8 Medical images

Fig. 9 Original image

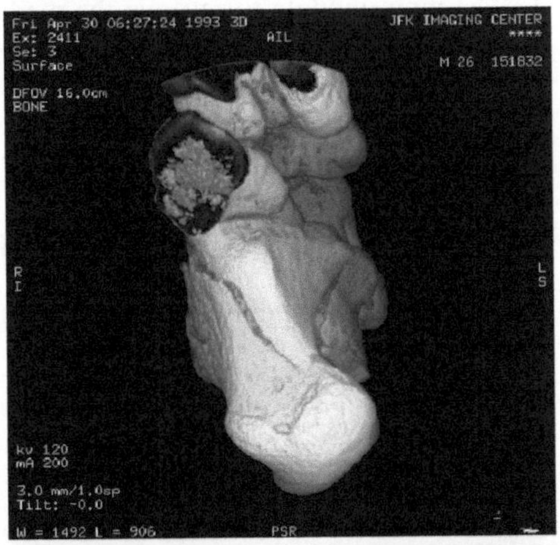

Fig. 10 Image without text area

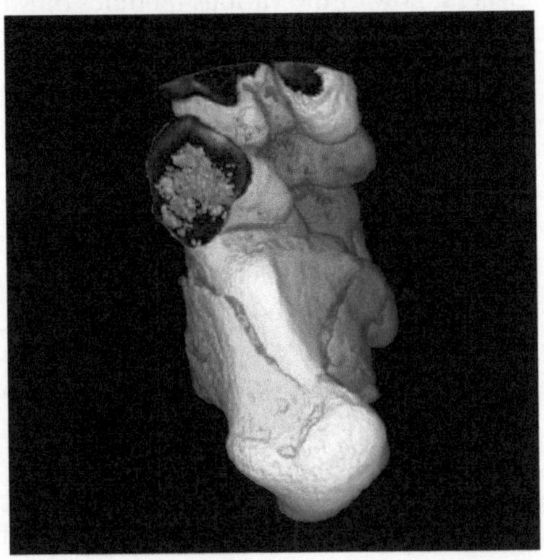

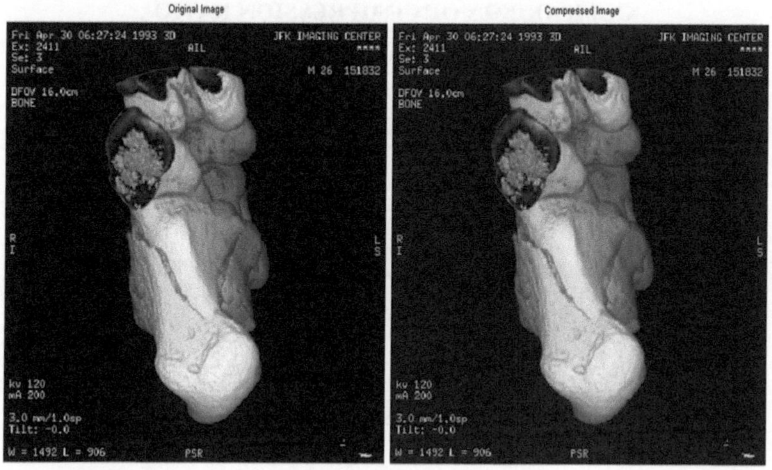

Fig. 11 Original and compressed images

Table 1 Calculation of bit rate, compression ratio, mean square error, peak signal to noise ratio

Image	Bit rate	Compression ratio	Mean square error	Peak signal to noise ratio
Image 1	0.58	1.73	0.19	103.63
Image 2	0.12	8.08	0.78	97.39
Image 3	1.00	1.00	0.0000038	150.51
Image 4	0.81	1.23	0.04	86.70
Image 5	0.25	4.02	0.57	74.68
Image 6	0.50	2.00	0.25	102.35
Image 7	0.06	16.38	0.92	96.68
Image 8	0.08	12.48	0.89	96.85
Image 9	0.67	1.48	0.01	117.45
Image 10	0.46	2.18	0.31	101.48

Simulation Results and Discussion

Simulation:

The images used in this project are as shown in Fig. 8. The Images for transformation are scanned directly from IPRO GE SYTEC 1800-i CT SCANNER. These Images are in DICOM format and are then converted into DCM.

Results:

Step 1: **Read an image from a DICOM file into the MATLAB workspace** (Fig. 9).

Step 2: **Read the metadata from the same DICOM file**—Create info as object to retrieve SeriesInstanceUID of the same Image. On applying the below command the following output appears:

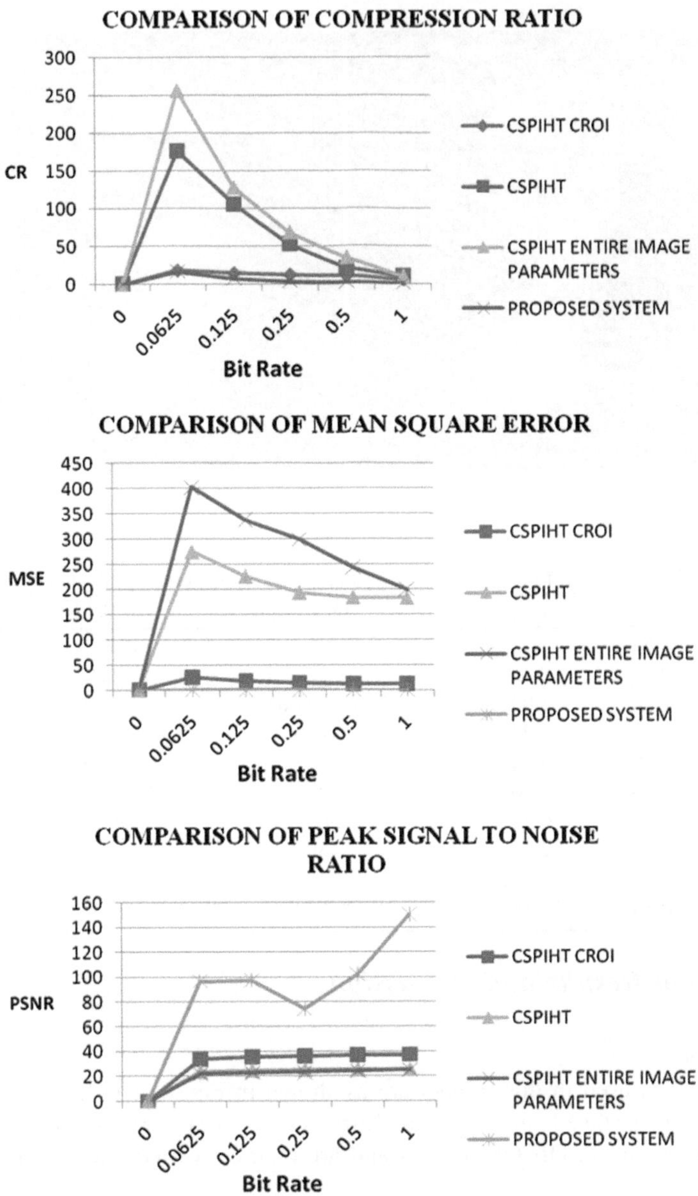

Fig. 12 Graphs showing comparison of various parameters for existing (CSPIHT) and proposed system (wavelet transform with run length encoding)

info.SeriesInstanceUID
ans = 1.2.840.113619.2.1.2411.1031152382.365.736169244

Step 3: **Remove all the text from the image (Enhancing Security)**—Finds the maximum and minimum values of all pixels in the image by using max and min functions. The pixels that form the white text characters are set to the maximum pixel value. The output screen appears as: (Fig. 10).
Step 4: **Generate a new DICOM UID using the dicomuid function**—Create UID as variable to store the value of new DICOM UID

uid = 1.3.6.1.4.1.9590.100.1.1.39331690911270240817931391323566307755

Step 5: **Set the value of the SeriesInstanceUID field in the metadata associated with the original DICOM file to the generated value**
Step 6: **Write the modified image to a new DICOM file, specifying the modified metadata structure, info, as an argument**
Step 7: **Apply wavelet-based lossless compression technique**—Apply wavelet transform and run length encoding. Output appears as: (Fig. 11)

Discussion:
On the basis of the parameters of image, the following calculations and results are shown: (Table 1) (Fig. 12).

Results

In this chapter, various techniques for wavelet transforms are developed with run length coding algorithm; wavelet transform makes it attractive both in terms of speed and memory needs and also enhances security features. It is found that the proposed method gives more than 34 % average improvement in the PSNR value in the bpp range of 0.0625–1.00 and high reduction in mean square error with a better quality of the reconstructed medical image judged on the basis of the human visual system (HVS).

Hence, finally, we can conclude that the proposed wavelet-based method is very suitable for low bit rate compression, high compression ratios, can perform lossless coding, high PSNR, low MSEs, as well as good visual quality of the reconstructed medical image at low bit rates. It can also maintain the high diagnostic quality of the compressed image and hence can reduce heavily the transmission and storage costs of the huge medical data generated everyday. Wavelet can also be used in Image registration, edge detection and segmentation, and denoising.

Acknowledgments I sincerely express indebtedness to my esteemed and revered guide Prof. Mukta Bhatele for her invaluable guidance, supervision, and encouragement throughout the work. I also thank MP, CT scan, and MRI Center, Jabalpur, for its contribution to the collection of images used. This study would not have been possible if compression researchers did not routinely place their code and papers on the Internet for public access.

References

1. Etemad K, Doerman D, Chellappa R (1994) Page segmentation using decision integration and wavelet packet basis. In: Proceedings of international conference on pattern recognition, IEEE
2. Lalitha YS, Latte MV (2010) Lossless and lossy compression of DICOM images with scalable ROI. IJCSNS Int J Comput Sci Netw Secur 10(7):276–281
3. Al Muhit A (2008) Error resilient transmission of quality scalable images over wireless channels. Digital Signal Processing, 18:588–597
4. Dr. Janet J, Mohandass D, Meenalosini S (2010) Lossless compression techniques for medical images in telemedicine. 2(7):112. ISSN print: 2076-2739
5. Kivijarvi J, Ojala TA (1998) A comparison of lossless compression methods for medical images. Comput Med Imaging Graph 22:323–339

Study of Science and Engineering in Biomedical

Manprit Kaur and Ratna Verma

Abstract In this paper the various applications of science, in particular, mathematics and various engineering principles in the field of biomedical and also the impact of biomedical on business and society are discussed. This paper also highlights the application of mathematics in medical imaging such as 3D-tomography, EPRI, TEM, and so on.

Keywords Approximation · Biomedical · Parameter · Robotic · Transmission · Tomography · Transform

Introduction

Biomedical Engineering is the application of engineering principles and design concepts to medicine and biology. This field seeks to close the gap between engineering and medicine. It combines the design and problem solving skills of engineering with medical and biological sciences to improve health care diagnosis, monitoring, and therapy.

Modern society has seen many changes in economy, health care, technology, education, lifestyle of people, and so on. These advancements and changes have contributed immensely to the different advances in providing health and medical

M. Kaur (✉) · R. Verma
Department of Mathematics, Gyan Ganga College of Technology, Jabalpur, India
e-mail: manpreet2410@gmail.com

R. Verma
e-mail: ratnaverma8@gmail.com

V. Kumar and M. Bhatele (eds.), *Proceedings of All India Seminar on Biomedical Engineering 2012 (AISOBE 2012)*, Lecture Notes in Bioengineering,
DOI: 10.1007/978-81-322-0970-6_15, © Springer India 2013

care to patients, both inside and outside medical institutions. Changes in science and technology have led to the achievement in offering a new perception in providing both sound mental and physical care to patients.

Advancements in Health Care

Health care advancements in many different forms such as e-prescribing, drug monitoring, reporting, and a broad variety of other information sources are now available which are saving lives and civilizing the health care field. Technology enables medical practitioners to treat their patients and prescribe medications more effectively, efficiently, and with fewer chances of error ever before. Digitized records, robotic surgeries, and new innovative methods for tracking diseases are continuously advancing. From robotic surgeries to micro-surgery and IVR, medical technology and health care are making patient care better and better everyday and continuously, in a progressive manner.

Advancements in Medical Technology

Over time, excellent medical advances have been made. With this progress have come some new medical procedures that can change society. Such medical techniques include plastic surgery and human cloning. As technology advances, the dimensions of communication and society change. Likewise, technology has appreciably served to redesign the business world and competitiveness in numerous ways. Different improvements and advancements in medical technology can be observed nowadays. Some of them include advancement in information technology (IT), telecommunications, such as through the use of the Internet, digital TV, personal digital assistants (PDAs), wireless application protocol (WAP) phones that provide Internet access for health care practitioners; telemedicine for medical consultations that can be carried out long distance through this technology. In the area of molecular biology, improvements are being made in medical technology which includes genetic screening. Another major advancement in medical technology is tissue engineering that may include implantation or transplantation of artificial body parts like skin and other internal organs of the body. Advancement also includes robotic surgery and radio surgery which make minimal invasive surgeries on patients, and require minimum support of surgeons during surgeries, as they will be using robots for surgeries. In this manner, the advancements in medical technology can be used in the medical field which relate to different applications of science and technology. Such developments in science and technology provide the medical field with new and innovative plans and ideas that would further deliver faster, efficient, and effective medical processes, which would considerably contribute to the suitable, effective, and efficient treatment and appreciable patient care. Health technologies are developed to cure all health problems and improve the quality and standard of life of the patient. These advancements in medical technologies form a very important component of the health services systems and can help in the diagnosis, prevention, and treatment of disease.

This rapid improvment in technology is revolutionizing a vast area of health care. Also, advancement in medical technologies provides a smooth cake walk for patients to reboot their life to the normal position. Advancement of new medical technology will help doctors to cure the health of ill people. New innovative technologies like this can make their job a lot easier. These new machines and treatments are helping to give quality and good treatment for the patient and also new drugs are being created which will help patients to have more resistance to viruses. These advancements are also useful for other third world countries to become knowledgable in fighting diseases. Today, there are various technological advances which provide support to doctors in serving the public better. Medical advancement can be achieved only if there is support from government, public, and other private organizations.

Recent Advancements in Medical Field

The hand-sized ultrasound machine allows doctors in remote locations to image a person's kidneys, liver, bladder, eyes, veins, and arteries in order to find out any problem. This could be a noteworthy breakthrough for developing nations especially countries like India, where over 70 % of the population has no access to needed medical equipment such as MRI scans or CT scanners.

Contact Lenses for Treating Diabetes

Instead of drawing blood in order to test blood/sugar levels, this advancement in technology made by Chemical and Biochemical Engineering professor at the University of Western Ontario, Jin Zhang, embeds nanoparticles into hydrogel lenses, which react with glucose molecules found in tears and cause a chemical reaction that changes one's eye color. These specially made contact lenses for diabetic patients would continuously alert them to variations in their glucose levels simply by looking in a mirror.

Future Scope and Targets in Medical Technology

1. *The Impact of advancements in Medical Technology on Business*:

There is a huge and considerable impact of advancements in medical technology on business communities. As there are two faces to a coins, similarly these advancements in medical technology have positive as well as negative impacts to mention. But when compared to the positive impact, the negative impact can be ignored. The two fundamental commercialization issues which are being faced by the academic and business communities are as follows:

(a) The ability of the academic groups to change the culture of scientists to commercialize their technology.
(b) The ability of the business groups to communicate successfully with scientists.

The new advancements in science usually come from the government supported, funded academic research. The academic-industrialists, entrepreneurs, and capitalists must either license the technology or become more knowledgable about commercializing their patented ideas. One such example which can be quoted is "A scientist and a businessman in San Francisco were able to successfully communicate with each other and sketch out a common goal that is the commercialization of insulin" a medical product which was the catalyst for the development of the biotech industry worldwide.

The business communities should get support from the government bodies in establishing their own research and development centers so that they can help in pacing up the advancements in medical technology which ultimately result in reaching the people more effectively, and in turn these technologies would generate huge revenues and incomes for the business bodies. As expenditure incurred on health care is increasing day by day, business bodies can expect good revenues if they are successful in finding out any new device or technology that could steer patient needs while giving treatment to them. With advancement in technology and patient care, engineers have to stay on their toes to provide the supporting M/E infrastructure, and often on a limited budget. Thus, ultimately this can help other business systems also to sustain and progress in the market. These advancements can provide to many a lot of job opportunities.

These advancements are changing the competitive business landscape, i.e., through increasing efficiency and reducing costs. Advancement in medical technology systems can decrease the employee training processes time, saving time and allowing personnel to work in other areas. Utilizing the time and resources in an effective manner is important to the success of a business. Advanced information systems may observe vital signs on critical patients over wireless networks; this technology not only improves care but also supports cost-efficiency and competitiveness within the health care industry. These advancements could help in reducing the intervention of humans in medical care as machines and robots could take care under minimal guidance of humans ultimately reducing the cost to the company on each employee.

2. *The Impact of Advancements in Medical Technology on Society*:

This is a fast developing branch of knowledge binding together science and engineering in a world of expertise to assist problem solving and innovative design and helping medics and physicians to make incredible advancements in people's lives.

The impacts of medical technology advancements on society include the development of new treatments for incurable illnesses, coming up with new ideas for long-term association of patients, and development of new procedures for better care of patients. As a result of advancements in medical technology, new varieties of drugs and numbers and types of machineries used in the medical field are increasing which are offering new occupations in hospitals, including safety engineers, respiratory therapists, bioengineers, and radiology technicians, and thus providing opportunities for employment and making the society more civilized. In other words, the impacts of medical technology advancements provide overall ease to patients in terms of treatment and management through the advancement in procedures and ideas in relation to their care. The final diagnosis of the patient would not be possible without the medical technology advancement results, like MRI and complicated neuronal and laboratory examinations. Such devices and processes are part of the advancements in medical technology, and without using them, diagnosis of the patient would not have been achieved.

In this way, the advancement in medical technologies has made its impact on society. This has made quality health care reach the common man. In developing countries like India, these advancements have made health care reach the poor more closely than ever before.

Some advancements like genetic screening have helped to identify people at risk of a particular disease and allow suitable interventions to be introduced before the disease advances. Minimally insidious surgery reduces postoperative stay of patients in hospitals. This helps them in saving a lot of money. Remote diagnosis and treatment is possible for the patient through these advancements.

The negative impacts of these advancements on the society are over-dependence on machines and technology which may result in helplessness and problems when technology malfunctions, the lack of knowledge of advancements that results in making wrong decisions, the lack of secured political and legal regulations, the unavailability of medical and technical innovations to all patients, and the high costs accompanying the use of medical technology advancements in patient care.

Application of Mathematics in the Field of Medical Sciences

The application of mathematics in the field of science has been in place since time immemorial. However, its actual importance and applicability in medical sciences have become more visible in today's world. To understand it medically, one can say that the application of mathematics in medical sciences is sporadic. The study of mathematics and the subject, in general, is contributing to biology and the study of life sciences in many ways.

Today, biologists and professionals in the field of medical sciences use the concepts of mathematical theorems and formula, among others, for obtaining quantitative measures and analyzing their studies in quantity along with quality. Many scientific medical equipments and machines have been designed keeping the applications of mathematics in view. Biologists use mathematics to derive quantitative data from medical studies, such as estimating the number of genes that are involved in inheriting a particular trail from the parents to the child.

Today, the concepts and theories of mathematics are being applied to almost all aspects of medical sciences. However, there are some fields of study under medical sciences where mathematics has found greater scope. These fields are clinical research, biotechnology, and genetics. In general, mathematics and its sub-branches play an important role in the study of genetics.

In the study of genetics, the two most important subsections of mathematics that play a major role are statistics and probability. Probability, its formula, and its applications are used by people working in genetics to understand the mechanism of meiosis, forming of egg cells and the sperm, and the process of inheritance, among others. They also get an understanding of how phenotypes (observable diseases) and genotypes (the DNA sequences) are related to each other through the study of probability distributions. They also conduct the analysis and study of genetic determinants through the applications of statistics and its methods and principles.

Another advantage that the study of mathematics in medicine and biology provides is to mathematical modeling. Mathematical modeling refers to looking and studying the biological systems and the medical phenomena through the study of mathematics by applying its principles and theorems. Mathematics has also shown its worth in testing out new ideas in the field of medicine. This has been of high importance in the study of cancerous and tumor cells. Medical practitioners have been successful in understanding the direction in which cancerous cells potentially grow inside the living body with the help of a model strictly based on mathematics.

Many health organizations are now using online systems and software applications to manage their patient records and keep a check on the remedial steps for each patient, coordinating with practitioners and other hospital staff on a regular basis along with many more things. All these online systems and software applications are developed keeping mathematics as the platform.

In biotechnology as well, mathematics is seen to play a major role. The study of mathematics is needed to understand concepts such as concentration/dilution, calibration, molarity, molality, solution preparation, serial dilution, radioactive decay and decomposition, absorption, and cell growth, among others. In clinical research, the understanding of DNA, thumb impressions, and markups, among others are also carried out based on the study of mathematics.

Mathematics in Medical Imaging

Tomography

Tomography refers to imaging by sections or sectioning, through the use of any kind of penetrating wave. A device used in tomography is called a tomograph, while the

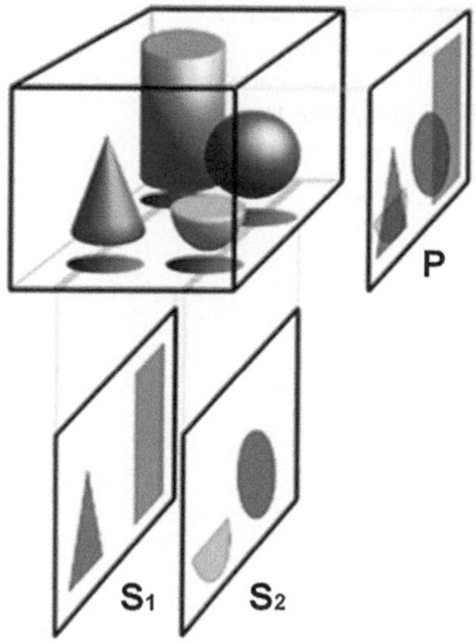

Fig. 1 Tomography superposition with projected image P

image produced is a tomogram. The method is used in radiology, archeology, biology, geophysics, oceanography, materials science, astrophysics, quantum information, and other sciences. In most cases, it is based on the mathematical procedure called tomographic reconstruction. Figure 1 represents the basic principle of tomography; superposition-free tomographic cross sections S1 and S2 compared with the projected image P.

Medical Imaging–Perspective

The perspective in medical imaging is dominated by the development of newer measuring technologies:

1. *3D tomography*: In nondestructive material testing, 3D X-ray CT is widely used in connection with a circular scanning geometry; i.e., the X-ray tube is moved on a circle in a plane around the examined object with the detector plane positioned at the opposite side. Helical geometry is favored in medical applications, but the necessary variable shift of the patient has not yet been solved satisfactorily in existing algorithms. In principle, X-ray tube and detector can be moved along arbitrary trajectories around the patient. The determination of trajectories that are optimal with respect to resolution and stability remains a mathematical challenge. Figure 2a represents the X-ray source trajectory.

   Figure 2b and c is the mathematical representations of X-ray source trajectory.

2. *Electron paramagnetic resonance imaging*: In this technique, a decoupling of the fourth dimension is not possible, since there, besides the three spatial

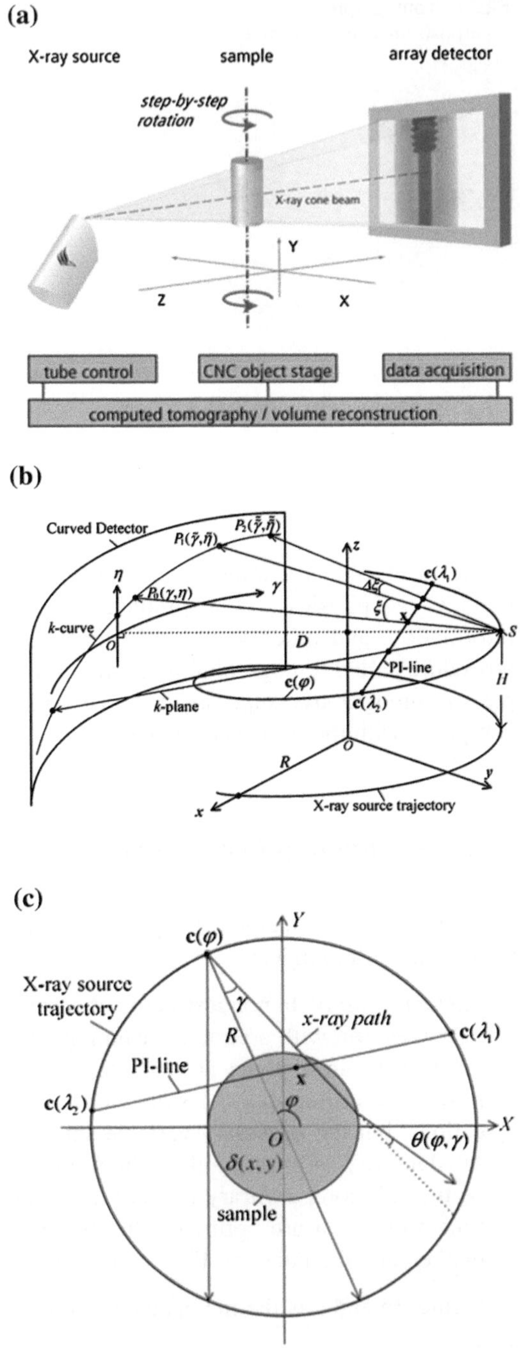

Fig. 2 **a** X-ray source trajectory, **b** and **c** mathematical representation of X-ray source trajectory

dimensions, a spectral dimension shows up additionally. The corresponding mathematical model is the Radon transform in four dimensions. This technology is presently studied in the stages of pharmaceutical research and animal experiments. However, due to the limitations in field strength, the data in Radon space cannot be sampled completely with the consequence that a limited angle problem has to be solved. Theoretically, the desired distribution would be uniquely determined, if all data in the restricted range were available, but instabilities and strong artifacts complicate the reconstruction problem.

3. *Ultrasound CT*: In this approach, the sender and receiver are spatially separated, the corresponding mathematical model is an inverse scattering problem for the determination of the spatially varying sound impedance and the scattering properties. The difficulty here is that, in contrast to CT, the paths of the waves depend upon the variable to be computed, which makes the problem highly nonlinear. A linearization of the problem via Born or Rytov approximation neglects the effects of multiple scattering, and is therefore not sufficiently accurate. That is why ultrasound tomography today is still a challenge to mathematics and algorithm development.
4. *Transmission electron microscopy (TEM)*: For the visualization of biomolecules by TEM, various approaches are pursued. If one does not aim at averaging over many probes of the same kind, again a limited angle problem arises. In addition, wave phenomena enter for small-sized objects, leading, as in ultrasound tomography, to nonlinear inverse scattering problems. Fortunately, linearization is feasible here, which facilitates the development of algorithms significantly.
5. *Phase-contrast tomography*: In this technology, where complex-valued sizes have to be reconstructed, linearizations are also applicable. The phase supplies information even when the density differences within the object are extremely small. Due to different scanning geometries, medical application still generates challenging problems for the development of algorithms.
6. *Diffusion tensor MRI*: This method provides a tensor at each reconstruction point, thus bearing information concerning the diffusivity of water molecules in tissue. In this, reconstruction and regularization are performed separately. Only after having computed tensors, properties of the tensor like symmetry or positive definiteness are produced point by point.

The above list of imaging techniques under present development is by no means complete. Methods like impedance tomography are studied as well as those applying light to detect objects close to the skin. In all of the mentioned measuring techniques, the technological development is so advanced that the solution of the associated mathematical problems like modeling, determination of achievable resolution, and development of efficient algorithms will yield a considerable innovation thrust.

A Novel Approach for Finding Frequent Medicine Set Using Maximal Apriori for Medical Application

Shailendra Chourasia, Rashmi Vishwakarma, Meghna Utmal and Neeraj Shukla

Abstract Frequent itemsets play an essential role in many data mining tasks that try to find interesting patterns from databases, such as association rules, correlations, sequences, classifiers, clusters, and many more of which the mining of association rules is one of the most popular problems. Frequent itemsets mining plays an important role in association rules mining. This chapter addresses the special features of data mining with medical data. So in this chapter, data mining with medical data is referred to as "Finding Frequent Medicine Set". Medicine is primarily directed at patient-care activity, and only secondarily as a research resource; almost the only justification for collecting medical data is to benefit the individual patient. Finally, medical data have a special status based upon their applicability to all people; their urgency (including life or death); and a moral obligation to be used for beneficial purposes.

Keywords Data mining · Frequent itemsets · Frequent medicine set · SRMine algorithm

Note: Frequent itemset = Frequent medicine set.

S. Chourasia (✉) · M. Utmal · N. Shukla
Gyan Ganga College of Technology, Jabalpur, Madhya Pradesh 482003, India
e-mail: shailendrachourasia@rediffmail.com

M. Utmal
e-mail: meghnautmal@ggits.org

N. Shukla
e-mail: neerajshukla28@yahoo.com

R. Vishwakarma
Gyan Ganga Institute of Technology and Sciences, Jabalpur, Madhya Pradesh 482003, India
e-mail: ray.of.light1985@gmail.com

V. Kumar and M. Bhatele (eds.), *Proceedings of All India Seminar on Biomedical Engineering 2012 (AISOBE 2012)*, Lecture Notes in Bioengineering,
DOI: 10.1007/978-81-322-0970-6_16,

Introduction

This chapter emphasizes the uniqueness of medical data mining. Raw medical data are voluminous and heterogeneous. Medical data may be collected from various images, interviews with the patient, laboratory data, the physician's observations and interpretations, and physician's recommendations for disease. All these components may bear upon the diagnosis, prognosis, and treatment of the patient, and cannot be ignored. All recommendations of medicine given by the physician can be used to analyze frequently used medicine (Frequent Medicine Set). This information can be used by the physician, Medical Store's owner, and pharmacy companies for decision making, regarding human health. Here, we are trying to implement SRMine Algorithm to find "**Frequent Medicine Set**".

This chapter includes three sections: first, SRMine Algorithm, second, example, and lastly conclusion.

SRMine Algorithm

Input: Transactional Database D, minimum support count [1].

Step 1: The algorithm scans the database in order to count the number of occurrences of each item to find the candidate 1-itemset with their support count.

Step 2: The set of frequent 1-itemset L1 can then be determined by removing the items having less than the minimum support count. It consists of the candidate 1-itemsets satisfying minimum support. Let the number of frequent 1-itemset be "n".

Step 3: Removes the infrequent items from each transaction and counts the number of items in each transaction (item_count).

Step 4: The transactions are sorted in descending order based on the item count.

Step 5: Call SRMine(Database).

Step 6: Stop.

(A) SRMine(Database) Procedure

Step 1: Take 2-D array; put the transaction into 2-D array with their count of repetition.

Step 2: Find maximal transactions (k-itemset) from the array whose count is greater than or equal to the minimum support known as maximal frequent itemsets or transactions. If k-itemsets count is less than minimum support, then look for k-itemsets and (k − 1)-itemsets jointly for next (k − 1) maximal itemsets and so on until no itemsets count is found greater than minimum support.

Table 1 Transactional database D

TID	List of medicines	Item count
T001	SARIDON, DISPRIN, ADVIL, CROCINE	4
T002	DISPRIN, PANADOL	2
T003	DISPRIN, NIMUSULIDE, IBOBRUFIN	3
T004	SARIDON, DISPRIN, PANADOL	3
T005	SARIDON, NIMUSULIDE	2
T006	DISPRIN, NIMUSULIDE	2
T007	SARIDON, NIMUSULIDE	2
T008	SARIDON, DISPRIN, NIMUSULIDE, ADVIL	4
T009	SARIDON, DISPRIN, NIMUSULIDE	3

Step 3: Once the maximal frequent transaction is found, then according to apriori property, consider all its nonempty subsets are frequent.

Step 4: There are itemsets remaining which are not included in maximal frequent itemset, but are frequent. Therefore, find all frequent 1-itemsets and pruning the database consider only those transactions which contain frequent 1-itemset element but are not included in the maximal frequent transaction.

Step 5: If no such transaction is found, then return to step 7.

Step 6: Call SRMine(PruneDatabase) Procedure.

Output: Prune Database and All frequent itemsets

Example

Suppose Table 1 is transactional database with Transactional Identity Number(TID), List of Medicines, and number of items in each transaction. There are nine transactions. Suppose the minimum support is two.

Scan the transactional database D for count of each candidate items. It is shown in Table 2.

Compare the candidate support count with minimum support count and remove the infrequent medicine from Table 2 and the result is shown in Table 3

Remove infrequent items from each transactions, update item count, and sort the transactions. as shown in Table 4.

Table 2 Candidate items, C1

Medicine set	Support count
{SARIDON}	6
{DISPRIN}	7
{NIMUSULIDE}	6
{PANADOL}	2
{ADVIL}	2
{CROCINE}	1
{IBOBRUFIN}	1

Table 3 Frequent 1-itemsets, L1

Medicine set	Support count
{SARIDON}	6
{DISPRIN}	7
{NIMUSULIDE}	6
{PANADOL}	2
{ADVIL}	2

Table 4 Sorted database

TID	List of medicines	Item count
T008	SARIDON, DISPRIN, NIMUSULIDE, ADVIL	4
T001	SARIDON, DISPRIN, ADVIL,CROCINE	4
T004	SARIDON, DISPRIN, PANADOL	3
T009	SARIDON, DISPRIN, NIMUSULIDE	3
T002	DISPRIN, PANADOL	2
T003	DISPRIN, NIMUSULIDE	3
T005	SARIDON, NIMUSULIDE	2
T006	DISPRIN, NIMUSULIDE	2
T007	SARIDON, NIMUSULIDE	2

Take 2-D array; put the transaction into 2-D array with their count of repetition.

2 Medicine set	Count	3 Medicine set	Count	4 Medicine set	Count
{SARIDON, NIMUSULIDE}	2	{SARIDON, DISPRIN, ADVIL}	1	{SARIDON, DISPRIN, NIMUSULIDE, ADVIL}	1
{DISPRIN, NIMUSULIDE}	2	{SARIDON, DISPRIN, PANADOL}	1		
{DISPRIN, PANADOL}	1	{SARIDON, DISPRIN, NIMUSULIDE}	1		

Find the maximal 4-itemset its count is 1. In our case, which is less than the given minimum support; therefore, this transaction is not considered as maximal frequent; therefore, now we scan 3-itemsets and 4-itemsets in array for maximal 3-itemsets jointly. This will result in two maximal 3-itemsets

{SARIDON, DISPRIN, NIMUSULIDE} {SARIDON, DISPRIN, ADVIL}

According to apriori property, subset of maximal frequent itemsets is also considered as all frequent subsets. They are

{SARIDON, DISPRIN, NIMUSULIDE} {SARIDON, DISPRIN, ADVIL} {DISPRIN, NIMUSULIDE} {DISPRIN, ADVIL} {SARIDON, DISPRIN} {SARIDON, NIMUSULIDE} {SARIDON, ADVIL} {SARIDON} {DISPRIN} {NIMUSULIDE} {ADVIL}.

Find the frequent 1-itemset from database—it is found that {PANADOL} is frequent but is not included in maximal itemsets

There are itemsets remaining which are not included in maximal frequent itemset, but they are frequent. Therefore, find all frequent 1-itemsets and reduce the database; consider only those transactions which contain frequent 1-itemset element but are not included in the maximal frequent transaction.

Reduce the database by considering only the transaction which contains {PANADOL} itemset

TID	List of medicines
T002	DISPRIN, PANADOL
T004	SARIDON, DISPRIN, PANADOL

Go to next step because we have a reduced database

By calling SortRecursiveMine (ReducedDatabase)

After scanning, prune puts items in 2-D array with the count of repetition

2 Medicine set	Count	3 Medicine set	Count
{DISPRIN, PANADOL}	1	{SARIDON, DISPRIN, PANADOL}	1

Find the maximal 3-itemset its count is 1. In our case, which is less than the given support; therefore, this transaction is not considered as maximal frequent. Therefore, now we scan 2-itemsets and 3-itemsets in array for maximal 2-itemsets jointly. This will result in one maximal 2-itemsets

{DISPRIN, PANADOL}

The final result of the frequent itemsets ({SARIDON, DISPRIN, ADVIL} {DISPRIN, NIMUSULIDE, ADVIL} {DISPRIN, NIMUSULIDE} {DISPRIN, PANADOL} {DISPRIN, ADVIL} {SARIDON, DISPRIN} {SARIDON, NIMUSULIDE} {SARIDON, ADVIL} {SARIDON} {DISPRIN} {NIMUSULIDE} {PANADOL}{ADVIL})

Conclusion

In this research work, the attempt has been to evaluate the SRMine algorithm with medical data which is generating **Frequent Medicine Set.** This Frequent Medicine Set can be used in various regions and is helpful for easy approach to health.

Reference

1. Chourasia S, Vishwakarma R, Utmal M, Shukla N (2012) An innovative approach for finding frequent item sets using maximal apriori and fusion process and its evaluation. Int J Comput Appl (IJCA), Foundation of computer science, New York, USA (0975–8887), 40(4)

Security Issues in Monitoring Medical Disease Through Vehicular Ad hoc Network

Priyanka Deodi, Shruti Shrivastava and Mukta Bhatele

Abstract Several diseases and medical conditions require constant monitoring of physiological signals and vital signs on daily bases, such as diabetics, hypertension, etc. In order to make these patients capable of living their daily life, it is necessary to provide a platform and infrastructure that allows the constant collection of physiological data even when the patient is not inside the coverage area. Ad hoc networks are a new wireless networking paradigm for mobile hosts. Unlike traditional mobile wireless networks, ad hoc networks do not rely on any fixed infrastructure. Instead, hosts rely on each other to keep the network connected. The medical, military, tactical, and other security-sensitive operations are still the main applications of ad hoc networks, although there is a trend to adopt ad hoc networks for commercial uses due to their unique properties. One main challenge in design of these networks is their vulnerability to security attacks. In this chapter, we study the threats an ad hoc network faces and the security goals to be achieved. We identify the new challenges and opportunities posed by this new networking environment and explore new approaches to secure its communication.

Keywords Security · Ad hoc network · Routing protocols · Error detection and correction

P. Deodi (✉) · S. Shrivastava · M. Bhatele
Gyan Ganga College of Technology, Jabalpur, India

V. Kumar and M. Bhatele (eds.), *Proceedings of All India Seminar on Biomedical Engineering 2012 (AISOBE 2012)*, Lecture Notes in Bioengineering,
DOI: 10.1007/978-81-322-0970-6_17, © Springer India 2013

Introduction

Ad hoc networks are a new paradigm of wireless communication for mobile hosts (which we call nodes). In an ad hoc network [1], there is no fixed infrastructure such as base stations or mobile switching centers. Mobile nodes that are within each other's radio range communicate directly via wireless links, while those that are far apart rely on other nodes to relay messages as routers (Fig. 1).

The embedded architecture can be seen in a variety of applications such as invasive sensing, urban sensing, automotive, air and space, and the health care industry. Different platforms have been introduced which can be used to monitor medical data while the patient is out of hospital. These architectures can be used for two classes of applications, some are life critical (ECG Monitoring) and some are not (monitoring the pressure on the feet or the way people are walking after post-knee surgery). Some of the applications that are life critical must have the capability of reporting medical data to physicians with fixed schedules periodically. In addition, these classes of applications must be able to notify the paramedics in case of any emergency to get immediate response. In all the cases when an application intends to transfer data to its appropriate destination, the patient must either be under coverage of a Wi-Fi wireless access point or its on-body terminal must have the capability of using the cellular network. However, in some cases (emergencies, attacks, etc.), neither the Wi-Fi nor the cellular network is available. This fact introduces a major reliability issue regarding the extension of these applications to mobile patients. Vehicles collect data from patients and transfer them to their final destination using ad hoc networks, where each mobile node is a vehicle. The vehicles communicate with each other and with nearby local roadside base stations. Vehicles move in an organized fashion and their range of motion is somehow restricted. For example, they mostly drive in the streets and highways. Moreover, a commuter drives everyday at almost about the same time to work and returns home almost following the same path. Security is an important issue for ad hoc networks, especially for those security-sensitive applications.

Mobile nodes that are within each other's radio range communicate directly via wireless links, while those that are far apart rely on other nodes to relay messages as routers. Node mobility in an ad hoc network causes frequent changes of the network topology. Figure 2 shows such an example: initially, nodes 1 and 4 have a direct link between them. When 4 moves out of 1's radio range, the link is broken. However, the network is still connected, because 1 can reach 4 through 3, 5, and 6.

Ad hoc networks can also be used for emergency, law enforcement, and rescue missions. Since an ad hoc network can be deployed rapidly at relatively low cost, it becomes an attractive option for commercial uses such as sensor networks or virtual classrooms [2, 3].

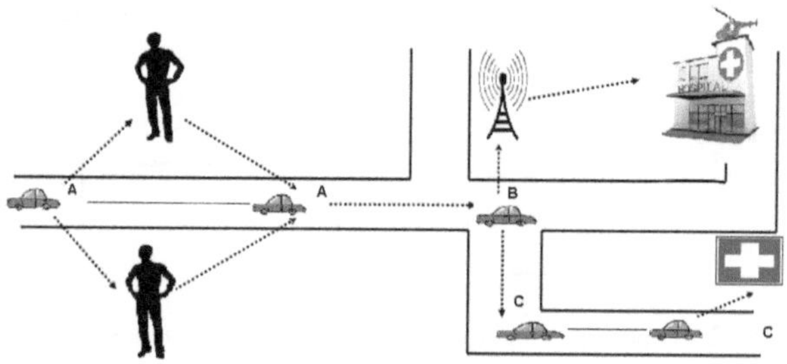

Fig. 1 Vehicles collect data from patients and transfer them to their final destination

Security Goals

To secure an ad hoc network, we consider the following attributes: availability, confidentiality, integrity, authentication, and nonrepudiation. Availability ensures the survivability of network services despite denial of service attacks. A denial of service attack could be launched at any layer of an ad hoc network. On the physical and media access control layers, an adversary could employ jamming to interfere with communication on physical channels. On the network layer, an adversary could disrupt the routing protocol and disconnect the network. On the higher layers, an adversary could bring down high-level services. One such target is the key management service, an essential service for any security framework. Confidentiality ensures that certain information is never disclosed to unauthorized entities. Network transmission of sensitive information, such as strategic or tactical, medical, military information, requires confidentiality. Leakage of such information to enemies could have devastating consequences. Routing information must also remain confidential in certain cases, because the information might be valuable for enemies to identify and to locate their targets in a battlefield. Integrity guarantees that a message being transferred is never corrupted. A message could be corrupted because of benign failures, such as radio propagation impairment, or because of malicious attacks on the network. Authentication enables a node to ensure the identity of the peer node it is communicating with. Without authentication, an adversary could masquerade a node, thus gaining unauthorized access to resource and sensitive information and interfering with the operation of other nodes. Finally, nonrepudiation ensures that the origin of a message cannot deny having sent the message. No repudiation is useful for detection and isolation of compromised nodes. When a node A receives an erroneous message from a node B, nonrepudiation allows A to accuse B using this message and to convince other nodes that B is compromised. There are other security goals (e.g., authorization) that are of concern to certain applications, but we will not pursue these issues in this chapter.

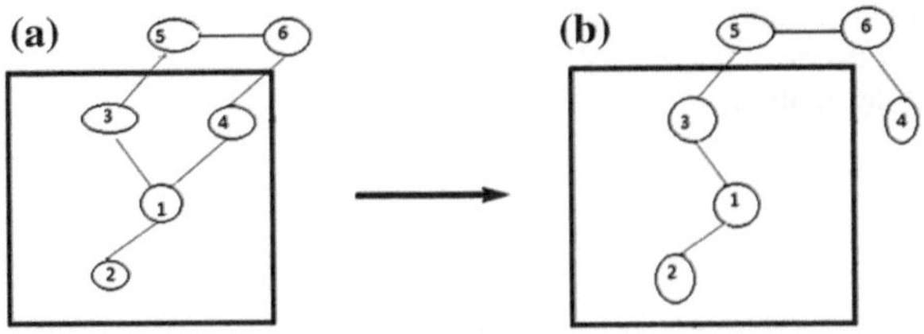

Fig. 2 Topology change in ad hoc networks: nodes 1, 2, 3, 4, 5, and 6 constitute an ad hoc network. The circle represents the radio range of node 1. The network initially has the topology in (**a**). When node 4 moves out of the radio range of 1, the network topology changes to the one in (**b**)

Routing

To achieve availability, routing protocols [4, 5] should be robust against both dynamically changing topology and malicious attacks. Routing protocols proposed for ad hoc networks cope well with the dynamically changing topology [6]. However, none of them, to our knowledge, have accommodated mechanisms to defend against malicious attacks. Routing protocols for ad hoc networks are still under active research. There is no single standard routing protocol. Therefore, we aim to capture the common security threats [7] and to provide guidelines to secure routing protocols. In most routing protocols, routers exchange information on the topology of the network in order to establish routes between nodes. Such information could become a target for malicious adversaries who intend to bring the network down. There are two sources of threats to routing protocols. The first comes from external attackers. By injecting erroneous routing information, replaying old routing information, or distorting routing information, an attacker could successfully partition a network or introduce excessive traffic load into the network by causing retransmission and inefficient routing. The second and also the more severe kind of threats come from compromised nodes, which might advertise incorrect routing information to other nodes. Detection of such incorrect information is difficult: merely requiring routing information to be signed by each node would not work, because compromised nodes are able to generate valid signatures using their private keys. To defend against the first kind of threats, nodes can protect routing information in the same way they protect data traffic, i.e., through the use of cryptographic schemes such as digital signature. However, this defense is ineffective against attacks from compromised servers. Worse yet, as we have argued, we cannot neglect the possibility of nodes being compromised in an ad hoc network. Detection of compromised nodes through routing information is also difficult in an ad hoc network because of its dynamically changing topology: when a piece of routing information is found invalid, the information could be generated by a compromised node, or it could have become invalid as a result of topology changes. It is difficult to distinguish between the two cases. On the other hand, we can exploit certain properties of ad hoc networks to achieve secure routing. Note that routing protocols for ad hoc networks must handle outdated routing information to accommodate the dynamically changing topology. False routing information generated by compromised nodes could, to some extent, be considered outdated information. As long as there are sufficiently many correct nodes, the routing protocol should be able to find routes that go around these compromised nodes. Such capability of the routing protocols usually relies on the inherent redundancies—multiple, possibly disjoint, routes between nodes—in ad hoc networks. If routing protocols can discover multiple routes (e.g., protocols in ZRP, DSR, TORA, and AODV all can achieve this), nodes can switch to an alternative route when the primary route appears to have failed. Diversity coding takes advantage of multiple paths in an efficient way without message retransmission. The basic idea is to transmit redundant information through additional routes for error detection and correction. For example, if there are n disjoint routes between two nodes, then we can use n−r channels to transmit data and use the other r channels to transmit redundant information. Even if certain routes are compromised, the receiver may still be able to validate messages and to recover messages from errors using the redundant information from the additional r channels. Secure routing in networks such as the Internet has been extensively studied. Many proposed approaches are also applicable to secure routing in ad hoc networks. To deal with external attacks, standard schemes such as digital signatures to protect information authenticity and integrity have been considered. For example, Sirios and Kent propose the use of a keyed one-way hash function with windowed sequence number for data integrity in point-to-point communication and the use of digital signatures to protect messages sent to multiple destinations. Kumar recognizes the problem of compromised routers as a hard problem, but provides no solution. Other works give only partial solutions. The basic idea underlying these solutions is to detect inconsistency using redundant information and to isolate compromised routers. For example, in where methods to secure distance-vector routing protocols are proposed, extra information of a predecessor in a path to a destination is added into each entry in the routing table. Using this piece of information, a path traversal technique (by following the predecessor link) can be used to verify the correctness of a path. Such mechanisms usually come with a high cost and are avoided because routers on networks such as the Internet are usually well protected and rarely compromised.

Conclusion

In this chapter, we have analyzed the security threats an ad hoc network faces and presented the security objectives that need to be achieved. On one hand, the security-sensitive applications of ad hoc networks require high degree of security; on the other hand, ad hoc networks are inherently vulnerable to security attacks. Therefore, security mechanisms are indispensable for ad hoc networks. The idiosyncrasy of ad hoc networks poses both challenges and opportunities for these mechanisms.

References

1. Haas ZJ, Liang B (1999) Ad hoc mobility management using quorum systems. IEEE/ACM Trans Networking 7:2
2. Lee U, Magistretti E, Zhou B, Gerla M, Bellavista P, Corradi A (2006) Mobeyes: smart mobs for urban monitoring with a vehicular sensor network. IEEE Wirel Commun 13(5):52
3. Feldman P (1987) A practical scheme for non-interactive verifiable secret sharing. In: Proceedings of the 28th annual symposium on the foundations of computer science, pp 427–437. IEEE, 12–14 Oct 1987
4. Hauser R, Przygienda T, Tsudik G (1999) Lowering security overhead in link state routing. Comput Netw 31(8):885–894
5. Kumar B (1993) Integration of security in network routing protocols. SIGSAC Rev 11(2):18–25
6. Desmedt Y, Jajodia S (1997) Redistributing secret shares to new access structures and its applications. Technical report ISSE TR-97-01, George Mason University
7. Gong L (1993) Increasing availability and security of an authentication service. IEEE J Sel Areas Commun 11(5):657–662

Remote Blood Pressure Monitoring Using a Wireless Sensor Network

Tomsy Varghese, Tissy Varghese and Mukta Bhatele

Abstract A remotely monitored system to measure patient's blood pressure (BP) is described. The data are transferred to a central monitoring station using a wireless sensor network for display and storage. One mote was interfaced to the BP monitor for data acquisition and the others were utilized to route the BP data to the monitoring station. A user friendly graphical user interface (GUI) is designed for monitoring current and past measurements for all observed patients. Test results indicated high accuracy in BP measurements. Power consumption by the BP monitor interfaced mote was minimized by forcing it into a low-power sleep mode when not in use.

Keywords Wireless sensor network · Blood pressure monitor (BPM) · Base station

Introduction

Recent advancements in information and communication technologies are paving the way for new paradigms in embedded computing systems. This, allied with an increasing eagerness for monitoring and controlling everything, everywhere, is pushing forward the design of new Wireless Sensor Network (WSN) infrastructures

M. Bhatele
Department of Computer Science, Gyan Ganga College of Technology, Jabalpur, India

T. Varghese (✉)
Department of Digital Communication, Gyan Ganga College of Technology, Jabalpur, India
e-mail: tomsyvarghese@yahoo.co.in

T. Varghese
Oriental Engineering College, Jabalpur, India

V. Kumar and M. Bhatele (eds.), *Proceedings of All India Seminar on Biomedical Engineering 2012 (AISOBE 2012)*, Lecture Notes in Bioengineering,
DOI: 10.1007/978-81-322-0970-6_18,

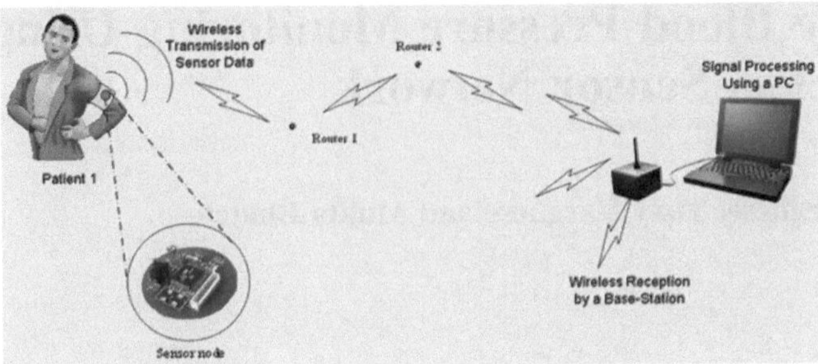

Fig. 1 Remote monitoring system

that will tightly interact with the physical environment in a ubiquitous and pervasive fashion [1]. The technology has several potential applications in the medical industry. In particular, the ability to remotely monitor patient vital signs in real time from a centralized location is a growing area of interest. Interest in WSNs is fueled by the fact that the nodes are cost effective, compact, and can be energy efficient.

Alternatives include WiFi and Bluetooth, which are focused on applications that normally require higher bandwidth. This chapter describes a system using Crossbow 2.4 GHz MICAz wireless sensor nodes [2], a commercial blood pressure monitor (BPM), and an internally developed Graphical User Interface (GUI) to design a prototype system that can monitor vital signs from a large number of patients simultaneously.

Description

A conceptual view of the system is shown in Fig. 1. Each patient is connected to a remote monitoring system, which allows the medical staff to track the patient's vital signs and transmit the readings wirelessly from the patient through a fixed infrastructure of routing nodes to the base station. Depending on the patient's distance from the base station, messages can pass through multiple router nodes to reach the base station. The base station is connected to a host computer running a Java-based GUI to interpret and display the data.

The three main areas of the system interface are sensor to BPM, sensor base station to host computer, and the human interface to the host computer (via GUI).

Sensor to Blood Pressure Monitor Interface

A commercially available A&D UA-767PC BPM is used to provide sensor readings for the system. The BPM takes simultaneous blood pressure measurements. It includes a serial port connection that facilitates bi-directional communication at

9,600 kbps. A sensor node communicates with the BPM on this serial link to start the reading process and receive the patient's blood pressure readings. Once the readings are received, the sensor node communicates with the network and transmits them to the base station.

The communication process in Fig. 2 initializes the sensor node by sending start signal to the BPM to switch it to communication mode. Once the BPM is in communication mode, the sensor node sends a command to open the communication port, then BPM is ready to receive commands. A command to take a measurement is then issued. This causes the BPM to inflate the arm cuff and acquire the blood pressure measurements. When reading process completes, the readings are sent to the sensor node. Limited processing is performed by the sensor node on the reading data before transmitting it through the network to the base station. All communication with the BPM is in ASCII format.

Sensor Base Station to Host Computer Interface

Java is used to implement the interface between the base station and the host computer. All communication between the base station and the PC is done through the UART. A separate thread from the main GUI thread is used to maintain constant monitoring of the serial port. When a message is received, the message type is determined. If the message is a data message sent from a sensor node (i.e., a measurement from one of the medical monitors), the data are extracted and stored according to the ID of the sensor node that took the reading. If the message is a control message, then the information is passed directly to the program thread running the GUI. Control messages contain network information used to generate a network view for the user. A control message from a sensor node includes the ID of the sensor node and the ID of the router node used as the initial entry point into the network. A control message generated by a router node contains the ID of the originating router node itself and the ID of the router's partner node. The information contained in the control message is used to generate a map of the network. In the current implementation, the map is a simple tree depicting the network structure.

The GUI

The GUI can be a Java-based program running on the host computer. All readings received by the PC from the patient's sensor node will be stored in an object corresponding to the patient. All stored readings can be viewed by selecting the desired patient name in the list and selecting the "View" option. It allows the user

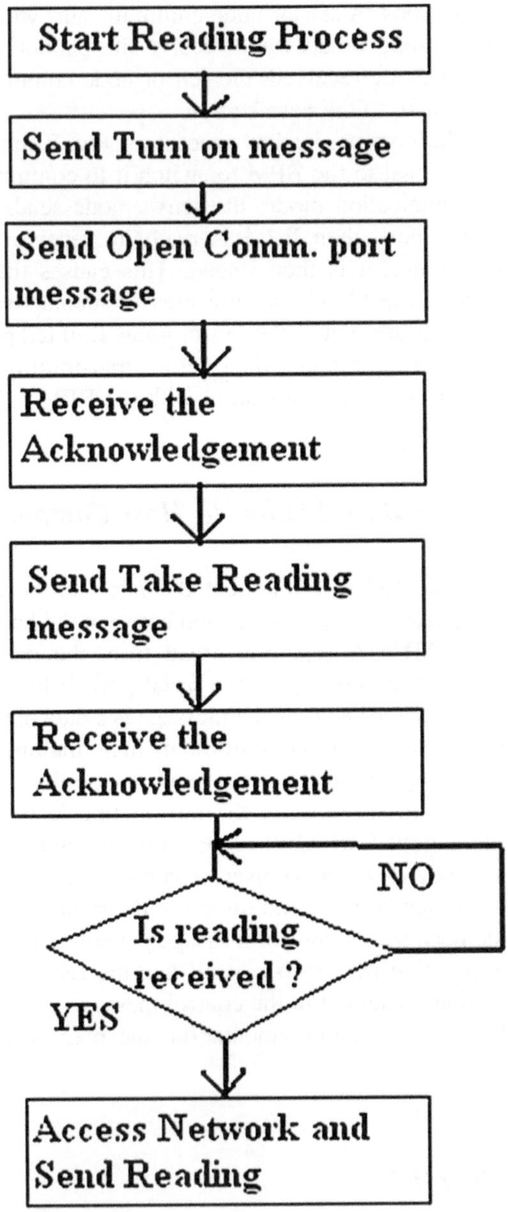

Fig. 2 Communication flowchart

to view various readings and edit patient information. It displays a text-only readout of the measurements. The received reading is checked against threshold limits and if it is beyond, a warning message appears to notify the user of the newest reading.

Network Description

The topology of our wireless network is that of a static routing infrastructure with mobile sensor nodes. Energy scavenging is employed at the router nodes so that connection to a permanent power supply is not needed [3]. The need for batteries is eliminated. Scavenging energy from indoor light sources is an inefficient process and results in limited amounts of energy to power the router nodes. To compensate for this, the router nodes operate in synchronized pairs and at a 50 % duty cycle. This allows sufficient time during the off-cycle for each node to scavenge the energy required for its next on-cycle.

The process of the router node in the network is as:

- Initialize Router Node Parameters
- Locate the Network
- Shortest path to base station is determined
- If ID is received and route partner is available, then Wake a Routine
- If not, then acquire ID from base station and find a route partner
- Message is forwarded
- If network connection is lost, then locate the network again.

Once the routing infrastructure is set up, a sensor node can easily access the network by choosing the shortest path. The sensor node processes as follows:

- Sensor node parameters are initialized
- Reading is taken
- Network is located
- Shortest path to base station is determined
- Sensor reading is sent to base station
- Sensor goes to sleep mode
- When it wakes, again reading is taken.

Sensor nodes are designed to be mobile to allow patient movement. Thus, each subsequent reading requires the sensor node to reconnect to the network in a potentially different location. This pattern also allows the sensor node to sleep between readings, thereby extending battery life [4].

Future Work

Future enhancements to the system may possess a graphical display of the incoming data replacing the text display. Additional medical instruments like a portable ECG, temperature measuring transducer can be interfaced. Increased integration with existing hospital systems and databases can be done. Apart from the medical field, it has wide applications in sensing forest fire, etc.

Conclusion

A prototype BP monitoring system using WSNs has been designed and developed. The system allows health personnel to monitor a patient's BP from a remote location without requiring the physician to be physically present to take the measurements. The system concept can be used for routing vital sign information to a central location within the hospital premises as well as in applications that require monitoring from within a patient's home.

Utilizing a sensor node tied to the BPM, we have successfully initiated a reading, gathered the data, and can forward it through the network to the base station. The measurements are then forwarded through the serial port to the host computer and the GUI displays the data correctly. Multiple sensor nodes are programmed to represent multiple patients. The patients have their own unique sensor node IDs whose measurements were successfully transmitted to the base station and then forwarded to the GUI for display

The BP measurements of patients were fairly accurate and equaled the measurements displayed on the monitor LCD display. Further research will focus toward integrating smaller OEM medical sensor boards to the Crossbow sensor nodes to miniaturize their size and make the system more practical.

References

1. Lorincz K et al (2004) Sensor networks for emergency response: challenges and opportunities. IEEE Pervasive Comput 3(4):16–23
2. Crossbow Technology Inc. (2005) MPR/MIB User's Manual, Rev. B, Document 7430-0021-06.http://www.xbow.com/Support/Support_pdf_files/MPR MIB_Series_Users_Manual.pdf
3. Karl H, Willig A (2005) Protocols and architectures for wireless sensor networks. Wiley
4. Akyildiz IF, Su W, Sankarasubramaniam Y, Cayirci E (2002) A survey on sensor networks. IEEE Commun Mag 40(8):102–114

A Reliable Sensor Data Collection Network for Health Monitoring

Shruti Shrivastava, Priyanka Deodi and Mukta Bhatele

Abstract In this paper we propose system architecture for smart healthcare based on an advanced wireless sensor network (WSN). This paper presents a method for reliably collecting data events from sensors and forwarding the data via a mobile ad hoc network (MANET) to sensor monitoring stations located on an external network. At the core is a MANET concept that consists of ground and unmanned aircraft (UA) nodes. UA enable a model whereby widely spaced sensors are intermittently connected to the network and data are sent in stages as connections become available along each stage. This paper describes our efforts to build such a network for a real application. The paper describes the sensor data collection model, the reliable multicast data delivery mechanism, and our experiences so far in this project. In particular, it describes our existing network test bed and the control of an UA through a MANET. It specifically targets assisted living residents and others who may benefit from continuous, remote health monitoring. We present the advantages, objectives, and status of the design.

Keywords Ad hoc networks · Unmanned aircraft · Sensor data collection

Introduction

This paper considers the role of a mobile ad hoc network (MANET) to support sensor data collection [1]. In this model an area has intelligence, surveillance, and reconnaissance (ISR), environmental monitoring, or other sensors that can range

M. Bhatele
Gyan Ganga College of Technology, Jabalpur, India

S. Shrivastava (✉) · P. Deodi
Department of Digital Communication, Gyan Ganga College of Technology, Jabalpur, India
e-mail: shrutishrivastava95@gmail.com

V. Kumar and M. Bhatele (eds.), *Proceedings of All India Seminar on Biomedical Engineering 2012 (AISOBE 2012)*, Lecture Notes in Bioengineering,
DOI: 10.1007/978-81-322-0970-6_19, © Springer India 2013

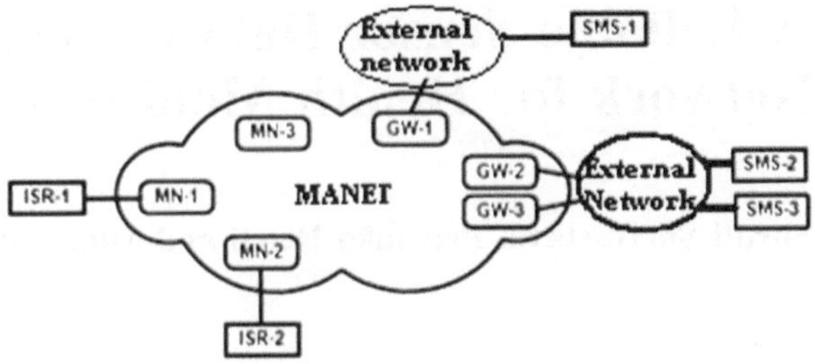

Fig. 1 Sensor data collection concept showing ISR sensors delivering data through a MANET to multiple gateways and sensor monitoring stations

from small and simple thermometers to large and highly functional RF scanners. Sensors need to report results in near real-time to one or more sensor monitoring stations (SMS) located at remote locations. A sensor reports events either periodically or upon some triggering condition. The sensor interfaces with a MANET node (MN) which in turn delivers the sensor event to a gateway node (GW) which connects to an external backhaul network to the SMS. The MANET can have stationary ground nodes to support this communication. A ground node typically has short-range and cannot support sensors over a wide area. Therefore, in order to provide a node capable of long-range communication and also having wide ranging coverage, unmanned aircraft (UA) are out with radio interfaces. The concept diagram is shown in Fig. 1. As the world's population ages, those suffering from diseases of the elderly will increase. In homes and nursing homes pervasive networks may assist residents and their caregivers by providing continuous medical monitoring, memory enhancement, control of home appliances, medical data access, and emergency communication. Researchers in computer, networking, and medical fields are working to make the broad vision of smart health care possible.

This concept has several issues to be resolved in routing, addressing, and the interaction between the UA mobility and communication. Each sensor event is considered valuable and requires a reliable delivery mechanism through the dynamic network to multiple SMS [5]. Mobility in the MANET may lead to a temporary lack of routes to the GW. The gateways may connect to external networks via satellite or cellular links which have occasional link outages. The distribution of the sensors and available MANET resources may be such that there is never an end to end route from the sensor and all the SMSs. The sensor is assumed to be simple and should be isolated from network specifics such as the number and network location of the SMS. The addresses of the sensors, MN, and external network nodes must be managed not only to enable the multicast delivery of sensor data to each SMS, but also to enable an individual SMS to make queries to specific sensors. The MN, in turn, should be isolated from the specifics of the GW to SMS backhaul network.

Major Goals

We are developing network architecture for smart health care that will open up new opportunities for continuous monitoring of assisted and independent living residents while preserving resident comfort and privacy. The network manages a

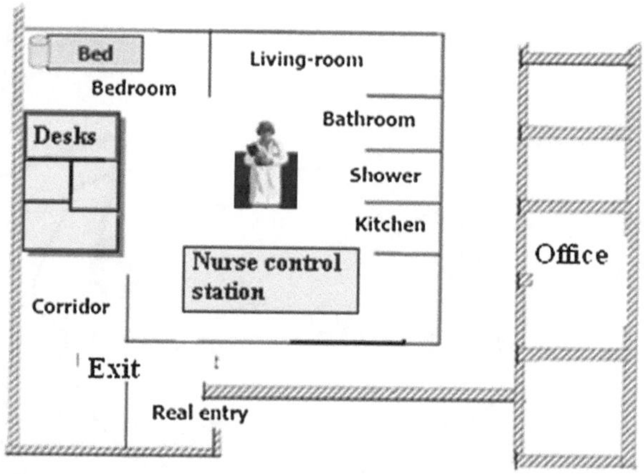

Fig. 2 Layout of the experimental smart health home at UVA

continuous medical history. Unobtrusive area and environmental sensors combine with wearable interactive devices to evaluate the health of spaces and the people who inhabit them. Authorized care providers may monitor resident's health and life habits and watch for chronic pathologies. Multiple patients and their resident family members as well as visitors are differentiated for sensing tasks and access privileges.

High costs of installation and retrofit are avoided by using ad hoc, self-managing networks [2, 3]. Based on the fundamental elements of future medical applications (integration with existing medical practice and technology, real-time and long-term monitoring, wearable sensors and assistance to chronic patients, elders or handicapped people), our wireless system will extend health care from the traditional clinical hospital setting to nursing and retirement homes, enabling telecare without the prohibitive costs of retrofitting existing structures. Figure 2 shows the layout of the experimental laboratory. The architecture is multitiered, with heterogeneous devices ranging from lightweight sensors, to mobile components, and more powerful stationary devices.

The advantages of a WSN are numerous for smart health care, as it provides the following important properties:

1. **Portability and unobtrusiveness**: Small devices collect data and communicate wirelessly, operating with minimal patient input. They may be carried on the body or deeply embedded in the environment. Unobtrusiveness helps with patient acceptance and minimizes confounding measurement effects. Since monitoring is done in the living space, the patient travels less often; this is safer and more convenient.
2. **Ease of deployment and scalability**: Devices can be deployed in potentially large quantities with dramatically less complexity and cost compared to wired networks. Existing structures, particularly dilapidated ones, can be easily augmented with a WSN network, whereas wired installations would be expensive and impractical. Devices are placed in the living space and turned on, self-organizing and calibrating automatically.

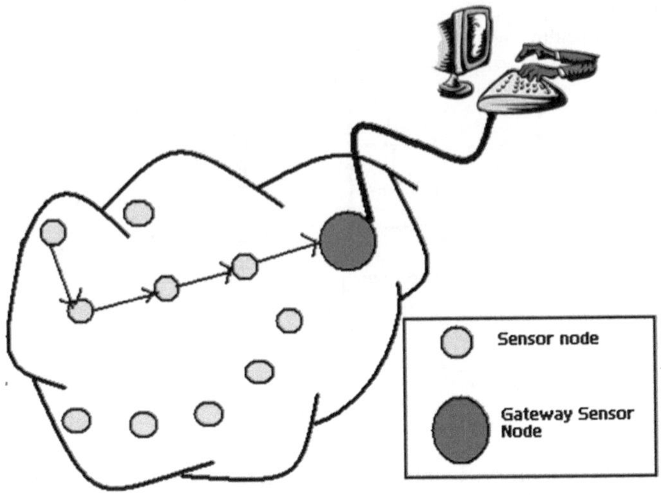

Fig. 3 Typical multihop wireless sensor network architecture

3. **Real-time and always on**: Physiological and environmental data can be monitored continuously, allowing real-time response by emergency or health care workers. The data collected form a health journal, and are valuable for filling in gaps in the traditional patient history. Although the network as a whole is always on, individual sensors still must conserve energy through smart power management and on-demand activation.
4. **Reconfiguration and self-organization**: Since there is no fixed installation, adding and removing sensors instantly reconfigures the network. Doctors may retarget the mission of the network as medical needs change. Sensors self-organize to form routing paths, collaborate on data processing, and establish hierarchies (Fig. 3).

The WSN is built of "nodes"—from a few to several hundreds or even thousands, where each node is connected to one (or sometimes several) sensors. Each such sensor network node has typically several parts: a radio transceiver with an internal antenna or connection to an external antenna, a microcontroller, an electronic circuit for interfacing with the sensors, and an energy source, usually a battery or an embedded form of energy harvesting. A sensor node might vary in size from that of a shoebox down to the size of a grain of dust, although functioning "motes" of genuine microscopic dimensions have yet to be created. The cost of sensor nodes is similarly variable, ranging from a few to hundreds of dollars, depending on the complexity of the individual sensor nodes. Size and cost constraints on sensor nodes result in corresponding constraints on resources such as energy, memory, computational speed, and communications bandwidth. The topology of the WSNs can vary from a simple star network to an advanced multihop wireless mesh network. The propagation technique between the hops of the network can be routing or flooding.

Communication Architecture

This section develops the detailed architecture and describes the protocols and addressing schemes that are used. It further explains how the network meets the design criteria and how it deals with network anomalies to guarantee packet delivery.

System Overview and Elements

The overall system architecture is shown in Fig. 3. An ISR sensor [6, 7] produces events that are sent to a nearby MN via a wired Ethernet connection to mitigate interference. This MN manages communication for the ISR and is designated the terminus. The terminus uses the MANET to connect to GW nodes which forward the data to the external networks and on to the SMSs. This ISR initiated event multicast is designated as Event communication. Conversely, an SMS can send commands on the reverse path to a specific sensor. This SMS initiated Command and Query Exchanges are designated as Command communication. Event communication sends sensor readings from one ISR to all active SMSs. Command communication enables a single SMS to control and query one ISR. Both communication paths are based on the same reliable forwarding protocol [4] as described in the next section.

Reliable Forwarding Approach

The design criteria dictate high reliability, but at the same time operation over an intermittently connected network, as well as minimal event message delivery time and overhead. Two primary mechanisms are used to provide reliable delivery: staged delivery and reliable transport. The first mechanism is that the packets are delivered in stages from the ISR to the Terminus, from the Terminus to the GW, and from the GW to the SMS. At each stage, the source node uses a reliable mechanism to deliver the packet to the destination node. Once delivered, the destination node becomes the source node for the next stage and is responsible for advancing the node to the next stage's destination. This breaks down the delivery problem so that the nodes in one stage are isolated from the network-specific issues in other stages. For instance, the ISR is only concerned with delivering its packets to the terminus and does not need to be aware of any of the MANET or satellite link protocols in the networks beyond the terminus. The second mechanism is a reliable delivery protocol, implemented by all communicating entities. As seen in earlier AUGNet experimentation, an ad hoc network with fast moving nodes possess a considerable challenge to existing reliable transport protocols like TCP. Since the goal is purely message transport, compared to data streaming, the UDP protocol was chosen and augmented with functionality to guarantee data delivery. The RUDP protocol provides windowing, congestion control, in order delivery, and over buffering. These are not necessary features in our data collection scenario and we instead chose a simpler UDP mechanism.

Conclusion

This paper describes the design and implementation of a reliable sensor data collection network for sparsely deployed sensors. A meshed ad hoc network of ground nodes and small, fast moving UA is used to gather sensor information and hand them over to SMS. The unique contributions of the conducted research are the control of the UA solely through a meshed ad hoc network, the reliable forwarding of single event packets from sensors to multiple monitoring stations through the intermittently connected network, and the demonstration of autonomous plane operations based on network and environmental parameters. The baseline of the system is implemented. A one-week experiment showed a robust system with some straightforward communications from front to backend of the system. The modularity of this system should enable progressive development of the research areas. We believe this system design will greatly enhance quality of life, health, and security for those in assisted living communities.

References

1. Basheer MR, Rao VS, Derriso MM (2003) Self-organizing wireless sensor networks for structural health monitoring. In: Proceeding of SPIE, vol 5049, pp 515–525
2. Basu P, Redi J (2004) Movement control algorithms for realization of fault-tolerant ad hoc robot networks. IEEE Netw pp 36–44
3. Brown TX, Argrow B, Dixon C, Doshi S, Thekkekunnel R-G, Henkel D (2004) Ad hoc UAV-ground network (AUGNet). In: AIAA 3rd unmanned unlimited technical conference, Chicago, IL (Sept 2004)
4. Doshi S, Bhandare S, Brown TX (2002) An on demand minimum energy routing protocol for a wireless ad hoc network. Mob Comput Commun Rev 6(3):50–66
5. Johnson D, Maltz D (1996) Dynamic source routing in Ad Hoc wireless networks, mobile computing, chapter 5, Kluwer Academic Publishers, Dordrecht, pp 153–181
6. Harvard University. CodeBlue project: Wireless Sensor Networks for Medical Care
7. Wiñeld AF (2000) Distributed sensing and data collection via broken ad hoc wireless connected networks of mobile robots, vol 4 of Distributed Autonomous Robotics Systems, Springer, New York (82) pp 273–282

An Efficient Approach to Categorize Data Using Improved Dendritic Cell Algorithm with Dempster Belief Theory

Kalpana Kumari, Anurag Jain and Aakriti Jain

Abstract One of the central challenges with computer security is determining the difference between normal and potentially harmful activity. Intrusions, in particular, Web-based ones, have become increasing threats for important information. The unique features of AIS encourage researchers to employ their techniques in a variety of applications and especially in intrusion detection systems. Among the wide range of available approaches, it is always challenging to select the optimal algorithm for intrusion detection. In this paper we compare the performance one of the algorithms of an artificial immune system called dendritic cell algorithm based on Dempster belief theory with the dendritic cell algorithm and Support vector machine. In terms of accuracy and computational complexity we observe that DCA-BF has a strong detection ability and good generalization performance.

Keywords Artificial immune system · Intrusion detection system · Human immune system · Negative selection algorithm · DCA · Dempster–belief theory

K. Kumari (✉) · A. Jain
Department of CSE, RITS, Bhopal, India
e-mail: kalpana04cs21@gmail.com

A. Jain
e-mail: anurag.akjain@gmail.com

A. Jain
Department of CSE, SIRT-S, Bhopal, India
e-mail: aakriti.jain@gmail.com

V. Kumar and M. Bhatele (eds.), *Proceedings of All India Seminar on Biomedical Engineering 2012 (AISOBE 2012)*, Lecture Notes in Bioengineering,
DOI: 10.1007/978-81-322-0970-6_20,

Introduction

Intrusion Detection Systems are one of the important building blocks of a secure, reliable network, and are used widely along with other security programs and concepts. There are several methods used to implement intrusion detection such as statistical analysis expert systems, state transition approaches, etc., and these several approaches are based on the immune system that were proposed in the recent years. The goal of Intrusion Detection is to detect illicit access and abuse of computer systems by both system insiders and external intruders, and guarantee the system integrity, confidentiality, and usability. Several techniques are used to achieve intrusion detection such as expert systems, state transition approaches, and statistical analysis. However, they are inefficient to detect the unknown intrusions. Therefore, several approaches based on the immune system were proposed in the recent years [1].

Artificial immune system for detecting intrusion has become a new approach in security research. Artificial immunology is an interdisciplinary between biology and information security. AIS is inspired from the human immune system (HIS) which is a system of structures in the human body that recognizes the foreign pathogens and cells from human body cells and protects the body against those disease [2].

In this paper we compare two popular algorithms that represent two different intrusion detection techniques. One is dendritic cell algorithm based on belief theory (DCA-BE) and the other is the DCA classification algorithm. The experiment's data come from the KDD CUP competition data set. These data are part of the data collected from the MIT Lincoln Labs 1998 DARPA Intrusion Detection Evaluation Program and are considered as benchmark data for evaluating the intrusion detection system [3]. The performance of an intrusion detection system may be evaluated in terms of TP rate and FP rate.

The rest of the paper is organized as follows. Section two deals with the Related Work. Section three briefly describes two algorithms, Dendritic Cell Algorithm Based on Dempster Belief Theory and Dendritic Cell Algorithm. Section four is about Experiment Result Discussion and finally section five is the Conclusion of this experiment.

Related Work

In recent years, use of Artificial Immune System (AIS) has been favored by the researcher to build Intrusion Detection Systems based on it. AIS is a new branch of computational intelligence. The primitive theoretical study on artificial immunology was conducted by Farmer in 1986 [4]. They put forward a new link between biological and computing science [1]. Forrest et al. in 1994, proposed the most effective idea in utilization of immunity in computer security for self and non-self discrimination. Aickelin [5] firstintroduced the theory to solve the recognition problem in existing AISs. Matzinger [6] in 2002 applied the Danger theory as an alternative approach for self-surrounding high false positive, poor adaptation, and short self-monitored. Danger Theory is becoming an efficient way to solve problems such as classifications, and anomaly detections.

They developed a negative selection algorithm (NSA) based on the principles of self/non-self discrimination in the human immune system [7].

This algorithm defines 'self' as normal behavior patterns of a monitored system. It generates a number of random patterns. If any randomly generated pattern matches a self-pattern, it fails to become a detector and will be removed. Otherwise, it becomes a 'detector' and is used to monitor subsequent access patterns. This algorithm operates on binary string, and adopts R-Contiguous Matching Function (RCMF) to determine a match degree between antibody and antigen [5].

Kim et al. shows that it is costly to only use negative selection. Inspired by human immune system, an artificial immune system model used for network intrusion detection has been presented by authors. This two-level (physical level and logical level) intrusion detection system has a primary part and secondary selection, and includes three stages: gene library evolution, negative selection, and clonal selection. These three processes are coordinated across the network to accommodate an effective intrusion detection system which is distributed, self-organizing, and lightweight. In 2002, Kim et al. proposed dynamic clonal selection algorithm. Via the lifecycle mechanism of the immune cells, the detectors identify the abnormal behavior that was normal in the past.

Algorithm Description

The current intrusion detection system is used to extract the characteristics of ordinary users' behaviors. Any unmatched behavior orders are considered as abnormal and would be alarming. The central challenge with computer security is developing systems which have the ability to differentiate between the normal and an intrusion which represents potentially harmful activity. A promising solution is emerging in the form of biologically inspired computing, and in particular, artificial immune systems (AIS). Both Dendritic Cell Algorithm (DCA) based on Belief theory and DCA are popular algorithms in the field of artificial immunology.

Dendritic Cell Algorithm

The DCA is a population-based algorithm, designed for tackling anomaly based detection tasks. It is inspired by functions of natural DCs of the innate immune system, which form part of the body's first line of defence against invaders. DCs have the ability to combine a multitude of molecular information and to interpret this information for T-cells of the adaptive immune system, to induce appropriate immune responses toward perceived threats. Therefore, DCs can be seen as detectors for different policing sites of the body as well as mediators for inducing a variety of immune responses. Signals are normally precategorized as "PAMP", "Danger" or "Safe" in the DCA.

The co-occurrence of antigen and high/low signal values forms the basis of categorization for the antigen data [4].

The primary components of a DC-based algorithm are as follows:

- Individual DCs with the capability to perform multisignal processing.
- Antigen collection and presentation.

Dendritic Cell Algorithm (DCA) Based on Belief Theory

The basic idea of the Dendritic Cell Algorithm (DCA) based on Belief theory is to solve the problem of correlation and resolve the problem of unknown and rapidly evolving harmful attacks [5]. The basic steps of the algorithm are given below:

Step1: With the help of Dendritic Cell Algorithm we categorized data, whether the data are normal or affected with anomaly or in other words, abnormal.

Step2: Dempster-Belief theory is used to compute the probability of evidences that indicate support to the attack or normal class. The use of Dempster Belief theory steadily spreads out, mostly because it is used to cope with large amounts of uncertainties that are inherent of natural environments. This new approach considers sets of propositions and assigns to each of them an interval [*Belief, Plausibility*] [8].

Step3: After the classification we calculate the entropy of the attack treated as signal. For the calculation of entropy let us consider a set having possible event Now measured entropy, represented by *H*(*x*) which is calculated with the help of the given formula [9]:

$$H(x) = \sum_{i=1}^{N} P(xi) \log\left(\frac{1}{pi}\right) \text{Bit/message} \tag{1}$$

where $p(xi)$ the probability of event.

Experimental Setup and Result

The experiment's data comes from the KDD CUP competition data set. These data are part of the data collected from the MIT Lincoln Labs 1998 DARPA Intrusion Detection Evaluation Program and are considered benchmark data for evaluating intrusion detection system.

Since 1999, KDD'99 [3] has been the most wildly used data set for the evaluation of anomaly detection methods. This data set is prepared by Stolfo et al. and is built based on the data captured in DARPA'98 IDS evaluation program. There are about 4,900,000 records and has 41 attributes [3].

The performance of an intrusion detection system may be evaluated in terms of TP rate and FP rate.True Positive(TP) rate is calculated as the number of abnormal patterns detected by the system, divided by the total number of abnormal patterns. Here, A represents attack and I represents Intrusion.

$$\mathrm{TPR} = \frac{\mathrm{TP}}{\mathrm{TP} + \mathrm{FN}} = \mathrm{P}(A|I) \tag{2}$$

Similarly, True negative (TN) rate can be calculated as

$$\mathrm{TNR} = \frac{\mathrm{TN}}{\mathrm{TP} + \mathrm{TN}} = \mathrm{P}(\leftharpoondown A \leftharpoondown I) \tag{3}$$

False Positive(FP) rate occurs when the system wrongfully classifies normal patterns as abnormal patterns. In this experiment, FP rate is calculated as the number of false positives created by the system, divided by the total number of self-antigens (Fig. 1).

$$\mathrm{FNR} = \frac{FP}{FP + TN} = \mathrm{P}(\leftharpoondown AI) \tag{4}$$

Similarly FN (False negative) rate can be calculated as

$$\mathrm{FNR} = \frac{FN}{TP + FN} = \mathrm{P}(\leftharpoondown AI) \tag{5}$$

The comparison of the simulation result is given in Fig. 2. It gives the comparison of the accuracy rate for the classification of attack using Dendritic Cell Algorithm (DCA) with Dendritic Cell Algorithm with belief function (DCA-BE). In simulation the generating function also called as the activated threshold value was set to 1.

The maximum accuracy rate of the algorithm is possible only by using DCA and the Belief function theory. Figure 2 shows when using DCA, classification of the accuracy of attack never reaches even 92.00 %, but by using DCA-BE approaches the accuracy rate reaches 96.00 %. The X-axes represents the accuracy rate and the Y-axes indicate detection generating value.

Table 1 shows the results of the experiment 1. From experiment 1 we conclude that the maximum accuracy of the detection of intrusion using DCA never reaches above 92 %, whereas by using DCA-BE the accuracy becomes even maximum 96 %.

In experiment 2, we can easily predicate that by using our proposed approaches the TPR, TNR, FPR, and FNR are minimal. Whereas with the help of DCA all the parameters show their maximum values. Figure 2 shows a comparison of the TPR, TNR, FPR, and FNR rates between DCA versus DCA-BE in training data set.

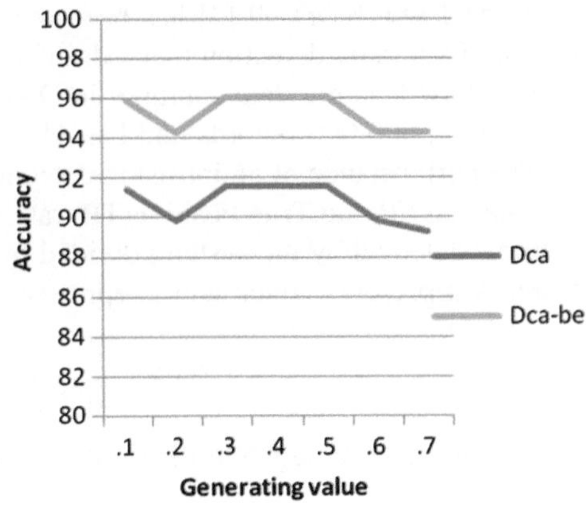

Fig. 1 Comparison of dendritic cell algorithm with dendritic cell algorithm and belief function (DCA-BE)

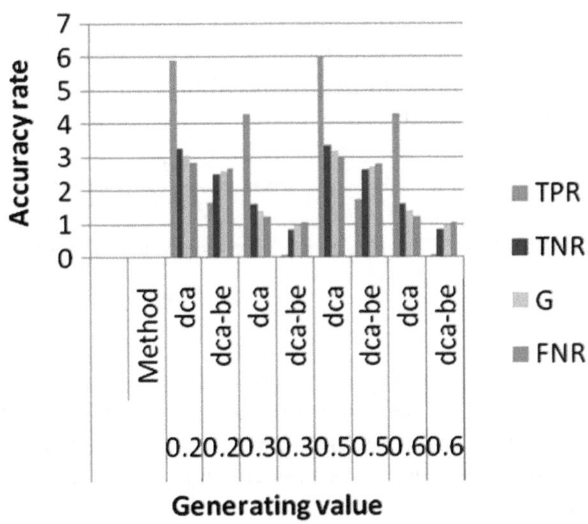

Fig. 2 Comparison of the TPR, TNR, FPR, and FNR rates between DCA versus DCA-BE in

Table 1 The results of experiment 1

Generating value	DCA	DCA-BE
0.2	91.4	95.9
0.3	89.79	94.3
0.5	91.55	96.06
0.7	91.53	96.04
0.8	91.55	96.06
0.9	89.79	94.3
0.1	89.29	94.3

Table 2 The results of experiment 2

Generating value	Method	TPR	TNR	FPR	FNR
0.2	DCA	5.91	3.25	3.05	2.85
0.2	DCA-BE	1.65	2.5	2.6	2.69
0.3	DCA	4.27	1.61	1.41	1.21
0.3	DCA-BE	0.08	0.86	0.96	1.05
0.5	DCA	6.03	3.37	3.17	2.97
0.5	DCA-BE	1.76	2.62	2.72	2.81
0.6	DCA	4.27	1.61	1.41	1.21
0.6	DCA-BE	0.08	0.86	0.96	1.05

Table 2 shows the results of experiment 2. From experiment 2 we conclude that the minimal TPR, TNR, FPR, and FNR are obtained with the help of experiment 2, we calculate minimal TPR, TNR, FPR, and FNR.

Our method gives better results compared with DCA. With the help of DCA all the parameters (TPR, TNR, FPR, and FNR) show their maximum values. However, in general, the method proposed in this paper is effective to detect the unknown intrusion.

From experiment 2, we conclude that DCA-BE gives better method for the classification of the data as well as minimum TPR, TNR, FPR, and FNR.

Conclusion and Future Work

This paper compares the two algorithms of Artificial Immune Systems (AIS) namely, Dendritic Cell Algorithm and Dendritic Cell Algorithm with belief theory. Integrating the Dendritic Cell Algorithm and Dempster-Belief theory solves the problem of correlation and Dempster–Belief theory resolves the problem of unknown and rapidly evolving harmful attacks more efficiently than the DCA. The simulation results show that the DCA-BE method has improved the correlation factor, minimizing the false +ve and false −ve alarm generation, and increases the rate of detection of intrusion as compared to the DCA.

However, the feature reduction process of KDD data set takes a large amount of time. Therefore, in the future work modifying the feature reduction optimization for the better selection of feature in KDD data set can be attempted.

References

1. Hosseinpour F, Bakar KA, Hardoroudi AH, Kazazi N (2010) Survey on artificial immune system as a bio-inspired technique for anomaly based intrusion detection systems. In: International conference on intelligent networking and collaborative systems, pp 158–189
2. Matzinger P (1994) Tolerance, danger and the extended family. Ann Rev Immunol 12:991–1045

3. Lippmann RP, Fried DJ, Graf I, Haines JW, Kendall KR, McClung D, Weber D, Webster SE, Wyschogrod D, Cunningham RK, Zissman MA (2000) Evaluating intrusion detection systems: the 1998 darpa off-line intrusion detection evaluation, discex, vol 02, pp 210–212
4. Dasgupta D (1999) Immunity-based intrusion detection system: a general framework. In: Proceeding of the 22nd national information systems security conference (NISSC), Arlington, Virgina, pp 147–160
5. Matzinger P (1994) Tolerance, danger and the extended family. Ann Rev Immunol 12(2004):991–1045
6. Aickelin U, Cayzer S (2002) The danger theory and its application to AIS. In: 1st international conference on AIS, 2002, pp 141–148
7. Chen G, Shuo P, Rong J, Chao L (2009) An anomaly detection system based on dendritic cell algorithm. In: Third international conference on genetic and evolutionary computing, pp 192–195
8. Kumari K, Prof. Jain A, Prof. Dongre S, Prof. Jain A (2012) Intrusion detection technique based on dendritic cell algorithm and dempster belief theory. Int Organ Sci Res 1(5): 38–43
9. Shafer G (1976) A Mathematical theory of evidence. Princeton University Press, NJ

Efficient Intrusion Detection with KNN Classification and DS Theory

Deepika Dave and Sumit Vashishtha

Abstract Intrusion detection is an appallingly exigent area of research in the existing scenario. Nowadays, to find a novel pattern of intrusions and detection is an exceedingly difficult job. Our aim is to affect a method for intrusion detection using KNN classification and Dempster theory of evidence. Using these modes, we devised a new pattern of intrusion and classified category of pattern and applied event evidence logic with the help of DS theory. Finned pattern of intrusion is compared with the existing pattern of intrusion which generates a new schema of pattern and updates a list of pattern of intrusion detection and improves the true rate of intrusion detection. We have also accomplished some experimental tasks with KDD99Cup and DARPA98 databases from MIT Lincoln Laboratory which show that the proposed method provides competitively high detection rates compared with other machine learning (ML) techniques and CRISP data mining. The experimental results clearly show that the proposed system achieved higher precision in identifying whether the records are abnormal or attacking ones.

Keywords Intrusion detection · KNN · DS theory · KDD data set 99

D. Dave · S. Vashishtha (✉)
Sagar Institute of Research, Technology and Science, Bhopal, Madhya Pradesh, INDIA
e-mail: sumitvbpl@gmail.com

D. Dave
e-mail: deepikadave.mds@gmail.com

V. Kumar and M. Bhatele (eds.), *Proceedings of All India Seminar on Biomedical Engineering 2012 (AISOBE 2012)*, Lecture Notes in Bioengineering,
DOI: 10.1007/978-81-322-0970-6_21, © Springer India 2013

Introduction

Intrusion detection systems (IDSs) are important elements for computer networks being one of the main security tools and organization of communication infrastructures. An IDS is a mechanism which quietly listens to network traffic in order to detect abnormal or suspicious activity. There are two distinct families of IDSs: (1) N-IDS (network based) which handles security at the network level and (2) H-IDS (host based) which handles security at host level. Intrusion detection is a technique for protecting the system when a network is being used by an unauthorized person.

Traditionally, the intrusion detection technique has been categorized in the following ways: (1) Misuse detection : Misuse detection technique focuses on developing a model of known attacks, i.e., in this we have predefined patterns of abnormal files which can be described by specific patterns or sequences of the data and elements. (2) Anomaly detection: The main aim of anomaly detection is to identify cases that are abnormal within data and that are apparently uniform. Anomaly detection is an important tool for detecting network intrusion and other rare events that may have great impact, but are difficult to find. Anomaly detection refers to the manner of finding patterns in data that are not conventional to the expected behavior. Intrusion detection has emerged as a significant field of research, because it is not theoretically possible to set up a system with no vulnerabilities. One main confrontation in intrusion detection is that we have to detect the concealed attacks from a large quantity of routine communication activities. Several machine learning (ML) algorithms, for instance Neural Network, Support Vector Machine, Genetic Algorithm, Fuzzy Logic, and Data Mining and more, have been extensively employed to detect intrusion activities, both known and unknown, from large quantities of complex and dynamic data sets. Generating rules is vital for IDSs to differentiate standard behaviors from strange behaviors by examining the data set which is a list of tasks created by the operating system that is registered into a file in historical sorted order. Various researches with data mining as the chief constituent has been carried out to detect newly encountered intrusions. The analysis of data to determine relationships and to discover concealed patterns of data which otherwise would go unobserved is known as data mining. Many researchers have used data mining to focus on the subject of database intrusion detection in databases.

We have designed intrusion detection using KNN Classification and Dempster–Shafer (DS) theory with fuzzy logic. The input to the proposed system is KDD Cup 1999 data set, which is separated into two subsets such as, training data set and testing data set. Initially, the training data set is classified into five subsets, so that four types of attacks—DoS (denial of service), R2L (remote to local), U2R (user to root), Probe—and normal data are separated. After that, we simply mine the one-length frequent items from attack data as well as normal data. These mined frequent items are used to find the important attributes of the input data set and the identified effective attributes are used to generate a set of definite and indefinite rules using deviation method. Then, we generate fuzzy rule in accordance with the definite rule by fuzzifying it in such a way that we obtain a set of fuzzy if–then rules with consequent parts that represent whether it is a normal data or an abnormal data. These rules are given to the fuzzy rule base to effectively learn the fuzzy system. In the testing phase, the test data is matched with fuzzy rules to detect whether the test data is an abnormal data or a normal data. We apply KNN classification and DS theory of evidence to classify data. Through these, we devised a new pattern of intrusion and classifieds category of pattern and apply event evidence logic with the help of DS theory. Finned pattern of intrusion is compared with the existing pattern of intrusion which generates a new schema of pattern and updates a list of pattern of intrusion detection and improves the true rate of intrusion detection. We used the concept of DS theory in this work on event evidence to find the validity of data and reduce the rate of intrusion. We also used the patterns of design of schema and data conversion in data conversion first-type intrusion detection in MATLAB, but for data of intrusion data in overall string format, now we have used the classification method. We faced various difficulties in classification of data conversion string through numeric format for suitability of classification. In the process of data conversion, we used the ratio mapping concept used by the machine learning (ML) receptory organization for mapping of data string to numeric format.

The rest of the chapter is organized as follows: In Literature Survey, some related works are reviewed, KNN (Known Nearest Neighbor) deals with KNN classifier, The Dempster–Shafer Theory overviews the DS theory, KDD Data Set 99 KDD data set, Method describes our method, Experimental Results and Performance Analysis shows performance and results, and Conclusion draws the conclusions.

Literature Survey

Classification Method by Fuzzy GNP-Based Class Association Rules

The work of Han and Kamber [1] in the field of intrusion detection with regard to the fuzzy GNP-based class association approach is designed for databases containing both discrete and continuous attribute as Network Connection Database. A specific classification method is described as follows: The definition of the matching degree between the continuous attribute A_i in rule r with q_i and testing data connection with value a_i is:

$$\text{MatchDegree}(q_i, a_i) = Fq_i(a_i) \tag{1}$$

where, Fq_i represents the membership function for linguistic term q_i.

and the matching between rule r (p continuous and q discrete attributes) and new unlabeled connection d is defined as:

$$\text{Match}_r(d) = \frac{1}{p+q}\left(\sum_{i\in \text{A}p} \text{MatchDegree}(q_i, a_i) + t\right) \quad (2)$$

where

i index of continuous attribute in rule r;
Ap set of suffixes of continuous attributes in rule r;
p number of continuous attributes in rule r;
q number of discrete attributes in r;
t number of discrete attributes in new unlabeled connection d satisfying rule r;

Match_r(d) ranges from 0 to 1. If $\text{Match}_r(d)$ equals 1.0, rule r matches connection data d completely. While $\text{Match}_r(d)$ equals 0, rule r does not match connection d at all. Then, the average matching between connection data d and all the rules in a certain rule pool is defined as:

$$\text{MATCH}_r(d) = \frac{1}{|Rp|}\sum_{r\in Rp} \text{Matchr}(d) \quad (3)$$

where R_p is the set of suffixes of extracted important class association rule in a certain rules pool.

A. **Classifier for misuse detection**

The average matching between connection data d and all the rules in the normal rule in pool $\text{MATCH}_n(d)$, and the average matching between connection data d and all the rules in the intrusion rule pool $\text{MATCH}_i(d)$ are calculated and compared.

If $\text{MATCH}_n(d) \geq \text{MATCH}_r(d)$, connection data d is labeled as normal. On the other hand, if $\text{MATCH}_n(d) < \text{MATCH}_i(d)$, connection data d is labeled as intrusion.

In summary, a new connection data is labeled according to their matching with normal and intrusion rule pools. Larger matching suggests the higher possibility of belonging to this class.

B. **Classifier for anomaly detection**

After getting matching between each connection data and rules in the normal rule pool, we can have the distribution of the matching with the mean value μ and standard deviation σ. The figure shows an example of the distribution.

In this testing period, when a new unlabeled connection data comes, the matching between the data and the rules in normal rule pool is calculated. If $\text{MATCH}_n(d) < (\mu - k\sigma)$, label the connection as intrusion. On the other hand, if $\text{MATCH}_n(d) \geq (\mu - k\sigma)$, the label is normal. By adjusting parameter k, we can balance the PFR (Positive False Rate) and NFR (Negative False Rate).

In all, by using the improved Fuzzy GNP-based class association rule mining, we can find a large number of rules related to normal behavior so as to explore the space of the normal connections, and any significant deviation from the normal space is viewed as an intrusion.

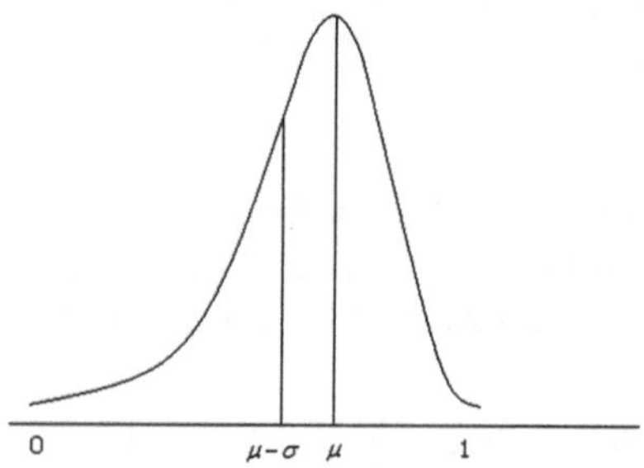

Probabilistic Classification

Freund [2] devised in the field of intrusion detection with the approach as: After extracting a number of important class association rules including normal and intrusion, a classifier is constructed to classify new connection data into normal, misuse, and anomaly intrusion correctly. The key points of probabilistic classification concern three aspects. First, the probability density function of the average matching degree of data with rules is used. Second, the probability that data is classified to anomaly intrusion is also considered. Third, in order to improve the classification accuracy.

$$\text{MatchDegree}_k(Q_i, a_i) = F_{Qi}(a_i)$$

where F_{Qi} represents the membership function of linguistic term $Q_{i.}$ Then, the matching degree between data and rule r (including p continuous attributes and q discrete attributes) is defined as:

$$\text{Match}_k(d, r) = \frac{1}{p+q}\left(\sum_{i \in CA} \text{MatchDegree}_k(Q_i, a_i) + t\right), \tag{5}$$

where, I is the suffix of continuous attributes in rule r; CA denotes the set of suffix of continuous attributes in rule r; p and q represent the number of continuous attributes and discrete attributes in rule r, respectively, and t is the number of matched discrete attributes in rule r with data. Then, the average matching degree can be defined as

$$m_k(d) = \frac{1}{|RK|}\left(\sum_{k \in C} \text{Match}_k(d, r), \right. \tag{6}$$

where, R_k is the set of suffixes of the extracted rules in class k in the rule pool (normal rules or misuse rules). Finally, the marginal probability density function $f_1(x_1), f_2(x_2), \ldots f_L(x_k)$ can be generated by calculating the distribution of the average matching degree of training data d ε $D_{train}(k)$ with r ε R_k, where, $D_{train}(k)$ is the set of suffixes of training data in class k. $K = 2$ is used in this paper.

A. **Building a Classifier**

After creating the probability density function $f_K(x_k)$ of the average matching degree between training data d ε $D_{train}(k)$ and rule r ε R_k, the probability that new connection data d ε D_{test} belongs to class k is represented as follows:

$$P_k(d) = \int_{mk(d)}^{1.0} f_K(x_K)\mathrm{d}x_k \ldots \sum\nolimits_{k\in C} f_K(x_K)\mathrm{d}x_K \ldots \int_{ml(d)}^{1.0} f_1(x_1)\mathrm{d}x_1, \quad (7)$$

where, D_{test} is the set of suffix of testing data. Actually, the probability that d Sigma D_{test} belongs to anomaly class is defined as:

$$P_0(d) = \sum_{k\in C} 1 - P_k(d) \quad (8)$$

where, C is the set of suffix of classes having training data. In the case of two classes, the probabilities of the first class and the second class can be calculated by the following equations.

$$P_1(d) = \int_{m2(d)}^{1.0} f_2(x_2)\mathrm{d}x_2 \int_0^{m1(d)} f_1(x_1)\mathrm{d}x_1 \quad (9)$$

$$P_2(d) = \int_0^{m2(d)} f_2(x_2)\mathrm{d}x_2 \int_{m1(d)}^{1.0} f_1(x_1)\mathrm{d}x_1 \quad (10)$$

Then, the probability that a new connection data belongs to anomaly class is calculated by $P_0(d) = 1 - \sum_{k\in C} P_k(d)$. Based on the calculation of these probabilities, d is assigned to the class with highest probability.

KNN (Known Nearest Neighbor)

KNN is a *nonparametric lazy learning* algorithm. That is a pretty concise statement. When you say a technique is nonparametric, it means that it does not make any assumptions on the underlying data distribution. This is pretty useful, as in the real world, most of the practical data do not obey the typical theoretical assumptions made (e.g Gaussian mixtures, linearly separable, etc.). Nonparametric algorithms like KNN come to the rescue here.

It is also a lazy algorithm. This means that it does not use the training data points to do any *generalization*. In other words, there is *no explicit training phase*, or it is very minimal. This means the training phase is pretty fast. Lack of generalization means that KNN keeps all the training data. More precisely, all the training data is needed during the testing phase. (Well this is an exaggeration, but

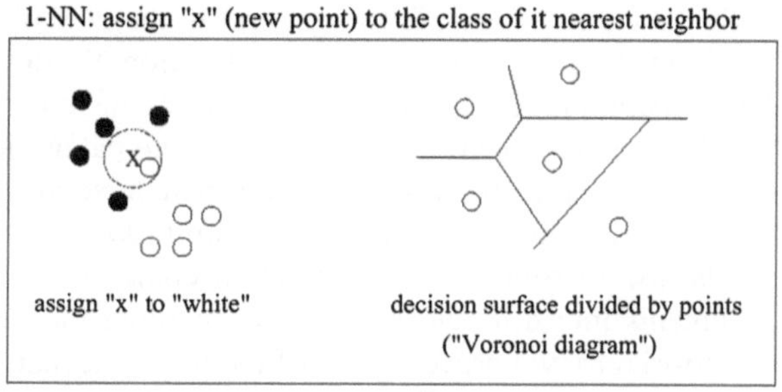

Fig. 1 Decision of nearest neighbor

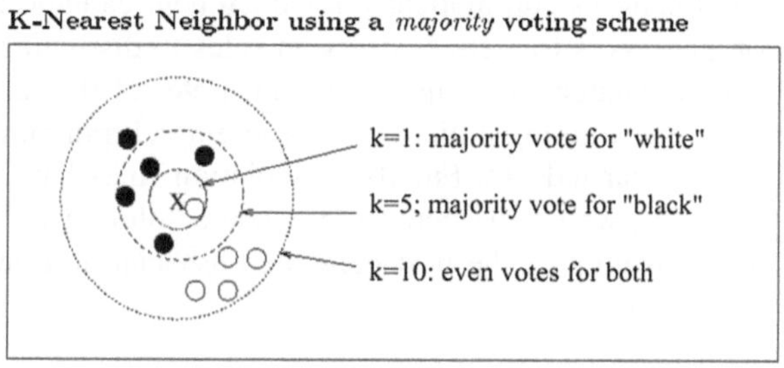

Fig. 2 Majority voting scheme

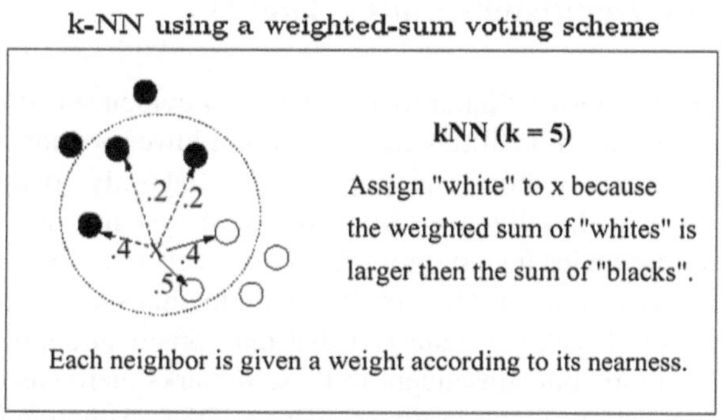

Fig. 3 Weighted-sum voting scheme

not far from the truth). This is in contrast to other techniques like SVM where you can discard all nonsupport vectors without any problems. Most of the lazy algorithms—especially KNN—makes decisions based on the entire training data set (in the best case a subset of them).

There are various methods which can be used to determine the nearest neighbor. Figure 1 shows the way in which decision is taken to decide the category of a new point.

Figures 2 and 3 shows various methods for deciding the nearest neighbor.

k-NN is a kind of example-based text categorization algorithm. However, the determination of the *k* has not yet obtained a good solution. Moreover, the good selection of *k* most similar texts also has a bigger effect on the categorization results. In addition, *k*-NN cannot effectively solve the problem of overlapped category borders.

Statistical rules are used in general in the classification of textual information, which include several tasks in Information Retrieval. It includes not only the determination of good documents in terms of relevance attending to user needs, but also the classification of documents into categories (topics) attending to prede ned classes [3]. In the following, we include studies found in the literature about both the retrieval and the categorization tasks.

The use of rules for categorization comes from a process of classification of documents into different categories regarding their topics in order to optimize a posteriori retrieval process. One of the most relevant works of categorization using rules is the one of [4]. The general idea of this work is the discovery of classification patterns automatically for document categorization. The aim of the induction process is for sets of decision rules to distinguish among different categories which documents belong to. The attributes of the rules can be a word or a pair of words constructing a dictionary where an elimination process of the less frequent words is carried out. Finally, association rules have also been used for categorization [5], where the authors propose a solution for text categorization based on the application of the best generated association rules to build a classifier.

The Dempster–Shafer Theory

The Dempster–Shafer theory (DST) of evidence originated in the work of [6, 7] on theory of probabilities with upper and lower bounds. It has since been extended by numerous authors and popularized, but only to a degree, in the literature on Artificial Intelligence (AI) and expert systems, as a technique for modeling reasoning under uncertainty. In this respect it can be seen to offer numerous advantages over the more "traditional" methods of Statistics and Bayesian decision theory. Hajek [8] remarked that real, practical applications of DST methods have been rare, but subsequent to these remarks there has been a marked increase in the applications incorporating the use of DST. Although DST is not in widespread use, it has been applied with some success to such topics as face recognition [9], statistical classification [10], and target identification [11]. Additional applications centered on multisource information, including medical diagnosis [12] and plan recognition [13]. An exception is the paper by Cortes-Rello and Golshani [14], which although written for a computing science–AI readership does deal with the "knowledge domain" of forecasting and Marketing Planning. For those with even limited knowledge of these domains the paper appears rather naive. Referring for example to rather venerable old editions of standard texts such as [15]. The aim of this paper is to suggest that there is a good deal of potential in the DST approach, which is as yet largely unexploited. The origins of the mathematical theory of probability date back at least to the work of the eighteenth century scholar, The Reversed Thomas [16], whose work was published posthumously in 1763. It provides the foundations for the theory of statistical inference (involving both estimation and testing of hypotheses) and for techniques of design making under certainty. The roots of decision analysis lie in the 1930s and 1940s. Wald [17], included the "complete class theorem", which stated that any procedure in a statistical decision problem can be beaten or at least matched in performance by Bayesian procedure, defined as procedure based on the adoption of some set of prior probabilities. The fact that numerous statistical principles and techniques may be developed without using prior and posterior probability distribution involves no loss of generality, given that the special case of a uniform or rectangular prior distribution may be adopted. Decision analysis relies more on a subjectivist view of the use of probability, whereby the probability of an event indicates the degree to which someone believes it, rather than the alternative frequents approach. The latter approach is based only on the number of times an event is observed to occur. As savage [18, 19] discusses, the subjectivists have been responsible for much of the theoretical work into statistical practice. He goes on to argue that the frequentists hold an uneasy upper hand over their Bayesian/ subjective colleagues in the domain of mathematical statistics. Bayesian statisticians may agree that their goal is to estimate objective probabilities from frequency data, but they advocate using subjective prior probabilities to improve the estimates [20]. French questions savages' theory of subjective expected utility, which suggests that each of us has within us an exact subjective probability for each possible event in the small world (model) under consideration. For a much fuller discussion of subjective and frequentists approaches see the collection of papers in [3] who notes that the three defining attributes of the Bayesian approach are:

1. Reliance on a complete probabilistic model of the domain or "frame of discernment".
2. Willingness to accept subjective judgment as an expedient substitute for empirical data.
3. The use of Bayes' Theorem (conditionality) the primary mechanism for updating beliefs in light of new information. However, the Bayesian technique is not without its critics including among others, Walleyl [21], as well as Caselton and Luo [4], who discussed the difficulty arising when conventional Bayesian analysis is presented only with weak information sources. In such cases we have the "Bayesian do mega of precision", whereby the information concerning uncertain statistical parameters, no matter how vague, must be represented by the conventional exactly specified, probability distribution.

Some of the difficulties can be understood through the "principle of Insufficient Reason" as illustrated by Wilson [5]. Suppose we are given a random device that randomly generates integer numbers between 1 and 6 (its "frame of discernment") but with unknown chances. What is our belief in "1" being the next number? A Bayesian will use a symmetry argument, or the Principle of insufficient Reason to say that the Bayesian belief in an "1" being the next number, says P(1) should be 1/6. In general, in a situation of ignorance a Bayesian is forced to use this principle to evenly allocate subjective (additive) probabilities over the frame of discernment.

To further understand the Bayesian approach, especially with regard to representation of ignorance, consider the following example, similar to that in [5]. Let there be a proposition that, "I live in Kings Road, Cardiff".

How could one construct P(a), a Bayesian belief in a? First, we must choose a frame of discernment, denoted by Θ and a subset A of Θ representing the proposition a; then would I need to use the Principle of Insufficient Reason to arrive at a Bayesian belief. The problem is there are a number of possible frames of discernment Θ that we could choose, depending effectively on how many Cardiff roads can be enumerated. If only two such streams are identifiable, then $\Theta = \{x_1, x_2\}$, $A = \{x_1\}$. The "Principle of Insufficient Reason" then gives P(a), to be 0.5, through evenly allocating subjective probabilities over the frame of discernment. If it is estimated that there are about 1,000 roads in Cardiff, then $\Theta = \{x_1, x_2, \ldots\ldots x_{1000}\}$ with again $A = \{x_i\}$ and other x_i 's representing the other roads. In this case the "theory of insufficient reason" gives $P(A) = 0.001$. Either of these frames may be reasonable, but the probability assigned to A is crucially dependent upon the frame chosen. Hence, once Bayesian belief is a function not only of the information given and one's background knowledge, but also of sometimes the arbitrary choice of frame of discernment. To put the point in another way, we need to distinguish between uncertainty and ignorance. Similar arguments hold where we are discussing not probabilities per se but weights which measure subjective assessments of relative importance. This issue arises in decision support models such as the Analytic Hierarchy Process (AHP), which requires certain weights on a given level of decision tree to unity, see [22].

KDD Data Set 99

In 1998, DARPA in concert with Lincoln Laboratory at MIT launched the DARPA 1998 data set for evaluating IDS [23]. The DARPA 1998 data set contains 7 weeks of training and also 2 weeks of testing data. In total, there are 38 attacks in training data as well as in testing data. The refined version of DARPA data set which contains only network data (i.e. Tcpdump data) is termed as KDD data set. The Third International Knowledge Discovery and Data Mining Tools Competition were held in colligation with KDD-99, the Fifth International Conference on Knowledge Discovery and Data Mining. KDD data set is a data set employed for this Third International Knowledge Discovery and Data Mining Tools Competition. KDD training data set consists of relatively 4,900,000 single connection vectors where each single connection vectors consist of 41 features and is marked as either normal or an attack, with exactly one particular attack type [23]. These features had all continuous and symbolic forms with extensively varying ranges falling into four categories:

- In a connection, the first category consists of the ***intrinsic*** features which comprises the fundamental features of each individual TCP connections.

Table 1 Various types of attacks described in four major categories

Denial of service attacks	Back, land, neptune, pod, smurf, teardrop
User to root attacks	Buffer_overflow, loadmodule, perl, rootkit
Remote to local attacks	Ftp_write, guess_passwd, imap, multihop, phf, spy, warezclient, warezmaster
Probes	Satan, ipsweep, nmap, portsweep

Some of the features for each individual TCP connections are the duration of the connection, the type of the protocol (TCP, UDP, etc.), and network service (http, telnet, etc.).
- The ***content*** features suggested by domain knowledge are used to assess the payload of the original TCP packets, such as the number of failed login attempts.
- Within a connection, the ***same host*** features observe the recognized connections that have the same destination host as present connection in the past 2 s and the statistics related to the protocol behavior, service, etc. are estimated.
- The ***similar same service*** features scrutinize the connections that have the same service as the current connection in the past 2 s.

A variety of attacks incorporated in the data set fall into the following four major categories: **Denial of Service Attacks**: A denial of service attack is an attack where the attacker constructs some computing or memory resource fully occupied or unavailable to manage legitimate requirements, or reject legitimate users' right to use a machine. **User to Root**

Attacks: User to Root exploits are a category of exploits where the attackers initiate by accessing a normal user account on the system (possibly achieved by tracking down the passwords, a dictionary attack, or social engineering) and take advantage of some susceptibility to achieve root access to the system.

Remote to User Attacks: A Remote to User attack takes place when an attacker who has the capability to send packets to a machine over a network but does not have an account on that machine, makes use of some vulnerability to achieve local access as a user of that machine. **Probes**: Probing is a category of attacks where an attacker examines a network to collect information or discover well-known vulnerabilities. These network investigations are reasonably valuable for an attacker who is staging an attack in future. An attacker who has a record, of which machines and services are accessible on a given network, can make use of this information to look for fragile points.

Table 1 illustrates a number of attacks falling into four major categories:

Method

The proposed system introduces intrusion detection system with KNN Classification and DS theory with fuzzy logic. The input to the proposed system is KDD Cup 1999 data set, which is separated into two subsets such as, training data set

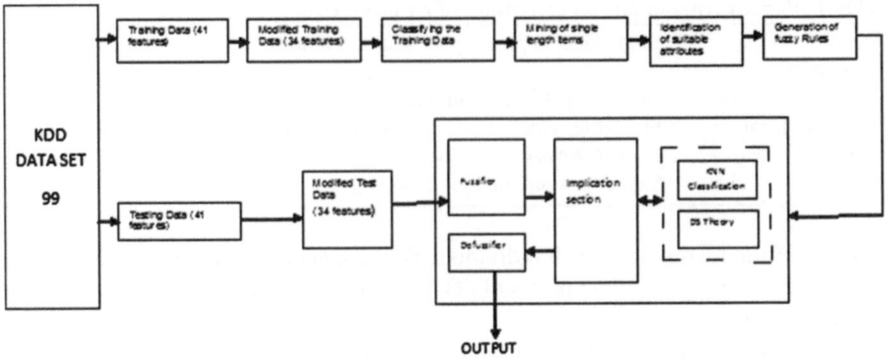

Fig. 4 The overall steps of the proposed intrusion detection system

and testing data set. Initially, the training data set is classified into five subsets so that, four types of attacks (DoS, R2L, U2R, Probe) and normal data are separated. After that, we simply mine the one-length frequent items from attack data as well as normal data. These mined frequent items are used to find the important attributes of the input data set and the identified effective attributes are used to generate a set of definite and indefinite rules using deviation method. Then, we generate fuzzy rule in accordance with the definite rule by fuzzifying it in such a way that we obtain a set of fuzzy if-then rules with consequent parts that represent whether it is a normal data or an abnormal data. These rules are given to the fuzzy rule base to effectively learn the fuzzy system. In the testing phase, the test data is matched with fuzzy rules to detect whether the test data is an abnormal data or a normal data. We apply KNN classification and Dempster theory of evidence on classified data. Through these we gathered a new discovered pattern of intrusion and classified category of pattern and apply event evidence logic with the help of DS theory. Finned pattern of intrusion compared with the existing pattern of intrusion generates a new schema of pattern and updates a list of patterns of intrusion detection and improved the true rate of intrusion detection. We used the concept of Dempster theory for this work on event evidence and found the validity of data and reduced the rate of intrusion. We also used the patterns of design of schema and data conversion, in data conversion first-type intrusion detection in MATLAB, but data of intrusion data in overall string format, now we has use classification method. We have faced various difficulties in classification of data conversion string through numeric format for suitability of classification. In the process of data conversion we used the ratio mapping concept used by the ML receptory organization for mapping of data string to numeric format. The above procedure is explained and depicted with the help of a flowchart in (Fig. 4);

Table 2 Result of tested data set

Category	Data set 1	Data set 2
Normal	680	673
Probs	44	46
DoS	118	121
R2R	100	103
R2L	57	57

Experimental Results and Performance Analysis

This section describes the experimental results and performance evaluation of the proposed system. The proposed system is implemented in MATLAB (R2010a) and the performance of the system is evaluated *False positive rate (FP), False negative rate (FN), True positive rate (TP), True negative rate (TN) ,and accuracy in respect of true positive and true negative rate.* For experimental evaluation, we have taken KDD cup 99 data set, which is mostly used for evaluating the performance of the intrusion detection system. Here, we have used only 1,000 instances of data of KDD Cup 99 data set for training and testing.

We have supervised different data sets with each 1,000 instances of data under the result of ratio of attacks as represented in tabular format in Table 2:

Performance Analysis

As seen from the output of performance on data sets it can be made out that when KNN is combined with DS method, the performance gets significantly improved.

Earlier application of isolated KNN on data set has much greater accuracy than later by integrating both KNN and DS Methods. Also, there is a considerable enhancement in the true positive and true negative detection ratios and false positive and false negative ratios. Thus, this gives the direct improvized accuracy in the result. In this paper, we are showing the result for the parameters—**Accuracy**, **FP, FN, TP, TN** only for one data set, i.e, for data set-1. Also, below is shown the graph for that particular data set, and how to calculate these parameters with suitable formulas.

$$\mathrm{FP} = \frac{\text{correct detection}}{\text{Total detection}}$$

$$\mathrm{FN} = \text{Total detection} - \text{false positive}$$

$$\text{Accuracy} = \frac{\mathrm{TP} + \mathrm{TN}}{\mathrm{TP} + \mathrm{FP} + \mathrm{TN} + \mathrm{FN}}$$

Table 3 Confusion matrix on test data of KNN and KNN-DS

Metric		Predicted		Total
		Normal	Attack	
Actual	Normal	TN	FP	TN + FP
	Attack	FN	TP	TP + FN
Total		TP + FN	TP + FP	Accuracy

Table 4 Parameter result of tested data sets

Metric		Accuracy (%)	Precision (%)	Recall (%)
Data set 1	KNN	92.14	87.24	84.43
	KNN-DS	97.14	96.11	94.10
Data set 2	KNN	89.90	84.32	83.23
	KNN-DS	95.23	92.14	91.21

$$\text{Precision} = \frac{\text{TP}}{\text{TP} + \text{FP}}$$

$$\text{Recall} = \frac{\text{TP}}{\text{TP} + \text{FN}}$$

where,
TP True Positive
TN True Negative
FP False Positive
FN False Negative

Confusion matrix: It is used to evaluate the general performance of the different classifiers and different metrics. These metrics were calculated using the confusion matrix, which shows the predict and actual classification; the tabular format of the confusion matrix is shown in Table 3. In the context of intrusion detection system, TP means correctly identified attack traffic and TN means correctly identified normal traffic. FP is the normal traffic being misclassified as an attack and FN are the attack instances being misclassified as normal (Table 4).

Comparative graph chart of KNN and KNN-DS result on given data set for Intrusion Detection System

DATA SET 1

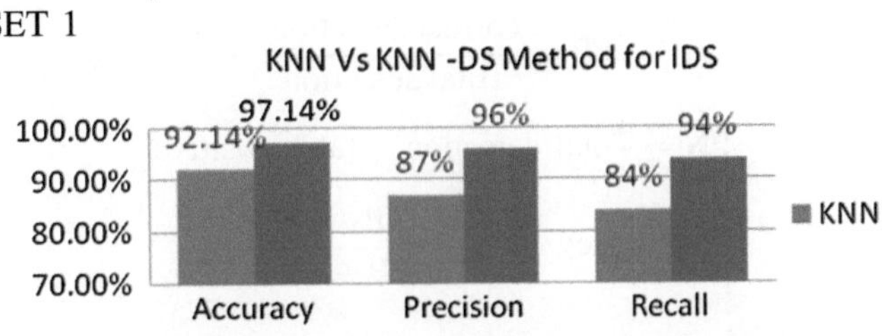

The above graph represents the assessment result of Data set 1as KNN and KNN-DS method as included parameters, i.e, Accuracy, Precision, Recall.

DATA SET 2

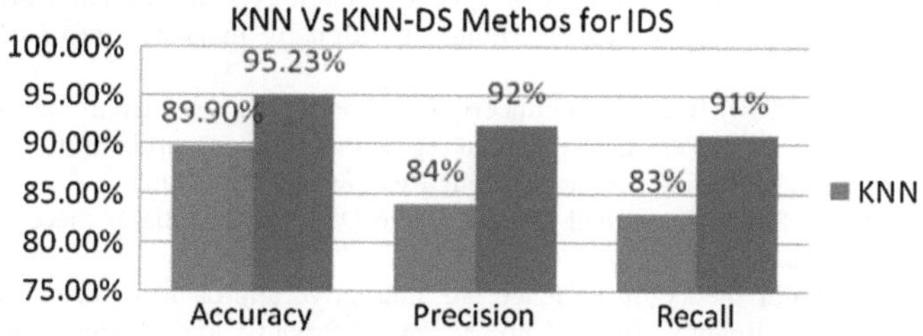

The above graph represents the assessment result of Data set 2as KNN and KNN-DS method as included parameters, i.e., Accuracy, Precision, Recall.

Conclusion

Our dissertation presents the performance of the intrusion detection system on application of our new design technique. We have designed an intrusion detection system using KNN classification and Dempster theory for detecting intrusion behavior within the network. As compared to the earlier technique used, the combined use of KNN and Dempster theory, it is found that, the performance gets considerably enhanced. This improvised design technique gives more efficient results. It was observe that KNN and Dempster can perform better in almost all situations, which is further proven by comparing the result on KDD Data set 99. Our Experiment on different data sets classifies the data using KNN classification (Normal Packet, DOS, R2L, U2R, Probes) and later the factor of evidence is formulated by using DS theory. The new pattern of intrusion is compared with the existing pattern of intrusion and generates a new schema of pattern and updates a list of pattern of intrusion detections and improves the true rate of intrusion detection.

Future Work

This work can be extended by studying the nitty-gritty of data mining techniques and the fundamentals of intrusion detection system and network behavior patterns. As a piece of future work, our design can be clubbed up with a more optimized classification technique. This improvised structure will increase the efficiency and will give improvised results; in addition the design can be made more comprehensive by supervising data from varied data sources and examining more complicated intrusion network scenarios.

References

1. Han J, Kamber M (2001) Data mining: concept and technology. China Machine Press, China (8)
2. Freund Y (1995) Boosting a weak learning algorithm by majority. Info Comput 121(2): 256–285
3. Shafer G, Pearl J (1990) Readings in uncertain reasoning. Morgan Kaufman, San Mateo
4. Caselton WF, Luo W (1992) Decision making with imprecise probabilities: Dempster ± Shafer theory and applications. Water Resour Res 28(12):3071–3083
5. Wilson PN (1992) Some theoretical aspects of the Dempster ± Shafer theory. PhD Thesis, Oxford Polytechnic
6. The Dempster Shafer theory of evidence: an alternative approach to multicriteria decision modelling Malcolm Beynon, Bruce Curry*, Peter Morgan Cardi Business School, Colum Drive, Cardi, CF1 3EU, UK Received 1 Dec 1998; accepted 1 June 1999
7. Dempster AP (1967) Upper and lower probabilities induced by a multi-valued mapping. Ann Math Stat 38:325–339
8. Hajek P (1994) Systems of conditional beliefs in Dempster Shafer theory and expert systems. Int J Gen Syst 22:113–124
9. HHS Ip, JMC Ng (1994) Human face recognition using Dempster ± Shafer theory. In: ICIP. 1st International Conference on Image Processing, vol. 2, p 292–295
10. Denoeux T (1995) A k-nearest neighbour classification rule based on Dempster ± Shafer theory. IEEE Transac Syst Man Cybern 25(5):804–813
11. Buede DM, Girardi P (1997) A target identification comparison of Bayesian and Dempster ± Shafer multisensor fusion. IEEE Trans Syst Man Cybern Part A Syst Hum 27(5):569–577
12. Yen J (1989) GERTIS a Dempster ± Shafer approach to diagnosing hierarchical hypotheses. Commun ACM 32(5):573–585
13. Bauer M (1996) A Dempster ± Shafer approach to modeling agent preferences for plan recognition. User Model User-Adap Inter 5:317–348
14. Cortes-Rello E, Golshani F (1990) Uncertain reasoning using the Dempster-Shafer method: an application in forecasting and marketing management. Expert Syst 7(1):9–17
15. Kotler P (1980) Marketing management: analysis, planning and control. Prentice Hall Englewood Cliffs, NJ
16. Bayes T (1763) An essay toward solving a problem in the doctrine of chances. Phil Trans Roy Soc (London) 53:370–418
17. Wald A (1950) Statistical decision functions. Wiley, New York
18. Savage LJ (1954) The foundations of statistics. Wiley, New York (2nd rev.ed., 1972 Dover)
19. Savage LJ (1961) The foundation of statistics reconsidered. In: Proceedings of the Fourth Berkeley Symposium on Mathematics and Probability 1. University of California Press, Berkeley
20. Good IJ (1983) Good thinking: the foundations of probability and its applications. University of Minnesota Press, Minneapolis
21. Walley P (1987) Belief-function representations of statistical evidence. Ann Stat 10:741–761
22. Saaty TL (1980) The Analytic Hierarchy Process: planning, priority setting, resource allocation. McGraw-Hill, New York
23. R. Shanmugavadivu, Dr.N.Nagarajan (1998) KDD CUP 99 DataSet Network intrusion detection system using fuzzy logic

An Improved ANN–BPN to Radial Distribution System Load Flow

Vaishali Holkar and Deepika Masand

Abstract This paper shows an application of artificial neural networks (ANNs) to determine the bus voltages and phase angles of a radial distribution system, without executing the load flow algorithm, for any given load. The performance of the conventional load flow methods such as Newtoh—Raphson load flow, Fast decoupled load flow is found to be very poor under critical conditions, such as high R/X ratio, heavily loading condition, etc. To overcome the limitations of these regularly used methods a simple and reliable ladder iterative technique is used for solving the power balance equations of radial distribution system (RDS). The proposed method makes use of a multilayer feed forward ANN with error back propagation learning algorithm for calculation of bus voltages and its angles. A sample IEEE 33-bus is extensively tested with the proposed ANN-based approach indicating its viability for RDS load flow assessment and results are presented.

Keywords Ladder iterative technique · R/X ratio · Artificial neural networks (ANNs) · Backpropagation network (BPN) · Radial distribution system (RDS) · Forward sweep · Backward sweep

V. Holkar (✉)
Department of Electrical and Electronics Engineering, Oriental Institute of Science and Technology, R.G.P.V, Bhopal, MP, India
e-mail: vaishaliholkar@yahoo.com

D. Masand
Head of Department of Electrical and Electronics Engineering, Oriental Institute of Science and Technology, R.G.P.V, Bhopal, MP, India
e-mail: deepikamasand@oriental.ac.in

V. Kumar and M. Bhatele (eds.), *Proceedings of All India Seminar on Biomedical Engineering 2012 (AISOBE 2012)*, Lecture Notes in Bioengineering,
DOI: 10.1007/978-81-322-0970-6_22,

Introduction

The load flow of distribution system is different from that of transmission system because of their high R/X ratio and radial topology. Convergence of load flow is utmost important. Matrix-based iterative methods do not lead themselves for radial distribution system owing to their poor performance under critical conditions and heavily loading conditions. A survey of literature shows that several methods for distribution system load flow have been proposed [1–3]. However, all these methods fail to obtain a solution in many instances because of matrices. Large RDS have complicated structure and are subjected to changes in their topology frequently for load balancing, maintenance, emergency operations under the umbrella of Supervisory Control and Data Acquisition (SCADA), SCADA requires a fast and reliable distribution load flow algorithm that computes the voltage solution very rapidly.

To overcome the limitations of these regularly used methods a simple and reliable ladder iterative technique is used for solving the power balance equations of radial distribution system (RDS) that is, ladder iterative technique is described for solving the radial system power balance equation treating every lateral and sub lateral line as an individual main line [4]. This method utilizes forward sweep and backward algorithm based on Kirchoff's current law (KCL) and Kirchoff's voltage law (KVL) for evaluating the bus voltage magnitude and angles iteratively. The computation of branch current depends only on the current injected at the neighboring node and the current in the adjacent branch. This approach starts from end nodes of sub lateral line, lateral line, and main line and moves toward the root node during branch current evaluation (Fig. 2). The node voltage calculation begins from the root node and moves toward the node situated at the far end of the main, lateral, and sub lateral lines [5] (Fig. 1).

Main line: Line emanating from the root node.
Lateral line: Line emanating from the main line.
Sub lateral line: Line emanating from the lateral line.
Minor line: Line emanating from the sub lateral line.

Artificial neural networks (ANNs) approach for determining the bus voltages and phase angles of a radial distribution system, without executing the load flow algorithm, for any given load. Artificial Neural Networks (ANNs) are nonlinear mapping structures based on the function of the human brains. They are powerful tools for modeling, especially when the underlying data relationship is unknown. ANNs can identify and learn correlated patterns between input data sets and the corresponding target values. After training, it can be used to predict the output of new independent input data. ANNs can imitate the process of learning as human brain and can process complex and nonlinear data even if data is imprecise and noisy. Therefore, here it is proposed to ideally suit the modeling of a balanced, complex, and often nonlinear radial distribution system as ANNs has the great capacity in predictive modeling and all the characters describing the unknown

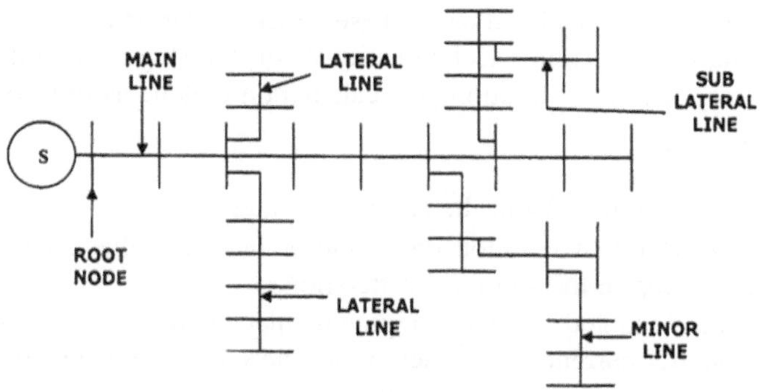

Fig. 1 Single line diagram of a radial distribution network

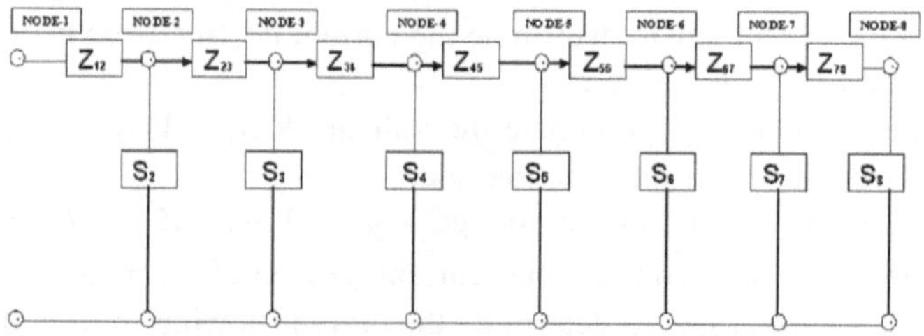

Fig. 2 A simple 8-bus ladder network

situation can be presented to the trained ANNs, and hence the prediction of RDS without any mathematical iterative and computational method is guaranteed.

In this paper, first a simple ladder iterative technique is described for solving the radial system power balance equation. The aim of using this technique is to reduce the data preparation and to assure computation for any type of numbering scheme for node and branch. A database providing information of the possible real and reactive power demands at different buses and their corresponding voltage magnitude and phase angles is created. Second, an ANN-Back Propagation Network is introduced with brief introduction of its architecture, training algorithm, and recognition phase. Third, an implementation of BPN for determining bus voltages and the corresponding angles is been shown, followed by the results of a sample IEEE test system studied by the proposed method. Finally, the conclusion is presented.

Ladder Network Technique

It is assumed that the ladder network parameters for lines, loads, and substation voltage V_S are known. If the line impedances, rated voltage, and the complex power at each node are known then the values of the current, voltage, active, and reactive power can be calculated using these called ladder iterative technique [6]. Iteration of the ladder iterative technique exists of two steps: forward sweep and backward sweep. IEEE-distribution grid calculation is done as follows:

A. *Forward sweep:*

- Assume rated voltage V_S at the end node voltage $\left(V_{(18)}, V_{(22)}, V_{(25)}, V_{(33)}\right)$ is $12660 + j0$ (for first iteration only) and equals the value computed in the backward sweep in the subsequent iteration.
- Start with the end node 33 and compute the node current $I_i = (S_i/V_i)^*$. Apply the Kirchhoff's current law to determine the current flowing from node 32 toward node 33: $I_{(32,33)} = I_{(33)} = \left(S_{(33)}/V_{(33)}\right)^*$.
- Compute with this current the voltage, $V_{(32)} = V_{(33)} + Z_{(32,33)}I_{(32,33)}$.
- Compute with this voltage the current, $I_{(32)} = \left(S_{(32)}/V_{(32)}\right)^*$. Apply the Kirchhoff's current law to determine the current flowing from node 31 toward node 32: $I_{(31,32)} = I_{(32,33)} + I_{(33)}$.
- Using the current $I_{(31,32)}$ compute the voltage, $V_{(31)} = V_{(32)} + Z_{(31,32)}I_{(31,32)}$.
- Similarly compute till the junction node.
- Compute with this current the voltage $V_{(26)} = V_{(27)} + Z_{(26,27)}I_{(26,27)}$.
- Compute with this voltage the current $I_{(26)} = \left(S_{(26)}/V_{(26)}\right)^*$. Apply the Kirchhoff's current law to determine the current flowing from node 6 toward node 26: $I_{(6,26)} = I_{(26,27)} + I_{(26)}$.
- Compute with this current the voltage, $V_{(6)} = V_{(26)} + Z_{(6,26)}I_{(6,26)}$. Node 6 is a junction node.
- Select node 18 and compute the node current $I_{(18)} = \left(S_{(18)}/V_{(18)}\right)^*$. Apply the Kirchhoff's current law to determine the current flowing from node 17 toward node 18: $I_{(17,18)} = I_{(18)}$.
- Compute with this current the voltage $V_{(17)} = V_{(18)} + Z_{(17,18)}I_{(17,18)}$.
- Compute with this voltage the current, $I_{(17)} = \left(S_{(17)}/V_{(17)}\right)^*$.
- Apply the Kirchhoff's current law to determine the current flowing from node 16 toward node 17, $I_{(16,17)}) = I_{(17,18)} + I_{(17)}$.
- Using the current $I_{(16,17)}$ compute the voltage, $V_{(16)} = V_{(17)} + Z_{(16,17)})I_{(16,17)}$.
- Similarly compute till the junction node.
- Compute with this current the voltage, $V_{(7)} = V_{(8)} + Z_{(7,8)}I_{(7,8)}$.
- Compute with this voltage the current, $I_{(7)} = \left(S_{(7)}/V_{(7)}\right)^*$. Apply the Kirchhoff's current law to determine the current flowing from node 6 toward node 7: $I_{(6,7)} = I_{(7,8)} + I_{(7)}$.
- Compute with this current the voltage, $V'_{(6)} = V_{(26)} + Z_{(6,26)}I_{(6,26)}$. This will be referred to as "the most recent voltage at node 6".

- Compute with the most recent voltage $\left(V'_{(6)}\right)$ at node 6 the current $I_{(6)} = \left(S_{(6)}/V_{(6)}\right)^*$. Apply the Kirchhoff's current law to determine the current, $I_{(5,6)} = I_{(6,7)} + I_{(6,26)} + I_{(6)}$.
- Similarly compute till the junction node.
- Using the current $I_{(1,2)}$ compute the voltage, $V_{(1)} = V_{(2)} + Z_{(1,2)}I_{(1,2)}$.

At the end of the forward sweep compare the calculated magnitude of the rated voltage at node 1 to the specified source voltage.

Voltage Difference (VD) $= ||V_s|-|V_1||$

Stop if the VD is less than a specified tolerance i.e., if VD < 0.001 pu ($\approx$ 12 V) else the backward sweep begins. The backward sweep begins at the node 1 with the rated voltage $V_S = V_1 = 12660 + j0$V.

B. *Backward sweep:*

- Start with node 1 and $V_{(1)} = V_{(S)}$.
- Compute the voltage $V_{(2)} = V_{(1)} - Z_{(1,2)}I_{(1,2)}$.
- Compute the voltage $V_3 = V2 - Z_{(2,3)}I_{(2,3)}$.
- Compute the voltage $V_{(4)}$ to $V_{(32)}$ similarly.
- Compute the voltage $V_{(33)} = V_{(32)} - Z_{(32,33)}I_{(32,33)}$.

After the backward sweep the first iteration is completed. At this point the forward sweep will be repeated, only this time starting with the new voltage at end nodes. These steps will be repeated until the error is less than the specified tolerance. At the substation, the voltage is mostly taken 5 % bigger than the rated voltage.

The key to understand the forward and backward sweep method is that

- The forward sweep is simply obtaining estimates of currents in each of the segments. In the forward sweep, voltage accuracy is not important.
- The backward sweep is concerned with accuracy of resulting voltages.

So the method is the same as previously given with the following additional rules:

1. Begin the algorithm by assuming nominal voltages at all far-end load nodes.
2. Compute all downstream currents (those currents flowing from a junction node toward the load) before moving upstream from the junction node.
3. Assign to the junction node a voltage computed base on the forward sweep done on the last downstream branch emanating from that junction node. (Note here that this is arbitrary—we could take the voltage computed base on the forward sweep from any of the downstream branches emanating from the junction node).
4. Use forward sweep currents in all backward sweep calculations.

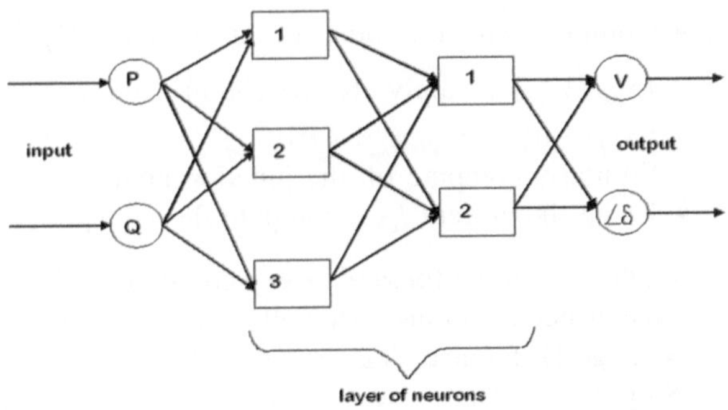

Fig. 3 Neural network

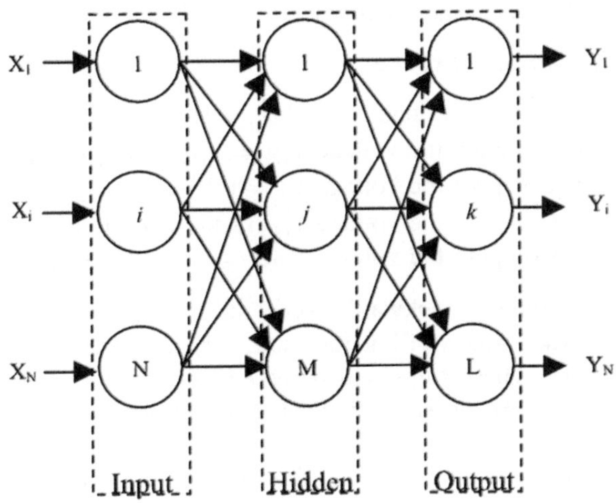

Fig. 4 Basic BPN architecture

ANN-BPN Architecture

The most widely used learning algorithm in an ANN, the Back propagation algorithm is presented in this context. The neural network structure defines its structure including number of hidden layers, number of hidden nodes, and number of output nodes (Fig. 3). Figure 4 shows the architecture of BPN to have three layers, namely—input, hidden, and the output layers.

The Multilayered perceptron (MLP) network is trained using one of the supervised learning algorithms of which is the best. It uses the data to adjust the network's weights and thresholds so as to minimize the error in its predictions on the training set. Many different sets of the input and their corresponding output vectors are considered during the training. To determine the weights between the input, hidden, and output layers, the training phase is used.

Typically in this study neurons used are the sigmoid activation function defined by the below equation:

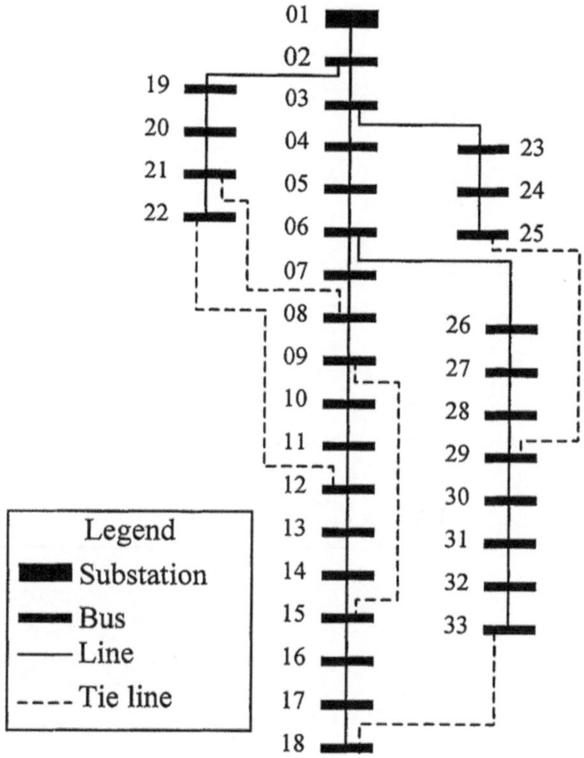

Fig. 5 The 33-bus radial distribution system

$$[\text{Neuron Input}] = \frac{1.0}{1.0 + e^{-\alpha v}} \tag{1}$$

Here, α is the abruptness of the sigmoid activation function and v is the total input to the neuron. Let the vector X represents an input layer as in Fig. 4. The net input at the hidden layers is computed by the matrix equation below:

$$V_H = [WH]X \tag{2}$$

where WH_{ji} denotes the weight between ith input layer node and jth hidden layer node. The output of the hidden layer node is given by,

$$Y_H = \phi(V_H) \tag{3}$$

here ϕ is the appropriate activation function. In a similar manner the total input at the output layer is given by the following equation:

$$V_o = [WO]V_H \tag{4}$$

The output of the output layer node is given by,

$$Y = \phi(V_O) \tag{5}$$

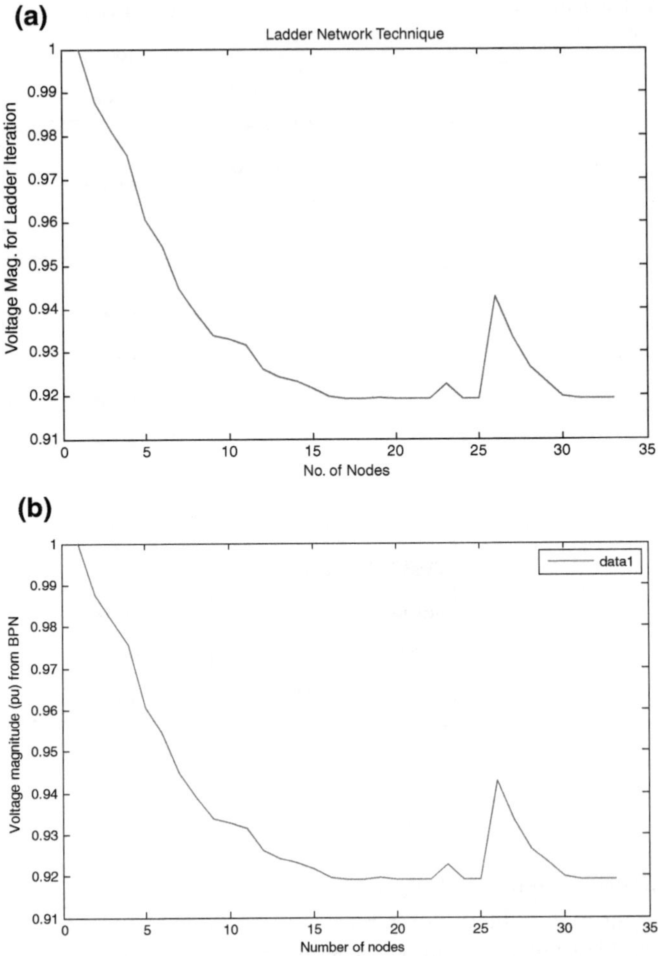

Fig. 6 **a** Ladder iterative voltage magnitude. **b** BPN voltage magnitudes after training

The steps of the well-established training algorithm based upon Network's steepest descent technique is as given below:

1. Read the training set and randomly initialize the weights. Set iteration index $n = 1$.
2. Set training set index $p = 1$.
3. Propagate X^P through the network.
4. Determine the error vector of the pth training set,

$$E^p = O^p - Y^p$$

where O^p is the vector of expected output.

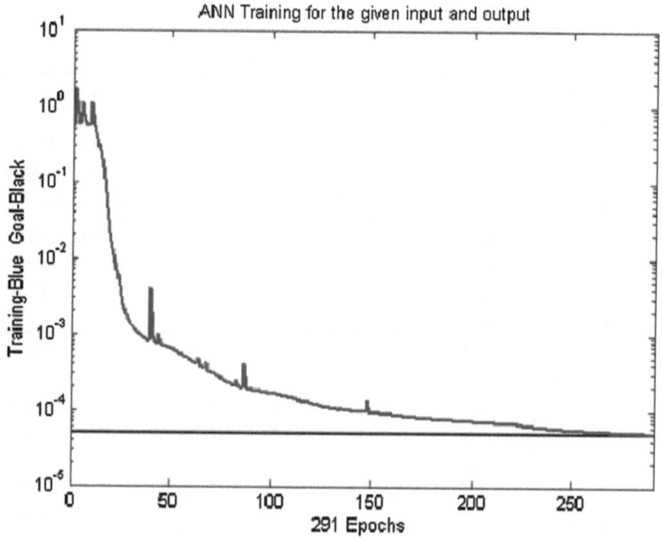

Fig. 7 Training results ANN-BPN

5. Correct the weights using Newton's steepest descent technique.
6. If $p <$ number training sets P, set $p = p + 1$ and go to step-3.
7. If $\sum_{p=1}^{P} |E^p|^2 >$ tolerance ϵ, increment the iteration index n and go to step-2.

The above method explained is tested successfully and requires the input and output to be from a continuous domain. Moreover, the input and the output set of vectors are non-contradictory for a successful training and operational function.

The following section explains the use of ANN-BPN to determine the voltages of a radial distribution system.

All paragraphs must be indented. All paragraphs must be justified, i.e. both left-justified and right-justified.

ANN-BPN Implementation for Determining Load Flow Solution

The input vector for the ANN-BPN is the reap power and reactive power loads at various buses of power system. Therefore,

$$X = [P_1, P_2, P_3, \ldots\ldots\ldots P_n; Q_1, Q_2, Q_3 \ldots\ldots\ldots Q_n] \tag{6}$$

here, P_i and Q_i are the real and reactive power loads at the ith bus of the RDS and 'n' is the number of buses in the RDS.

By using this scheme several sets of loads were created:

Table 1 Comparison of results from conventional method and ANN-BPN

Line No.	Sending bus	Receiving bus	Load at receiving end bus (test input)		Solution from BPN		Expected solution (solution from ladder iterative technique)		Accuracy (%)
			Real power (P) (kW)	Reactive power (Q) (kVAr)	Voltage mag. (pu)	Phase angle (rads)	Voltage mag. (pu)	Phase angle (rads)	
1	1 main SS	2	100	60	1.00	0.00	1.00	0.00	100
2	2	3	90	40	0.99	0.00	0.99	0.00	99.99
3	3	4	120	80	0.98	0.01	0.98	0.01	99.98
4	4	5	60	30	0.96	0.01	0.96	0.01	99.91
5	5	6	60	20	0.95	0.02	0.95	0.02	99.87
6	6	7	200	100	0.95	0.02	0.95	0.02	99.92
7	7	8	200	100	0.93	0.01	0.93	0.01	99.61
8	8	9	60	20	0.92	0.01	0.92	0.01	99.97
9	9	10	60	20	0.92	0.01	0.92	0.01	99.68
10	10	11	45	30	0.91	0.01	0.91	0.01	99.23
11	11	12	60	35	0.91	0.01	0.91	0.01	99.47
12	12	13	60	35	0.92	0.01	0.92	0.01	99.36
13	13	14	120	80	0.92	0.01	0.92	0.01	99.24
14	14	15	60	10	0.92	0.01	0.92	0.01	99.23
15	15	16	60	20	0.92	0.01	0.92	0.01	99.15
16	16	17	60	20	0.92	0.01	0.92	0.01	99.58
17	17	18	90	40	0.92	0.01	0.92	0.01	99.78
18	2	19	90	40	0.92	0.01	0.92	0.01	99.14
19	19	20	90	40	0.92	0.00	0.92	0.00	99.55
20	20	21	90	40	0.90	0.00	0.90	0.00	99.59
21	21	22	90	40	0.90	0.00	0.90	0.00	99.95
22	3	23	90	50	0.90	0.00	0.90	0.00	99.87
23	23	24	420	200	0.99	0.00	0.99	0.00	99.99
24	24	25	420	200	0.99	0.00	0.99	0.00	99.91
25	6	26	60	25	0.99	0.00	0.99	0.00	99.71
26	26	27	60	25	0.98	0.02	0.98	0.02	99.32
27	27	28	60	20	0.97	0.02	0.97	0.02	99.33
28	28	29	120	70	0.96	0.02	0.96	0.02	99.27
29	29	30	200	600	0.94	0.02	0.94	0.02	99.71
30	30	31	150	70	0.93	0.03	0.93	0.03	99.71
31	31	32	210	100	0.92	0.03	0.92	0.03	99.19
32	32	33	60	40	0.92	0.02	0.91	0.02	98.71

Substation voltage = 12.66 kV

1. By varying real and reactive power loads simultaneously at all load buses of RDS.
2. By varying both the real and reactive power loads simultaneously at a single load bus of the RDS.
3. By varying only the real power load at a single load bus of the RDS.
4. By only varying the reactive power load at single load bus of the RDS.

The *k*th such load so generated is referred to by the vector X^k. Similarly, the corresponding output vector for *k*th input referred to O^k. The output vector refers to the bus voltages magnitude and the corresponding angle. Summarizing, several of these sets of input and output vectors are generated using the above method and are stored. After the successful training of the ANN-BPN it should be able to produce the bus voltage magnitude and phase angle for any of the input load pattern with maximum accuracy and minimum time.

In the next section, the application of the analysis and the results of the proposed technique of determining load flow solution is discussed.

Results of the System Study

The proposed approach has been tested for 33-bus radial distribution system (Fig. 5) using MATLAB environment. By using the Ladder Iterative Technique as explained in section two, the power flow equations were solved. Approximately 150 input and output vector pairs were generated for considering 33-bus system, in order to achieve a broad representation of the power system in the ANN-BPN. The BPN was trained and the results are as shown in Fig. 6 and the output voltages of BPN can be seen in Fig. 7.

And hence, the ANN-BPN is ready to use. The results from the actual load flow solution and from the training ANN for a particular pattern is shown in Table 1. The method seems to be fast and found to be very efficient. It works well and smooth.

Conclusion

The novel approach in this paper presents a well-defined technique to determine the load flow solution of a radial distribution system, which is simple to implement and efficient in computation. Several load pairs were considered and their solution was assessed using the conventional method of Ladder Iterative technique. Then using these pairs of input and target vector sets, the ANN-Back propagation Network is trained. Thereafter, the BPN is ready for use wherein, given a load, it gives out the voltage solution in minimum time and maximum accuracy. The proposed reconfiguration method is tested on the standard 33-bus RDS and results demonstrate the effectiveness of the proposed method.

References

1. Kersting WH, Mendive DL (1976) An application of ladder network theory to the solution of three phase radial load flow problem. In: IEEE PES winter meeting, New Work
2. Kersting WH (1984) A method to design and operation of distribution system. IEEE Trans Power App Syst 103:1945–1952
3. Stevens RA, Rizy DT, Puruker SL (1986) Performance of conventional power flow routines for real time distribution automation application. In: Proceedings of 18th South Eastern symposium on system theory, IEEE computer society, pp 196–200
4. Arunagiri A, Venkatesh B, Ramasamy K (2006) Artificial neural network approach-an application to radial loadflow algorithm. IEICE Electornics Express,vol 3, pp 353–360
5. Vinoth Kumar K, Selvan MP (2008) A simplified approach for load flow analysis of radial distribution network. IJCIE 2:4
6. Kersting WH (2012) Distribution system modelling and analysis. New Mexico State University, Las Cruces, New Mexico, pp 269–276

Biologically Motivated Approaches for Complex Problem Solving

Sushil Kumar, Praneet Saurabh and Bhupendra Verma

Abstract Danger Theory is presented with particular predominance on analogies in the Artificial Immune Systems world. Artificial Immune System (AIS) is relatively naive paradigm for intelligent computations. The inspiration for AIS is derived from natural Immune System (IS). The idea is that the artificial cells release signals describing their status, e.g., safe signals and danger signals. The various artificial cells use the signals in order to adapt their behavior. This new theory suggests that the immune system reacts to threats based on the correlation of various (danger) signals and it provides a method of 'grounding' the immune response, i.e., linking it directly to the attacker. In this paper, we look at Danger Theory from the perspective of AIS practitioners and an overview of the Danger Theory is presented with particular emphasis on analogies in the Artificial Immune Systems world.

Keywords Artificial immune system · Danger theory · System cells

Introduction

Over the last decade, a new theory has become popular amongst immunologists. It is called the Danger Theory, and its chief advocate is Matzinger [1–3]. A variety of contextual clues may be essential for a meaningful danger signal, and

S. Kumar (✉) · P. Saurabh · B. Verma
Department of CSE, TIT, Bhopal, India
e-mail: asktosushil@gmail.com

P. Saurabh
e-mail: praneetsaurabh@gmail.com

B. Verma
e-mail: bk_verma3@gmail.com

V. Kumar and M. Bhatele (eds.), *Proceedings of All India Seminar on Biomedical Engineering 2012 (AISOBE 2012)*, Lecture Notes in Bioengineering,
DOI: 10.1007/978-81-322-0970-6_23,

immunological studies will provide a framework of ideas as to how ‘danger’ is assessed in the HIS. The danger signals should show up after limited attack to minimize damage and therefore have to be quickly and automatically measurable. Once the danger signal has been transmitted, the artificial immune systems (AIS) should react to those artificial antigens that are ‘near’ the emitter of the danger signal. A number of advantages are claimed for this theory; not least that it provides a method of ‘grounding’ the immune response. The theory is not complete, and there are some doubts about how much it actually changes behavior and or structure. Nevertheless, the theory contains enough potentially interesting ideas to make it worth assessing its relevance to AIS. Few other AIS practitioners are aware of the Danger Theory, notable exceptions being Burgess [4] and Willamson [5]. Hence, this deals directly with the Danger Theory. In the next section, we provide an overview of the Danger Theory, pointing out, where appropriate, some analogies in current AIS models. We then discuss about anomaly detection for AIS.

Danger Theory

The AIS are computational systems designed on the principles of natural Immune System (IS), which is highly distributed, adaptive and diverse system [6]. Danger Theory is presented with particular emphasis on analogies in the Artificial Immune Systems world [7, 8]. The idea is that the artificial cells release signals describing their status, e.g., safe signals and danger signals. The immune system is commonly thought to work at three levels: External barriers (skin, mucus), innate immunity, and the acquired or adaptive immune system. As part of the third and most complex level, B Lymphocytes secrete specific antibodies that recognize and react to stimuli. It is this pattern matching between antibodies and antigens that lie at the heart of most Artificial Immune System implementations. Another type of cell, the T (killer) lymphocyte, is also important in different types of immune reactions. Although not usually present in AIS models, the behavior of this cell is implicated in the Danger model and so it is included here. From the AIS practitioner’s point of view, the T killer cells match stimuli in much the same way as antibodies do. It is fundamental that only the ‘correct’ cells are matched as otherwise this could lead to a self-destructive autoimmune reaction. Classical immunology [9] stipulates that an immune response is triggered when the body encounters something non-self or foreign. It is not yet fully understood how this self-non-self discrimination is achieved, but many immunologists believe that the difference between them is learnt early in life. In particular it is thought that the maturation process plays an important role to achieve self-tolerance by eliminating those T and B cells that react to self. In addition, a ‘confirmation’ signal is required; that is, for either B cell or T (killer) cell activation, a T (helper) lymphocyte must also be activated. Matzinger’s Danger Theory debates this point of view (for a good introduction, see Matzinger [1]). Technical overviews can be found in Matzinger [2] and Matzinger [3]. Danger Theory clearly has many facets and intricacies, and we have touched on only a few.

It might be instructive to list a number of considerations for an Artificial Immune System practitioner regarding the suitability of the danger model for their application. The basic consideration is whether negative selection is important. If so, then these points may be relevant:

Negative selection is bound to be imperfect, and therefore auto-reactions (false positives) are inevitable.
The self-/non-self boundary is blurred since self- and non-self antigens often share common regions.
Self changes over time. Therefore, one can expect problems with memory cells, which later turn out to be inaccurate or even auto-reactive.

If these points are sufficient to make a practitioner consider incorporating the Danger Theory into their model, then the following considerations may be instructive:

1. A danger model requires an antigen-presenting cell, which can present an appropriate danger signal.
2. 'Danger' is an emotive term. The signal may have nothing to do with danger
3. The appropriate danger signal can be positive (presence of signal) or negative (absence).
4. The danger zone in biology is spatial. In Artificial Immune System applications, some other measure of proximity (for instance temporal) may be used.
5. If there is an analogue of an immune response, it should not lead to further danger signals. In biology, killer cells cause a normal cell death, not danger.
6. Matzinger proposes priming killer cells via antigen presenting cells for greater effect. Depending on the immune system used (it only makes sense for spatially distributed models) this proposal may be relevant.
7. There are a variety of considerations that are less directly related to the danger model. For example, migration—how many antibodies receive signal one/two from a given antigen-presenting cell? In addition, the Danger Theory relies on concentrations, i.e., continuous not binary matching.

This theory is borne out of the observation that there is no need to attack everything that is foreign, something that seems to be supported by the counter examples above. In this theory, danger is measured by damage to cells indicated by distress signals that are sent out when cells die an unnatural death (cell stress or lytic cell death, as opposed to programmed cell death, or apoptosis). Figure 1 depicts how we might picture an immune response according to the Danger Theory. A cell that is in distress sends out an alarm signal, whereupon antigens in the neighborhood are captured by antigen-presenting cells such as macrophages, which then travel to the local lymph node and present the antigens to lymphocytes. Essentially, the danger signal establishes a danger zone around itself. Thus, B cells producing antibodies that match antigens within the danger zone get stimulated and undergo the clonal expansion process. Those that do not match or are too far away do not get stimulated.

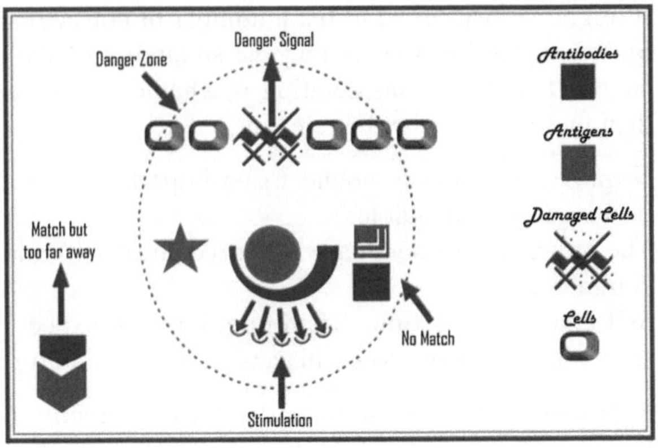

Fig. 1 Danger theory model

Another way of looking at the danger model is to see it as an extension of the Two-signal model by Bretscher and Cohn [10]. In this model, the two signals are antigen recognition (signal one) and co-stimulation (signal two).

Co-stimulation is a signal that means "this antigen really is foreign" or, in the Danger Theory, "this antigen really is dangerous". How the signal arises will be explained later. The Danger Theory then operates by applying three laws to lymphocyte behavior (the laws of lymphotics [11]):

Law 1. Become activated if you receive signals one and two together. Die if you receive signal one in the absence of signal two. Ignore signal two without signal one.

Law 2. Accept signal two from antigen-presenting cells only (or, for B cells, from T helper cells). B cells can act as antigen-presenting cells only for experienced (memory) T cells. Note that signal one can come from any cells, not just antigen-presenting cells.

Law 3. After activation (activated cells do not need signal two) revert to resting state after a short time.

For the mature lymphocyte, (whether virgin or experienced) these rules are adhered to. However, there are two exceptions in the lymphocyte lifecycle. First, immature cells are unable to accept signal two from any source. This enables an initial negative selection screening to occur. Second, activated (effector) cells respond only to signal one (ignoring signal two), but revert to the resting state shortly afterwards.

The Danger Theory and Some Affinity to AIS

Danger Theory clearly has many features and dilemmas, and we have touched on only a few. It might be instructive to list a number of considerations for an Artificial Immune System practitioner regarding the suitability of the danger model for their application. The basic consideration is whether negative selection is important. If so, then these points may be relevant:

- The self-/non-self boundary is blurred since self- and non-self antigens often share common regions.
- Self changes over time. Therefore, one can expect problems with memory cells, which later turn out to be inaccurate or even auto reactive.
- Negative selection is bound to be imperfect, and therefore auto reactions (false positives) are inevitable.

If these points are sufficient to make a practitioner consider incorporating the Danger Theory into their model, then the following considerations may be instructive:

1. A danger model requires an antigen-presenting cell, which can present an appropriate danger signal.
2. 'Danger' is an emotive term. The signal may have nothing to do with danger.
3. The appropriate danger signal can be positive (presence of signal) or negative (absence).
4. The danger zone in biology is spatial. In AIS applications, some other measure of proximity (for instance temporal) may be used.
5. If there is an analogue of an immune response, it should not lead to further danger signals. In biology, killer cells cause a normal cell death, not danger.
6. Matzinger proposes priming killer cells via antigen presenting cells for greater effect.

Depending on the immune system used (it only makes sense for spatially distributed models) this proposal may be relevant.

The Danger Theory and Anomaly Detection

In anomaly detection we watch not for a known intrusion—a signal—but rather for abnormalities in the traffic; we assume that something abnormal is probably suspicious. The construction of such a detector starts by forming an opinion on what constitutes normal for the observed subject (which can be a computer system, a particular user etc.), and then deciding on what percentage of the activity to flag as abnormal and how to make this particular decision (Fig. 2). This detection principle flags behavior that is unlikely to originate from the normal process, without needing actual intrusion scenarios [12].

In this section we will present indicative examples of such artificial systems, explain their current shortcomings, and show how the Danger Theory might help overcome some of these.

One of the first such approaches is presented by Forrest et al. [13] and extended by Hofmeyr and Forrest [15]. This work is concerned with building an AIS that is able to detect non-self in the area of network security where non-self is defined as

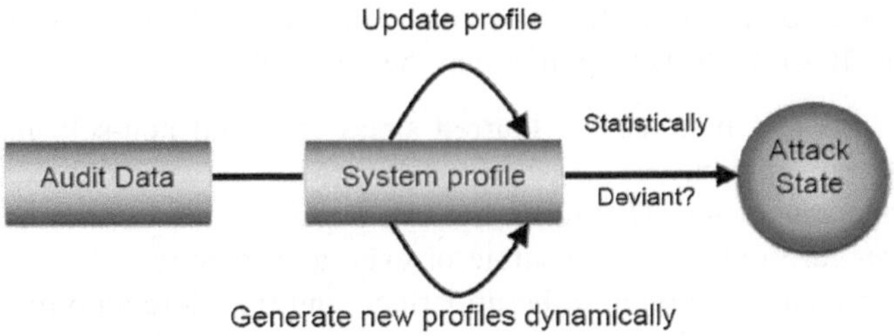

Fig. 2 A typical anomaly detection system

an undesired connection. All connections are modeled as binary strings and there is a set of known good and bad connections, which is used to train and evaluate the algorithm. To build the AIS, random binary strings are created called detectors. These detectors then undergo a maturation phase where they are presented with good, i.e., self, connections. If they match any of these they are eliminated otherwise they become mature, but not activated. If during their further lifetime these mature detectors match anything else, exceeding a certain threshold value, they become activated. This is then reported to a human operator who decides whether there is a true anomaly. If so the detectors are promoted to memory detectors with an indefinite life span and minimum activation threshold. Thus, this is similar to the secondary response in the natural immune system, for instance after immunization.

An approach such as the above is known in AIS as negative selection as only those detectors (antibodies) that do not match live on. It is thought that T cells mature in similar fashion in the thymus such that only those survive and mature that does not match any self cells after a certain amount of time.

An alternative approach to negative selection is that of positive selection as used for instance by Forrest et al. [14] and by Somayaji and Forrest [16]. These systems are a reversal of the negative selection algorithm described above with the difference that detectors for self are evolved. From a performance point of view there are advantages and disadvantages for both methods. A suspect non-self string would have to be compared with all self-detectors to establish that it is non-self, whilst with negative selection the first matching detector would stop the comparison. On the other hand, for a self-string this is reversed giving positive selection the upper hand. Thus, performance depends on the self to non-self ratio, which should generally favor positive selection.

However, there is another difference between the two approaches: the nature of false alarms. With negative selection inadequate detectors will result in false negatives (missed intrusions) whilst with positive selection there will be false positives (false alarms). The preference between the two in this case is likely to be problem specific.

What could such danger signals be? They should show up after limited infection to minimize damage and hence have to be quickly and automatically measurable. Suitable signals could include:

- Too low or too high memory usage.
- Inappropriate disk activity.
- Unexpected frequency of file changes as measured for example by checksums or file size.
- SIGABRT signal from abnormally terminated UNIX processes.
- Presence of non-self.

Of course, it would also be possible to use 'positive' signals, as discussed in the previous section, such as the absence of some normal 'health' signals.

Consequently, those antibodies or detectors that match (first signal) those antigens within a radius, defined by a measure such as the above (second signal), will proliferate. Having thereby identified the dangerous components, further confirmation could then be sought by sending it to a special part of the system simulating another attack. This would have the further advantage of not having to send all detectors to confirm danger. In conclusion, using these ideas from the Danger Theory has provided a better grounding of danger labels in comparison to self/non-self, whilst at the same time relying less on human competence.

Conclusion

To conclude, the Danger Theory is not about the way AIS represent data. Instead, it provides ideas about which data the AIS should represent and deal with. They should focus on dangerous, i.e., interesting data.

It could be argued that the shift from non-self to danger is merely a symbolic label change that achieves nothing. We do not believe this to be the case, since danger is a grounded signal, and non-self is (typically) a set of feature vectors with no further information about their meaning.

The danger signal helps us to identify which subset of feature vectors is of interest. A suitably defined danger signal thus overcomes many of the limitations of self–non-self selection. It restricts the domain of non-self to a manageable size, removes the need to screen against all self, and deals adaptively with scenarios where self (or non-self) changes over time.

The challenge is clearly to define a suitable danger signal, a choice that might prove as critical as the choice of fitness function for an evolutionary algorithm. In addition, the physical distance in the biological system should be translated into a suitable proxy measure for similarity or causality in an AIS. We have made some suggestions in this paper about how to tackle these challenges in a variety of domains, but the process is not likely to be trivial. Nevertheless, if these challenges are met, then future AIS applications might derive considerable benefit, and new insights, from the Danger Theory.

Acknowledgments We would like to thank the two anonymous reviewers, whose comments greatly improved this paper.

References

1. Matzinger P (1998) An Innate sense of danger, Seminars in Immunology, pp 399–415
2. Matzinger P (2001) The danger model in its historical context. Scand J Immunol 54:4–9
3. Matzinger P (1994) Tolerance danger and the extended family. Annu Rev Immunol 12:991–1045
4. Burgess M (1998) Computer Immunology. Proc LISA XII:283–297
5. Williamson M (2002) Biologically inspired approaches to computer security, HP labs technical reports HPL-2002, pp 131
6. Somayaji A, Hofmeyr S, Forrest S (1998) Principles of a computer immune system. In: Proceedings New Security Paradigms Workshop, Charlottesville, pp 75–82
7. Aickelin U, Cayzer S (2002) The danger theory and its application to artificial immune systems. In: Proceedings of the 1st internet conference on artificial immune systems. ICARIS, Springer, pp 141–148
8. Aickelin U, Bentley P, Cayzer S, Kim J, McLeod J (2003) Danger theory: the link between AIS and IDS? In: Proceedings ICARIS-2003, 2nd international conference on artificial immune systems. ICARIS, Springer, pp 147–155
9. Goldsby R, Kindt T, Osborne B (2000) Kuby immunology, 4th edn. W H Freeman, New York
10. Bretscher P, Cohn M (1970) A theory of self–nonself discrimination. Science 169:1042–1049
11. Matzinger P (1994) Tolerance, danger and the extended family. Annu Rev Immunol 12:991–1045
12. Sundaram A (1996) An introduction to intrusion detection, crossroads: the ACM student magazine 2(4)
13. Forrest S, Perelson A, Allen L, Cherukuri R (1994) Self non-self discrimination in a computer. In: Proceedings of the 1994 IEEE symposium on research in security and privacy, pp 202–212
14. Forrest S, Hofmeyr S, Somayaji A, Longstaff T (1996) A sense of self for unix processes. In: Proceedings of the 1996 IEEE symposium on research in security and privacy, pp 120–128
15. Hofmeyr S, Forrest S (2000) Architecture for an artificial immune system. Evolutionary Computation 8(4):443–473
16. Somayaji A, Forrest S (2000) Automated response using system-call delays. In: Proceedings of the ninth USENIX security symposium, pp 185–197

Improving High Embedding Capacity Using Artificial Immune System: A Novel Approach for Data Hiding

Kirti Bala Bahekar, Praneet Saurabh and Bhupendra Verma

Abstract Data hiding is a method of hiding secret messages into a cover media such that an unintended observer will not be aware of the existence of the hidden messages. Various embedding mechanisms are provided with different robustness capacity. This mechanism has two major categories of embedding data. In addition, it is observed that the unevenly distributed embedding capacity brings difficulty in data hiding. Thus, a comprehensive solution to this problem is addressing the considerations for choosing constant or variable embedding rate and enhancing the performance for each case. This chapter deal with Artificial Immune system technique to text, audio, image, and video data without embedding any information into the target content trained on frequency domain. Proposed method can detect a hidden bit codes from the content Hidden codes are retrieved from the AIS network only with the proper extraction key provided. The goal of this chapter is to be able to introduce Damage less information hiding scheme with no damage to the target content using Artificial Immune System.

Keywords Data hiding · AIS · Damage less information

K. B. Bahekar (✉) · P. Saurabh · B. Verma
Department of CSE, TIT, Bhopal, India
e-mail: kkirti06@gmail.com

P. Saurabh
e-mail: praneetsaurabh@gmail.com

B. Verma
e-mail: bk_verma3@gmail.com

V. Kumar and M. Bhatele (eds.), *Proceedings of All India Seminar on Biomedical Engineering 2012 (AISOBE 2012)*, Lecture Notes in Bioengineering,
DOI: 10.1007/978-81-322-0970-6_24,

Introduction

Digital representation of media facilitates access and potentially improves the portability, efficiency, and accuracy of the information presented. Undesirable effects of facile data access include an increased opportunity for violation of copyright and tampering with or modification of content. The motivation for this work includes the provision of protection of intellectual property rights, an indication of content manipulation, and a means of annotation.

Data hiding [1–4] is a method of hiding secret messages into a cover media such that an unintended observer will not be aware of the existence of the hidden messages. In this paper, 8-bit grayscale images are selected as the cover media. These images are called cover images. Cover images with the secret messages embedded in them are called stego images. For data hiding methods, the image quality refers to the quality of the stego images. The paper is mainly designed for providing security for the data. In this, the sender encrypts the data to some form. While encrypting the data into some form, the key file is entered by the sender. The purpose of the key file is to provide security to the system as it is known only to the sender and the receiver. Since the actual processing of the data takes place on the remote client the data has to be transported over the network, which requires a secured format of the transfer method. Present day transactions are considered to be "un-trusted" in terms of security, i.e., they are relatively easy to be hacked. And also we have to consider the transfer the large amount of data through the network will give errors while transferring. Nevertheless, sensitive data transfer is to be carried out even if there is lack of an alternative. Network security in the existing system is the motivation factor for a new system with higher level security standards for the information exchange [5]. This paper proposes the following features. It provides flexibility to the user to secure the data very easily. In this system, the data is also hided inside the JPEG Image and Video file. The user who received the file will do the operations like de-embedding, and decryption in their level of hierarchy. People for long time have tried to sort out the problems faced in the general digital communication system but as these problems exist even now, a secured and easy transfer system evolved and came to be known as the Encryption and Decryption of the data and converting the file to JPEG image and video format [6, 7] to be transferred using the cryptographic standards. The advantages are:

- High-level Security
- Cost-effective transfer

In this fast growing world where every individual free to access the information on the network and even the people are technically sound enough in hacking the information from the network for various reasons. The organizations have the process of information transfer in and out of their network at various levels, which need the process to be in a secured format for the organizational benefits. The

JPEG and Video file that the employee sends reach the destinations within no time in a JPEG and Video file format where the end user needs to de-embed the file, decrypt it, and use for the purpose.

Features and Applications

Data-hiding techniques [8, 9, 10] should be capable of embedding data in a host signal with the following restrictions and features:

1. The host signal should be nonobjectionably degraded and the embedded data should be minimally perceptible (The goal is for the data to remain hidden. As any magician will tell you, it is possible for something to be hidden while it remains in plain sight; you merely keep the person from looking at it. We will use the words hidden, inaudible, unperceivable, and invisible to mean that an observer does not notice the presence of the data, even if they are perceptible).
2. The embedded data should be directly encoded into the media, rather than into a header or wrapper, so that the data remain intact across varying data file formats.
3. The embedded data should be immune to modifications ranging from intentional and intelligent attempts at removal to anticipated manipulations, e.g., channel noise, filtering, resembling, cropping, encoding, lossy compressing, printing and scanning, digital-to-analog (D/A) conversion, and analog- to-digital (A/D) conversion, etc.
4. Asymmetrical coding of the embedded data is desirable, since the purpose of data hiding is to keep the data in the host signal, but not necessarily to make the data difficult to access.
5. Error correction coding 1 should be used to ensure data integrity. It is inevitable that there will be some degradation to the embedded data when the host signal is modified.
6. The embedded data should be self-clocking or arbitrarily re-entrant. This ensures that the embedded data can be recovered when only fragments of the host signal are available, e.g., if a sound bite is extracted from an interview, data embedded in the audio segment can be recovered. This feature also facilitates automatic decoding of the hidden data, since there is no need to refer to the original host signal.

Applications

Tradeoffs exists between the quantity of embedded data and the degree of immunity to host signal modification. By constraining the degree of host signal degradation, a data-hiding method can operate with either high embedded data rate, or high resistance to modification, but not both. As one increases, the other must decrease. While this can be shown mathematically for some data-hiding systems such as a spread spectrum, it seems to hold true for all data-hiding systems. In any system, you can trade bandwidth for robustness by exploiting redundancy. The quantity of embedded data and the degree of host signal modification vary from application to application. Consequently, different techniques are employed for different applications. Several prospective applications of data hiding. An application that requires a minimal amount of embedded data is the placement of digital watermark. The embedded data are used to place an indication of ownership in the host signal, serving the same purpose as an author's signature or a company logo. A second application for data hiding is tamper proofing. It is used to indicate that the host signal has been modified from its authored state. Modification to the embedded data indicates that the host signal has been changed in some way. A third application, feature location, requires more data to be embedded. In this application, the embedded data are hidden in specific locations within an image. It enables one to identify individual content features, e.g., the name of the person on the left versus the right side of an image. Typically, feature location data are not subject to intentional removal. However, it is expected that the host signal might be subjected to a certain degree of modification, e.g., images are routinely modified by scaling, cropping, and tone scale enhancement. As a result, feature location data-hiding techniques must be immune to geometric and nongeometric modifications of a host signal.

Data Hiding Various Streams

Data Hiding in Still Images

Data hiding in still images [11] presents a variety of challenges that arise due to the way the human visual system (HVS) works and the typical modifications that images undergo. Additionally, still images provide a relatively small host signal in which to hide data. A fairly typical 8-bit picture of 200 $\times$ 200 pixels provides approximately 40 kilobytes (kb) of data space in which to work. This is equivalent to only around 5 s of telephone-quality audio or less than a single frame of NTSC television. Also, it is reasonable to expect that still images will be subject to operations ranging from simple affine transforms to nonlinear transforms such as cropping, blurring, filtering, and lossy compression. Practical data-hiding techniques need to be resistant to as many of these transformations as possible. Despite these challenges, still images are likely candidates for data hiding. There are many attributes of the HVS that are potential candidates for exploitation in a data-hiding system, including our varying sensitivity to contrast as a function of spatial frequency and the masking effect of edges (both in luminance and The HVS has low sensitivity to small changes in luminance, being able to perceive changes of no less

Fig. 1 Data hiding in image

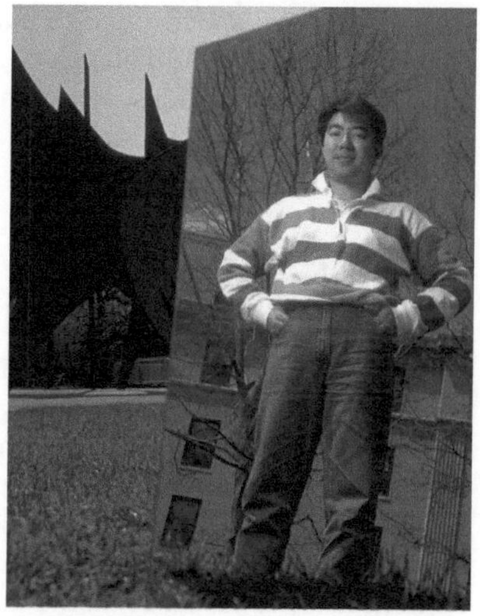

than one part in 30 for random patterns. However, in uniform regions of an image, the HVS is more sensitive to the change of the luminance, approximately one part in 240. A typical cathode ray tube (CRT) display or printer has a limited dynamic range. In an image representation of one part in 256, e.g., 8-bit gray levels, there is potentially room to hide data as pseudorandom changes to picture brightness. Another HVS "hole" is our relative insensitivity to very low spatial frequencies such as continuous changes in brightness across an image, i.e., vignetting.

An additional advantage of working with still images is that they are noncausal. Data-hiding techniques can have access to any pixel or block of pixels at random.

Using these observations, we have developed a variety of techniques for placing data in still images. Some techniques are more suited to dealing with small amounts of data, while others to large amounts. Some techniques are highly resistant to geometric modifications, while others are more resistant to nongeometric modifications, e.g., filtering. We present methods that explore both of these areas, as well as their combination (Fig. 1).

Data Hiding in Audio

Data hiding [12, 13] in audio signals is especially challenging, because the human auditory system (HAS) operates over a wide dynamic range. The HAS perceives over a range of power greater than 1 billion to one and a range of frequencies greater than one thousand to one, Sensitivity to additive random noise is also acute. The perturbations in a sound file can be detected as low as one part in 10 million (80 dB below ambient level). However, there are some "holes" available. While the HAS has a large dynamic range, it has a fairly small differential range.

As a result, loud sounds tend to mask out quiet sounds. Additionally, the HAS is unable to perceive absolute phase, only relative phase. Finally, there are some environmental distortions so common as to be ignored by the listener in most cases. We exploit many of these traits in the methods.

Data Hiding in Text

Soft-copy text is in many ways the most difficult place to hide data [14, 15]. (Hard-copy text can be treated as a highly structured image and is readily amenable to a variety of techniques such as slight variations in letter forms, kerning, baseline, etc.) This is due largely to the relative lack of redundant information in a text file as compared with a picture or a sound bite. While it is often possible to make imperceptible modifications to a picture, even an extra letter or period in text may be noticed by a casual reader. Data Hiding [16–19] in text is an exercise in the discovery of modifications that are not noticed by readers. We considered three major methods of encoding data: open space methods that encode through manipulation of white space (unused space on the printed page), syntactic methods that utilize punctuation, and semantic methods that encode using manipulation of the words themselves.

Data Hiding in Video

A video data embedding scheme in which the embedded signature data is reconstructed without knowing the original host video [20, 21]. The proposed method enables high rate of data embedding [22] and is robust to motion compensated coding, such as MPEG-2. Embedding is based on texture masking and utilizes a multidimensional lattice structure for encoding signature information. Signature data is embedded in individual video frames using the block DCT. The embedded frames are then MPEG-2 coded. At the receiver, both the host and signature images are recovered from the embedded bit stream [23, 24].

Tradition Method Used in Data Hiding

Least Significant Bit (LSB) Method

In computing, the least significant bit (LSB) [25–28] is the bit position in a binary integer giving the units value, that is, determining whether the number is even or odd. The lsb is sometimes referred to as the right-most bit, due to the convention in positional notation of writing less significant digit further to the right. It is analogous to the least significant digit of a decimal integer, which is the digit in the ones (right-most) position. In referencing specific bits within a binary number, it is common to assign each bit a bit number, ranging from zero upwards to one less than the number of bits in the number. However, the order used for this assignment may be in either direction. Both orderings are used (in different contexts), which is why "lsb" is often used to designate the units bit instead of a bit number, which has the potential for confusion.

Data Hiding by PVD

The pixel-value differencing (PVD) method proposed by Wu and Tsai [25] can successfully provide both high embedding capacity and outstanding imperceptibility for the stego image. The PVD method segments the cover image into nonoverlapping blocks containing two connecting pixels and modifies the pixel difference in each block (pair) for data embedding.

Data Hiding by GLM

In 2004, Potdar et al. [3] proposes gray level modification (GLM) technique which is used to map data by modifying the gray level of the image pixels. Gray level modification steganography is a technique to map data (not embed or hide it) by modifying the gray level values of the image pixels. GLM technique uses the concept of odd and even numbers to map data within an image. It is a one-to-one mapping between the binary data and the selected pixels in an image. From a given image, a set of pixels is selected based on a mathematical function. The gray level values of those pixels are examined and compared with the bit stream that is to be mapped in the image.

Artificial Immune Systems

Artificial immune systems (AIS) are a class of computationally intelligent systems inspired by the principles and processes of the vertebrate immune system. The algorithms typically exploit the immune system's characteristics of learning and memory to solve a problem.

The field of AIS is concerned with abstracting the structure and function of the immune system to computational systems, and investigating the application of these systems toward solving computational problems from mathematics, engineering, and information technology. AIS is a subfield of Biologically inspired computing, and Natural computation, with interests in Machine Learning and belonging to the broader field of Artificial Intelligence. AIS is distinct from computational immunology and theoretical biology that are concerned with simulating immunology using computational and mathematical models toward better understanding the immune system, although such models initiated the field of AIS and continue to provide a fertile ground for inspiration. Finally, the field of AIS is not concerned with the investigation of the immune system as a substrate computation, such as DNA computing. This latter approach has been by far the most popular while building Information Hiding System.

AIS Technique

The common techniques are inspired by specific immunological theories that explain the function and behavior of the mammalian adaptive immune system.

- **Clonal Selection Algorithm**: A class of algorithms inspired by the clonal selection theory of acquired immunity that explains how B and T lymphocytes improve their response to antigens over time called affinity maturation. These algorithms focus on the Darwinian attributes of the theory where selection is inspired by the affinity of antigen–antibody interactions, reproduction is inspired by cell division, and variation is inspired by somatic hyper mutation. Clonal selection algorithms are most commonly applied to optimization and pattern recognition domains, some of which resemble parallel hill climbing and the genetic algorithm without the recombination operator.
- **Negative Selection Algorithm**: Inspired by the positive and negative selection processes that occur during the maturation of T-cells in the thymus called T-cell tolerance. Negative selection refers to the identification and deletion (apoptosis) of self-reacting cells, that is T-cells that may select and attack self-tissues. This class of algorithms is typically used for classification and pattern recognition problem domains where the problem space is modeled in the complement of available knowledge.
- **Immune Network Algorithms**: Algorithms that describes the regulation of the immune system by anti-idiotypic antibodies (antibodies that select for other antibodies). This class of algorithms focus on the network graph structures involved where antibodies (or antibody producing cells) represent the nodes and the training algorithm involves growing or pruning edges between the nodes based on affinity (similarity in the problems representation space). Immune network algorithms have been used in clustering, data visualization, control, and optimization domains, and share properties with artificial neural networks.
- **Dendritic Cell Algorithms (DCA)**: The DCA is an example of an immune inspired algorithm developed using a multiscale approach. This algorithm is based on an abstract model of dendritic cells (DCs). The DCA is abstracted and implemented through a process of examining and modeling various aspects of

DC function, from the molecular networks present within the cell to the behavior exhibited by a population of cells as a whole. Within the DCA information is granulated at different layers, achieved through multiscale processing.

Proposed Method

Negative Selection Algorithm for Information Hiding System

The Negative selection algorithms [26, 27] are inspired by the main mechanism in the thymus that produces a set of mature T-cells capable of binding only non-self-antigens. The first negative selection algorithm was proposed by Forrest et al. [20] (1994) to detect data manipulation caused by a virus in a computer system. The starting point of this algorithm is to produce a set of self-strings, *S*, that define the normal state of the system. The task then is to generate a set of detectors, *D*, that only bind/recognize the complement of *S*. These detectors can then be applied to new data in order to classify them as being self or non-self, thus in the case of the original work by Forrest et al. [22], highlighting the fact that data have been manipulated. The algorithm of Forrest et al. [29] produces the set of detectors via the process outlined below.

The Procedure for Negative Selection algorithm is as follows
Input: S_{seen} = set of seen known self elements
Output: D = set of generated detectors

Begin

Repeat

- Randomly generate potential detectors and place them in a set *P*
- Determine the affinity of each member of *P* with each member of the self-set S_{seen}
- If at least one element in *S* recognizes a detector in *P* according to a recognition threshold,
- then the detector is rejected, otherwise it is added to the set of available detectors *D*
- until Stopping criteria have been met

end

The Negative Selection Algorithm was designed for change detection, novelty detection, intrusion detection and similar pattern recognition, and two-class classification problem domains. The algorithm can be configured to balance between detector convergence (quality of the matches) and the space complexity (number of detectors). The lack of dependence between detectors means that detector preparation and application is inherently parallel and suited for a distributed and parallel implementation, respectively.

Conclusion

The security of data is of extreme importance in today's information-based society, including the fields of military, diplomacy, corporation, medicine, and even the individual, the information have to be safeguarded to avoid the unauthorized or illegal accesses and prevent the misuses and abuses. Any system, method or technique that deal with, processing information (data), and put this data in shapes or forms of media under the condition that it must not be visible in its new form to human observer. All such systems are called hiding systems for information. In this paper, several techniques are as possible methods for embedding data in host text, image, and audio signals [6, 30, 31]. While we have had some degree of success, all of the proposed methods have limitations The goal of achieving protection of large amounts of embedded data against intentional attempts at removal may be unobtainable. Proposed method uses Negative Selection Algorithm for classifying the input patterns to corresponding hidden signals. The most important point for this technique is that humans cannot see any information in the bit planes of a image if it is very complex.

References

1. Katzenbeisser S, Fabien AP (eds) (2000) Information hiding techniques for steganography and digital watermarking. Artech House Publishers, p 1
2. Cox I, Miller M, Bloom J, Fridrich J, Kalker T (2007) Digital watermarking and steganography, 2nd edn. Morgan Kaufmann, p 11
3. Chang CC, Tseng HW (2009) Data hiding in images by hybrid LSB substitution. In: 3rd international conference on multimedia and ubiquitous engineering, article no. 5318917, pp 360–363
4. Li X, Wang J (2007) A steganographic method based upon JPEG and particle swarm optimization algorithm. Inf Sci 177(15):3099–3109
5. Sasaki H (ed) (2007) Intellectual Property Protection For Multimedia Information Technology. IGI Global, p 12
6. Johnson NF, Jajodia S (1998) Exploring steganography: seeing the unseen. IEEE Comp J 31(2):26–34
7. Fridrich J, Goljan M (2001) Practical steganalysis of digital images—state of the art
8. Wang RZ, Lin CF, Lin JC (2001) Image hiding by optimal LSB substitution and genetic algorithm. Pattern Recognition Letter 34:671–683
9. Hwang MS, Chang CC, Hwang KF (2000) Digital watermarking of images using neural networks. J Electron Imaging 9:548–555
10. Yu PT, Tsai HH, Lin JS (2001) Digital watermarking based on neural networks for color images. Signal processing 81:663–671

11. Aveibas I, Memon N, Sankur B (2001) Steganalysis based on image quality metrics. In: IEEE fourth workshop on multimedia signal processing, pp 517–522
12. Wang RZ, Lin CF, Lin JC (2000) Hiding data in images by optimal moderately significant-bit replacement. IEE Electronics Letter 36:2069–2070
13. Chan CK, Cheng LM (2001) Improved hiding data in images by optimal moderately significant-bit replacement. IEE Electronics Letter 37:1017–1018
14. Chen B, Wornell GW (2001) Implementations of quantization index modulation methods for digital watermarking and information embedding of multimedia. Special Issue Multimedia Signal Processing 27:7–33
15. Voloshynovskiy S, Herrigel A, Rytsar Y (2002) StegoWall: blind statistical detection of hidden data. Proceedings SPIE 4675:57–68
16. Rumelhart D, McClelland J (1986) Parallel distributed processing: explorations in the microstructure of cognition, vol 1: Foundations. MIT Press Cambridge, MA
17. Bender W, Morimoto N, Lu A (1996) Techniques for data hiding. IBM Syst J 35(3/4):313–336
18. Chan CK, Cheng LM (2004) Hiding data in images by simple LSB substitution. Pattern Recogn 37(3):469–474
19. Chang CC, Hsiaob JY, Chan CS (2003) Finding optimal least-significant-bit substitution in image hiding by dynamic programming strategy. Pattern Recognit 36:1583–1595
20. Johnson NF, Jajodia S (1998) Steganalysis of images created using current steganography software. Lecture notes in computer science, vol 1525. Springer-Verlag, Berlin, pp 273–289
21. Fridrich J, Goljan M, Du R (2001) Steganalysis based on JPEG compatibility, SPIE multimedia systems and applications IV, 20–24 Aug 2001
22. Kahn D (1996) The history of steganography. In: Proceedings of the first international workshop on information hiding. Springer-Verlag, London, pp 1–5
23. Kelley J (2001) Terror groups hide behind Webencryption. USA Today, Feburary 2001. http://www.usatoday.com/life/cyber/tech/2001-02-05-binladen.htm
24. Johnson NF, Jajodia S (1998) Steganalysis: "the investigation of hidden information". Proceedings of the IEEE Information Technology Conference, Syracuse, New York, USA
25. Marvel LM, Boncelet CG, Retter CT (1999) Spread spectrum image steganography. IEEE Trans Image Process 8(8):1075–1083
26. Schneier B (1996) Applied cryptography second edition: protocols, algorithms, and source code in C. Wiley,
27. Wang RZ, Lin CF, Lin JC (2000) Hiding data in images by optimal moderately significant-bit replacement. IEE Electron Lett 36(25):2069–2070
28. Wang RZ, Lin CF, Lin JC (2001) Image hiding by optimal LSB substitution and genetic algorithm. Pattern Recogn 34(3):671–683
29. Rosenblatt F (1958) The perceptron a probabilistic model for information storage and organization. Brain Psych Rev 62:386–408
30. Chen TS, Chang CC, Hwang MS (1998) A virtual image cryptosystem based upon vector quantization. IEEE Trans Image Process 7(10):1485–1488
31. Chung KL, Shen CH, Chang LC (2001) A novel SVD- and VQ-based image hiding scheme. Pattern Recognit Lett 22(9):1051–1058

A Novel Approach for Intrusion Detection System Using Artificial Immune System

Akanksha Parashar, Praneet Saurabh and Bhupendra Verma

Abstract Intrusion detection, a topic that has evolved heavily due to the rising concern for information technology security, has endured numerous architecture abstractions. All of these architecture abstractions have strengths and weaknesses with regard to various factors like efficiency, security, integrity, durability, and cost-effectiveness, to name a few. In this chapter, we explore the appropriateness of the artificial immune system negative selection for intrusion detection and anomaly detection problems. Negative selection is appropriate for anomaly detection problems, especially when compared to statistical K-mean clustering methods, and can detect unseen or unknown attack.

Keywords Intrusion detection system · Artificial immune system · Clustering

Introduction

Computer security is used frequently, but the content of a computer is vulnerable to few risks unless the computer is connected to other computers on a network. As the use of computer networks, especially the Internet, has become pervasive, the concept of computer security has expanded to denote issues pertaining to the

A. Parashar (✉) · P. Saurabh · B. Verma
Dept of CSE, TIT Bhopal, Bhopal, India
e-mail: akanksha.parashar1@gmail.com

P. Saurabh
e-mail: praneetsaurabh@gmail.com

B. Verma
e-mail: bk_verma3@gmail.com

V. Kumar and M. Bhatele (eds.), *Proceedings of All India Seminar on Biomedical Engineering 2012 (AISOBE 2012)*, Lecture Notes in Bioengineering,
DOI: 10.1007/978-81-322-0970-6_25,

networked use of computers and their resources. The major technical areas of computer security are usually represented by the initials confidentiality, integrity, and authentication or availability. Confidentiality means that information cannot be access by unauthorized parties. Confidentiality is also known as secrecy or privacy; breaches of confidentiality range from the embarrassing to the disastrous. Integrity means that information is protected against unauthorized changes that are not detectable to authorized users; many incidents of hacking compromise the integrity of databases and other resources. Authentication means that users are who they claim to be. Availability means that resources are accessible by authorized parties; "denial of service" attacks, which are sometimes the topic of national news, are attacks against availability. Other important concerns of computer security professionals are access control and no repudiation. The main goal of intrusion detection is to detect unauthorized use, misuse, and abuse of computer systems by both system insiders and external intruders. Among automated intrusion detection systems (IDSs), a particular system for network intrusion detection, known as a network-based IDS, monitors any number of hosts on a network by scrutinizing the audit trails of multiple hosts and network traffic. It is usually comprised of two main components: an anomaly detector and a misuse detector [1, 2]. The anomaly detector establishes the profiles of normal activities of users, systems, system resources, network traffic, and/or services and detects intrusions by identifying significant deviations from the normal behavior patterns observed from profiles. The misuse detector defines suspicious misuse signatures based on known system vulnerabilities and a security policy. This component probes whether these misuse signatures are present or not in the auditing trails. Currently, many network-based IDSs have been developed using diverse approaches. Nevertheless, there still remain unresolved problems to build an effective network-based IDS [3]. As one approach of providing the solutions of these problems, the previous work [4] identified a set of general requirements for successful network-based IDS and three design goals to satisfy these requirements: being distributed, self-organizing, and lightweight. In addition, [5] introduced a number of remarkable features of human immune systems (HISs) that satisfy these three design goals. It is anticipated that the adoption of these features should help the construction of an effective network-based IDS [6]. This chapter proposes the use of negative selection and niching of artificial immune system (AIS) for developing an effective network-based ID. An overall artificial immune model for network intrusion detection presented in [7] consists of three different evolutionary stages: negative selection, clonal selection, and gene library evolution. Among these stages, the first stage, negative selection, is investigated in this chapter. We present a more efficient implementation of negative selection using a niching feature of AISs [8].

Literature Survey

A lot of research works have been carried out in the literature for intrusion detection and some of them have motivated us to take up this research. Brief reviews of some of those recent significant researches are presented below: **Tich Phu oc Tran** have applied machine learning (ML) techniques to solve Intrusion Detection problems within computer networks. Due to complex and dynamic nature of computer networks and hacking techniques, identifying malicious activities remains a challenging task for security experts, that is, defence systems that were currently available suffer from low detection capability and high number of false alarms. **Ye Yuan et al**. proposed a method of evidence assignment in combination with Dempster-Shafer theory to identify network attack data. In this method, extracted features were identified by a multi-generalized regression neural network classifier, which determined the basic probability assignment. **Snehal A** proposed the decision-tree-based algorithm to build multiclass IDS. Support vector machines (SVM) were the classifiers which were initially designed for binary classification. Shun J and **Malki H. A.** presented a neural network-based intrusion detection method for the Internet-based attacks on a computer network. **Aida O. Ali** did a relative study between the performances of recent nine artificial neural networks (ANNs)-based classifiers was assessed, centered on a particular set of features. The outcomes showed that; the Multilayer perceptrons (MLPS)-based classifier yielded the best results; about 99.63 % true positive (TP) attacks were detected. **Pohsiang Tsai** suggested a ML framework in which various types of intrusions would be detected with different classifiers, containing different attribute selections and learning algorithms. Appropriate voting techniques were used to combine the outputs of these classifiers.

The pattern-learning abilities of the IS have been modeled and described by [9] and [6] who successfully applied their AISs to recognize and classify tasks. Also **Byoung-Doo,** in 2006, built IDS that deals well with various mutated attacks, as well as well-known attacks by using Time Delay Neural Network classifier that discriminates between normal and abnormal packet flows. It seems that the area where the notion of AIS has been most widespread is in the area of computer security. **A. H. M. Rezaul Karim** proposed collaborative IDS for MANET using Bayesian method using a set of very useful features which guarantee the effectiveness of the IDS [10]. L. Khan et al. proposed a method with a scalable solution for detecting network-based anomalies [11]. They used SVM for classification. They used the dynamically growing self-organizing tree (DGSOT) algorithm for clustering. **Tsong** et al. introduced a three-tier architecture of IDS which consists of a blacklist, a white list, and a multiclass SVM classifier. They designed three-tier IDS based on the KDD'99 benchmark dataset. **Weiming Hu** proposed an intrusion detection algorithm based on the AdaBoost algorithm. The discrete AdaBoost algorithm was selected to learn the classifier. **Hu Zhengbing1** proposed an algorithm to use the known signature to find the signature of the related attack quickly. They used nine different-sized databases. **Amit Kumar Choudhary** proposed a neural network approach to improve the alert throughput of a network and making it attack prohibitive using IDS. For evolving and testing intrusions, the KDD CUP 99 dataset were used. **Stefano Zanero** proposed a novel architecture which implements a network-based anomaly detection system using unsupervised learning algorithms. They described how the pattern recognition features of a self-organizing Map algorithm can be used for intrusion detection purposes on the payload of TCP network World Journal of Science and Technology 2012, 2(3):127–133 131 packets.

Liberios Vokorokos presented IDS and design architecture of intrusion detection based on neural network self-organizing map. Result of the designed architecture is simulation in real conditions.

IDS and AIS Background

This section gives a brief introduction to two distinct fields of study—IDS and AIS, setting the background to and defining the terminology used in the sections that follow.

Intrusion Detection System

An IDS constantly monitors actions in a certain environment and decides whether they are part of a possible hostile attack or a legitimate use of the environment. The environment may be a computer, several computers connected in a network, or the network itself. The IDS analyzes various kinds of information about actions emanating from the environment and evaluates the probability that they are symptoms of intrusions. Such information includes, for example, configuration information about the current state of the system, audit information describing the events that occur in the system (e.g., event log in Windows XP), or network traffic. Several measures for evaluating IDS have been suggested [12–15]. These measures include accuracy, completeness, performance, efficiency, fault tolerance, timeliness, and adaptivity. The more widely used measures are:

The TP rate, that is, the percentage of intrusive actions (e.g., error-related pages) detected by the system, false positive (FP) rate which is the percentage of normal actions (e.g., pages viewed by normal users) the system incorrectly identifies as intrusive, and accuracy which is the percentage of alarms found to represent abnormal behavior out of the total number of alarms. In the current research, TP, FP, and Accuracy measures were adopted to evaluate the performance of the new methodology. There are IDS that simply monitor and alert, and there are IDS that perform an action or actions in response to a detected threat. We will cover each of these briefly.

Artificial Immune Systems

The HIS protects the body against damage from an extremely large number of harmful bacteria, viruses, parasites, and fungi, termed pathogens. It does this largely without prior knowledge of the structure of these pathogens. This property, along with the distributed, self-organized, and lightweight nature of the mechanisms by which it achieves this protection [11], has in recent years made it the focus of increased interest within the computer science and intrusion detection communities. Seen from such a perspective, the HIS can be viewed as a form of anomaly detector with very low false positive and false negative rates.

An increasing amount of work is being carried out attempting to understand and extract the key mechanisms through which the HIS is able to achieve its detection and protection capabilities. A number of AIS have been built for a wide range of applications including document classification, fraud detection, and network- and host-based intrusion detection [16]. These AIS have met with some success and in many cases have rivaled or bettered existing statistical and ML techniques. Two important mechanisms dominate AIS research: network-based models and negative selection models, although this distinction is somewhat artificial as many hybrid models also exist. The first of these mechanisms refers to systems which are largely based on Jerne's idiotypic network theory [17, 18] which recognizes that interactions occur between antibodies and antibodies as well as between antibodies and antigens. Negative selection models use the process of non-self matching selection, as seen with T-lymphocytes in the thymus as a method of generating a population of detectors. This latter approach (along with other newer algorithms) has been, by far, the most popular when building IDS, as can be seen from the work.

Problem Identification in IDS

Clustering Used in IDS

Clustering is an unsupervised learning technique which aims to find structure in a collection of unlabeled data. It is being used in many fields such as data mining, IDS [17, 19]. Traditional methods of network intrusion detection [17, 18, 20] are based on the saved patterns of known attacks. They detect intrusion by comparing the network connection features to the attack pattern that are provided by human experts. The main drawback of traditional methods is that they cannot detect unknown intrusion. Even if a new pattern of the attacks was discovered, this new pattern would have to be manually updated into system. It is also capable of identifying new attacks to some degree of resemblance to the learned ones, the neural networks are widely considered as an efficient approach to adaptively classify patterns (Boger) [21], but their high computation intensity and the long training cycles greatly hinder their applications, especially for the intrusion detection problem, where the amount of related data is very important.

K-means Algorithm

The *K*-means clustering [22, 23] is a classical clustering algorithm. After an initial random assignment of example to *K* clusters, the centers of clusters are computed and the examples are assigned to the clusters with the closest centres. The process is repeated until the cluster centers do not significantly change. Once the cluster assignment is fixed, the mean distance of an example to cluster centers is used as the score. Using the *K*-means clustering algorithm, different clusters were specified and generated for each output class. *Input*: The number of clusters *K* and a dataset for intrusion detection *Output*: A set of *K* clusters that minimizes the squared—error criterion.

Algorithm:

1. Initialize *K* clusters (randomly select *k* elements from the data).
2. While cluster structure changes, repeat from 2.
3. Determine the cluster to which source data belongs. Use Euclidean distance formula. Add element to cluster with min [Distance (xi, yj)].
4. Calculate the means of the clusters.
5. Change cluster centroids to means obtained using Step 3.

The main disadvantage of K-Mean algorithm is that it may take a large number of iterations through dense datasets, before it can converge to produce the optimal set of centroids. This can be inefficient on large datasets due to its unbounded convergence of cluster centroid.

Negative Selection Algorithm for Intrusion Detection

The negative selection algorithms [23, 24] are inspired by the main mechanism in the thymus that produces a set of mature T-cells capable of binding only non-self antigens. The first negative selection algorithm was proposed by [25] to detect data manipulation caused by a virus in a computer system. The starting point of this algorithm is to produce a set of self-strings, *S*, that define the normal state of the system. The task then is to generate a set of detectors, *D*, that only bind/recognize the complement of S. These detectors can then be applied to new data in order to classify them as being self or nonself, thus in the case of the original work by Forrest et al. highlighting the fact that data has been manipulated. The algorithm of Forrest et al. produces the set of detectors via the process outlined below.

Input: S_{seen} = set of seen known self-elements
output: D = set of generated detectors

Begin
Repeat

- Randomly generate potential detectors and place them in a set *P*
- Determine the affinity of each member of *P* with each member of the self-set S_{seen}
- If at least one element in *S* recognizes a detector in *P* according to a recognition threshold,
- then the detector is rejected, otherwise it is added to the set of available detectors *D*
- **until** Stopping criteria has been met

end

The negative selection algorithm was designed for change detection, novelty detection, intrusion detection, similar pattern recognition, and two-class classification problem domains. The algorithm can be configured to balance between detector convergence (quality of the matches) and the space complexity (number of detectors). The lack of dependence between detectors means that detector preparation and application is inherently parallel and suited for a distributed and parallel implementation, respectively.

Evaluation Measures

To evaluate the system performance, the following measures (based on [26]) were used.

True Positive Rate (TP) (also known as detection rate or completeness): the percentage of terrorist pages receiving a rating above the threshold in the experiments, terrorist pages will be obtained from the users simulating terrorists.

False Positive Rate (FP): the percentage of regular Internet access pages that the system incorrectly determined as related to terrorist activities, i.e., the percentage of nonterrorist pages receiving a rating above threshold and suspected falsely as terrorists.

Conclusion

This chapter has described the use of negative selection algorithm with niching for network intrusion detection. After an existing negative selection algorithm was analyzed, this chapter proposed a modified negative selection algorithm with niching and the anticipated advantages of this modified approach for network intrusion detection were discussed. Based on these studies, real network packet data used for this work were introduced. Finally, this chapter outlined a number of novel implementation aspects including a novel genotype allowing the evolution of clusters together with the evolution of detectors and a fitness function which evaluates at the phenotype level.

References

1. Cho SB (2003) Chapter 2: Artificial Life Technology for Adaptive Information Processing. In: Nikola K Fuzziness and soft computing. Future directions for intelligent systems and information sciences: the future of speech and image technologies, brain computers, WWW, and bioinformatics, 13.33, vol 45. Heidelberg, Germany: Physica, ISBN 3-7908-1276-5.
2. Dasgupta D (1999) Immunity-based intrusion detection system: a general framework. In: Proceedings of the 22nd national information systems security conference (NISSC). National Institute of Standards and Technology and National Computer Security Center, Hyatt Regency, Crystal City, Virginia, United States
3. Guan Y, Ghorbani AA, Belacel N (2003) Y-means: a clustering method for intrusion detection. In: Canadian conference on electrical and computer engineering, Montreal, Qubec, Canada, pp 1–4
4. Banfield JD, Raftery AE. Model-based gaussian and non-gaussian clustering
5. Kim J, Bentley P (1999a) The Human ImmuneSystem and Network Intrusion Detection, 7th European Conference on Intelligent Techniques and Soft Computing (EUFIT '99), Aachen, Germany
6. Dasgupta D, Cao Y, Yang C (2003) An immunogenetic approach to spectra recognition. In: Wolfgang B, Jason D, Agoston EE, Max HG, Vasant H, Mark J, Robert ES (eds) Proceedings of the genetic and evolutionary computation (GECCO) Conference, vol 1. Morgan Kaufmann, Orlando, p 149, 155, ISBN 1-55860-611-4
7. Kim J, Bentley P (1999b) The Artificial ImmuneModel for Network Intrusion Detection, 7th European Conference on Intelligent Techniques and Soft Computing (EUFIT99), Aachen, Germany
8. FAQ: network intrusion detection systems, Version 0.8.3, March 21, 2000 (Intrusion Detection)
9. Timmis J, Andrews P, Owens N Clark E (2008) An interdisciplinary perspective on artificial immune systems. Evolutionary Intelligence 1(1):5–26
10. Leonid P (2000) Intrusion detection with unlabeled data using clustering. Undergraduate thesis, Columbia University, NY
11. Lane T, Brodley CE (1999) Temporal sequence learning and data reduction for anomaly detection. ACM Trans Inf Syst Secur 2(3):295–331
12. Debar H, Dacier M, Wespi A (1999) Towards a taxonomy of intrusion-detection systems. Computer Networks 31:805–822
13. Richard C (1999) A learning, multi-layered, hardware artificial immune system. Genetic and Evolutionary Computation Conference 13:149–158
14. Spafford, Zamboni D (2002) Intrusion detection using autonomous agents detection. J Computer Security 10(1/2):23-70
15. Balasubramaniyan et al (1998) An Architecture For Intrusion Detection Using Autonomous Agents, Technical Report 98/05, coast laboratory—Purdue university
16. Michael Sobirey's intrusion detection systems http://www.rnks.informatik.tucot
17. Fan W, Lee W, Stolfo S, Miller M (2000) A multiple model cost sensitive approach for intrusion detection. In: 11th European conference on machine learning (ECML '00) 2000
18. Fan W, Miller M, Stolfo S, Lee W, Chan P (2001) Using artificial anomalies to detect unknown and known network intrusions, CA
19. Kohonen Teuvo (1997) Self-organizing map. Springer, New York

20. Stolfo SJ, Fan W, Lee W (2000) Cost-based modeling for fraud and intrusion detection: results from the JAM project. In: Proceedings of the 2000 DARPA information survivability conference and exposition, 2000
21. Kohonen T (1995) Self-organizing maps. In: Springer series in information sciences, vol 30. Springer, Berlin (Second Extended Edition 1997)
22. Lichodzijewski P, Zincir-Heywood AN, Heywood MI (2002) Host-based intrusion detection using neural gas. In: Proceedings of the 2002 IEEE world congress on computational intelligence, 2002 (in press)
23. Lee W, Stolfo S, Mok K (1999) Mining in a data environment: experience in network intrusion detection. In: Proceedings of 5th ACM SIGKDD international conference knowledge discovery and data mining, 124, San Diego, CA, p 114
24. Lee W, Stolfo S (1998) Data mining approaches for intrusion detection. In: Proceedings of the 7th USENIX security symposium (SECURITY '98), San Antonio, TX
25. Forrest, S. et al (1994) Self-Nonself Discrimination in a Computer, In: Proceedings of IEEE Symposium on Research in Security and Privacy, Los Alamos, CA: IEEE Computer Society Press
26. Sequeira and Zaki (2002) Anomaly Based Data Mining For Intrusion IJCSI PUBLICATION SP 800–31

A Performance-Centric Comparative Study of Hybrid Security Protocol Architectures

Kirtiraj Bhatele, Amit Sinhal and Mayank Pathak

Abstract This research paper contains a performance-based comparative study of a new Hybrid security protocol architecture for online transaction. This protocol is designed using combination of both symmetric and asymmetric cryptographic techniques known as Hybrid cryptography. This protocol serves three very important cryptographic primitives—integrity, confidentiality, and authentication. Each of the so-called cryptographic primitives is provided or fulfilled by the particular symmetric or asymmetric cryptographic techniques. The symmetric cryptographic algorithms are fast compared to asymmetric cryptographic algorithms, so when both symmetric and asymmetric algorithms are used in tandem or together in a proper way, the result is very encouraging in terms of providing high security with fast speed. This research paper simply showcases that the proposed protocol architecture is better than the relevant or recent protocol architecture in terms of execution time and security.

Keywords Hybrid cryptography · ECC · AES · Dual RSA · MD5

K. Bhatele (✉)
Department of IT, TIT College, Bhopal, India
e-mail: kirtirajbhatele8@gmail.com

A. Sinhal · M. Pathak
Department of CSE, TIT College, Bhopal, India
e-mail: amit_sinhal@rediffmail.com

M. Pathak
e-mail: pathak.mayank@rediffmail.com

V. Kumar and M. Bhatele (eds.), *Proceedings of All India Seminar on Biomedical Engineering 2012 (AISOBE 2012)*, Lecture Notes in Bioengineering,
DOI: 10.1007/978-81-322-0970-6_26,

Introduction

Cryptography is the science which uses mathematics to encrypt and decrypt data. This science enables you to store sensitive information or transmit it across insecure networks so that it cannot be read by anyone except the intended recipient. In conventional cryptography, also called secret-key or symmetric-key encryption, one key is used both for encryption and decryption. In asymmetric cryptography, the encryption and decryption keys are different on both the sides. Hybrid cryptography is a combination of both symmetric and asymmetric cryptographic techniques. Hybrid cryptography is very effective indeed in providing high degree of security because whatever the problems associated with symmetric-key cryptographic techniques were solved when asymmetric cryptographic mechanism is used. So when both the types of algorithm are used in the protocol architecture, the resulted new protocol architecture, is more immune against the attacks and hence providing the high degree of security [1].

E-commerce and M-commerce transactions are growing at an explosive rate. The success of these depends on how transactions are carried out in the most secured manner. The prime requirements for any e-commerce and m-commerce transactions are Privacy, Authentication, Integrity maintenance, and Non-Repudiation [2]. Cryptography helps us in achieving these prime requirements. Today, various cryptographic algorithms have been developed [3, 4].

The Cryptographic Algorithms Used

1. *Advance Encryption Standard (AES) Algorithm*

The Rijndael proposal for AES defined a cipher in which the block length and the key length can be independently specified to be 128, 192, and 256 bits [2].

AES algorithm contains the following four different stages: (1) Substitution bytes: Uses S box (substitution box) to perform byte-to-byte substitution. (2) Shift rows: A simple permutation (3) Mix columns: A diffusion layer that makes use of Finite field arithmetic. (4) Add Round Key: A simple bit-wise XOR of the current block with the expanded key [5]. The beauty of AES is that all known attacks are computationally infeasible to it.

2. *Dual RSA*

In practice, the RSA decryption computations are performed in p and q and then combined via the Chinese remainder theorem (CRT) to obtain the desired solution in Z N, instead of directly computing the exponentiation in Z N. This decreases the computational costs of decryption in two ways. First, computations in Z p and Z q are more efficient than the same computations in Z N since the elements are much smaller. Second, from Lagrange's Theorem, we can replace the private exponent d with $dp = d \bmod (p - 1)$ for the computation in Z p and with $dq = d \bmod (q - 1)$

for the computation in Z p, which reduces the cost for each exponentiation when d is larger than the primes. It is common to refer to dp and dq as the CRT-exponents. The first method to use the CRT for decryption was proposed by Quisquater and Couvreur [3, 6].

Since the method requires knowledge of p and q, the key generation algorithm needs to be modified to output the private key (d, p, q) instead of (d, N). Given the private key (d, p, q) and a valid ciphertext C Z N, the CRT decryption algorithm is as follows:

(a) Compute Cp = Cdp mod p.
(b) Compute Cq = Cdq mod q.
(c) Compute M0 = (Cq − Cp). p − 1 mod q.
(d) Compute the plaintext M = Cp + M0. p.

This version of CRT-decryption is simply Garner's Algorithm for the CRT applied to RSA. If the key generation algorithm is further modified to output the private key (dp, dq, p, q, p − 1 mod q), the computational cost of CRT-decryption is dominated by the modular exponentiations in steps (a) and (b) of the algorithm. When the primes p and q are roughly the same size (i.e., half the size of the modulus), the computational cost for decryption using CRT-decryption (without parallelism) is theoretically 1/4 the cost for decryption using the original method [7]. Using RSA along with CRT-decryption allows for extremely fast encryption and decryption that is at most four times faster than standard RSA [8].

3. *Message Digest 5 (MD5) Algorithm*

MD5 consists of 64 of these operations, grouped in four rounds of 16 operations. F is a nonlinear function; one function is used in each round. Mi denotes a 32-bit block of the message input, and Ki denotes a 32-bit constant, different for each operation. s is a shift value, which also varies for each operation [3].

MD5 processes a variable length message into a fixed-length output of 128 bits. The input message is broken up into chunks of 512-bit blocks; the message is padded so that its length is divisible by 512 [9]. The padding works as follows: first a single bit, 1, is appended to the end of the message. This is followed by as many zeros as are required to bring the length of the message up to 64 bits less than a multiple of 512. The remaining bits are filled up with a 64-bit integer representing the length of the original message [10].

The main MD5 algorithm operates on a 128-bit state, divided into four 32-bit words, and are denoted A, B, C, and D. These are initialized to certain fixed constants. The main algorithm then operates on each 512-bit message block in turn, each block modifying the state. The processing of a message block consists of four similar stages, termed rounds; each round is composed of 16 similar operations based on a nonlinear function F, modular addition, and left rotation. Many message digest functions have been proposed and are in use today. Here are just a few like HMAC, MD2, MD4, MD5, SHA, SHA-1. Here, we concentrate on MD5, one of the widely used digest functions [1].

The Recent Architecture

The recent architecture has been already discussed in the Research paper [11].

Proposed Architecture

In the proposed architecture, given plain text can be encrypted with the help of AES and the derived cipher text can be communicated to the destination through any secured channel. Simultaneously the Hash value is calculated through MD5 for the same plaintext, which already has been converted into the cipher text by AES. This Hash value has been encrypted with Dual RSA and the encrypted message of this Hash value is also sent to destination.

Now at the receiving end, hash value of Decrypted plaintext is calculated with MD5 and then it is compared with the hash value of original plaintext which is calculated at the sending end for its integrity. By this we are able to know whether the original text being altered or not during transmission in the communication medium.

The intruders may try to hack the original information from the encrypted messages. Although he may be able to trap both the encrypted messages of plaintext and the hash value, but he will not be able to decrypt these messages to get original one. Hence the message can be communicated to the destination in a highly secured manner. The design of proposed hybrid security protocol architecture is given in Fig. 1.

The proposed Hybrid security protocol architecture is superior from the previous security protocol architecture because of three reasons which are as follows:

1. The proposed security protocol architecture is more time efficient as compared to the recent security protocol architecture because its execution time is less compared to the execution time of recent security protocol architecture. It is evident from the performance evaluation matrix drawn below. The proposed security protocol architecture performance is better from its counterpart on most of the hardware platform available right from Pentium 4 to the latest i5 processors.
2. The proposed hybrid security protocol is more immune against the square attacks because of the inclusion of AES algorithm. The square attack on AES Rijndael can be extended to 7 rounds by guessing the 16 bytes of the last round key.

The attractiveness of AES is that it offers better security for smaller key size and thereby reducing processing overheads. The benefits of this higher strength per bit include higher speed low power consumption, bandwidth saving, storage efficiencies, smaller certificates. These advantages are beneficial in applications where bandwidth, processing capability, power availability, and storage are constrained. The hybrid security protocol architecture is as such it can be easily upgraded and

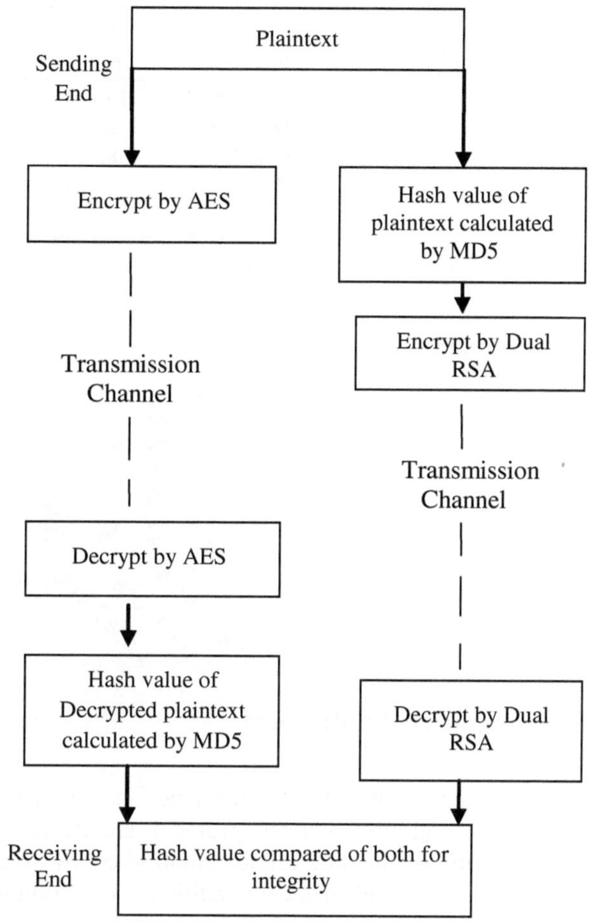

Fig. 1 The proposed hybrid security protocol architecture

hence the protocol becomes more immune against the attacks and at the same time it becomes more time efficient.

3. With the inclusion of AES Rijindael inside the security protocol architecture simply adds a quotient of standardization because in the United States, AES was announced by National Institute of Standards and Technology (NIST) as U.S. FIPS PUB 197 (FIPS 197) on November 26, 2001. This announcement followed a 5-year standardization process in which fifteen competing designs were presented and evaluated, before the Rijndael cipher was selected as the most suitable. It became effective as a Federal government standard on May 26, 2002 after approval by the Secretary of Commerce. AES is available in many different encryption packages, and is the first publicly accessible and open cipher approved by the National Security Agency (NSA) for top secret information when used in an NSA approved cryptographic module.

Table 1 A performance matrix based on execution time

Processor	Execution time (ms)	
	Recent architecture	Proposed architecture
Pentium 4	15,170	14,504
Dual core	9,876	9,408
Core 2 duo	8,660	8,142
i3	2,865	2,448
i5	2,504	2,308

Chart 1 A performance-based chart

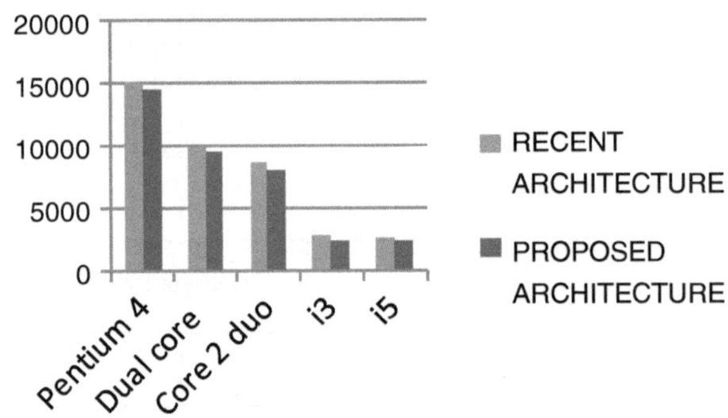

Performance Evaluation

In order to evaluate the performance of the proposed architecture, we first implement both the security protocol architecture's using Java 1.6 and then execute both architecture implementation codes over a number of hardware platform (processors) under ideal conditions. The common data set given as an input to both the architecture implementation in order to get the most accurate execution time as possible.

Table 1 contains the average execution time of both the architecture implementation. The average execution time is obtained by first making 1,000 hits to the security architecture implementation and then by dividing the total execution time we get faster the execution of architecture implementation by 1,000. The same methodology adopted in the software companies in order to know the performance of the code (Chart 1).

However, the selection of the programming language for implementing both the security protocol architecture is obvious Java programming language because of two simple reasons:

1. Java is platform-independent language, i.e., we can develop the code of the proposed architecture in it and then makes it run on any platform. The developed code will be platform independent which in turn increases the domain of its application in a variety of fields such as use of proposed hybrid security protocol in Mobile Adhoc network (MANET) also apart from E-commerce and M-commerce transactions [12].

2. Java programming language provides inbuilt security and cryptographic packages which proved to be very helpful while implementing both the security protocol architecture.

Conclusion

In this research paper, we proposed a new improved Hybrid security protocol architecture and carried out a comparative study in between the Proposed and the recent architecture. The comparative study simply proves that the proposed hybrid security protocol architecture scores high over the previous security protocol architecture in terms of being more time efficient and providing better security especially against square attacks because of the inclusion of AES algorithm. The square attack on AES Rijndael can be extended to 7 rounds by guessing the 16 bytes of the last round key.The proposed hybrid security protocol may solve many problems regarding practical implementation, provides short response time, efficient computation, and increases the strength of cryptosystems.

The performance matrix which contains the execution time of both the architecture's, the recent one and the proposed one on a number of hardware platforms (processors) under ideal conditions proves that the proposed hybrid security protocol architecture is faster or requires less execution time and is better in any working environment.

Future Work

As there is always room for improvement, the security as well as the performance of the proposed security protocol architecture can be improved by simply incorporating the improved versions of the constituent's cryptographic algorithms.

References

1. Stallings W (2003) Cryptography and network security—principles and practices, 3rd edn. Pearson Education Asia
2. Domingo-Ferrer J, Herrera-Joancomarti J (1996) New privacy homomorphism and applications. Inf Process Lett 60(5):277–282
3. Schneier B (1996) Applied cryptography, 2nd edn. Wiley, New York
4. Dabida GI, Wells DB, Kam JB (1981) A database encryption system with subkeys[J]. ACM Trans Database Syst 6(2):192–199

5. Jingmei L, Baodian W, Xiangguo C, et al (2005) An AES to increase complexity and cryptographic analysis[C]. In: 19th International conference on advanced information networking and applications, pp 724–728
6. Subasree S, Sakthivel NK (2010) Design of a new security protocol using hybrid cryptography algorithm, IJRRAS (2 Feb 2010)
7. Sun H-M (2007) Dual RSA and its security analysis. IEEE Trans Inf Theory 53(8):2922–2933
8. Bleichenbacher D, May A (2006) New attacks on RSA with small CRT exponent in public key cryptography, PKC 2006. Lecture notes in computer science, vol 3968. Springer, Heidelberg, pp 1–13
9. Rivest R (1992) The MD5 message-digest algorithm, RFC 1321
10. Ramaraj E, Karthikeyan S (2011) A design of enhanced security protocol for wireless communication using hybrid encryption technique (AES—Rijndael and RSA), India
11. Bhatele K, Sinhal A, Pathak M (2012) A novel approach to the design of a new Hybrid security protocol Architecture. IEEE ICACCCT conference at Ramanathapuram, Tamil Nadu, India
12. Dubal MJ, Mahesh TR, Ghosh PA (2011) Design of new security algorithm using hybrid cryptographic architecture. IEEE (ICECT 2011) 1:1–428

Social Engineering: A Psychological Hacking to Temper Medical Security

L. N. Pandey, Mukta Bhatele and Vivek Badhe

Abstract There are several techniques available to a hacker for infringe the information from persons using social networks. The human approach often called "Social Engineering" and is almost the most difficult one to handle. The hackers of today are using a hybrid approach combining social networking techniques and hacking methodologies to gain unauthorized access to computer systems. In general, the user is easy to fool—and that is why so many people get infected. Even if user knows about security, and knows that he have to be careful on the internet, no one is safe when something is really targeted at you. This paper describes some common Social Engineering techniques and their impact on the Medical Security. This paper describes the ways to protect the images or data from being tempered. It also discusses innovative ways for us to construct and utilizes scenarios for social engineering tests, and provides key strategies for successfully defeating these attacks.

Keywords Psychological hacking · Social engineering · Spam · Medical security

Introduction

As hacking attacks on systems have been increased, many security systems also developed to prevent them. As a result, attackers are shifting their focus and targeting peoples through social engineering methods to gain unnoticed access to

M. Bhatele · V. Badhe
Department of Computer Science, Gyan Ganga College of Technology, Jabalpur, India

L. N. Pandey (✉)
Computer Technology and Application, Gyan Ganga College of Technology, Jabalpur, India
e-mail: vklnpandey@gmail.com

V. Kumar and M. Bhatele (eds.), *Proceedings of All India Seminar on Biomedical Engineering 2012 (AISOBE 2012)*, Lecture Notes in Bioengineering,
DOI: 10.1007/978-81-322-0970-6_27,

computer systems and sensitive information. This is due to the widely accepted fact that people are the weakest links in a security framework to penetrate.

Teleradiology applications and universal availability of patient records using web-based technology are rapidly gaining importance. Consequently, digital medical image security has become an important issue when images and their pertinent patient information are transmitted across public networks, such as the Internet. Health mandates such as the Health Insurance Portability and Accountability Act require healthcare providers to adhere to security measures in order to protect sensitive patient information.

Social Engineering is a collection of techniques used to manipulate people in such a way that they unintentionally or unknowingly leak confidential information or do such actions that may lead to leave a way unauthorized access for hackers. It is similar to a confidence trick or a simple fraud, the term typically applies to trickery for information gathering or computer system access. In most of the cases, the attacker never comes face-to-face with the victims and the latter seldom realize that they have been manipulated.

A determined penetration tester or attacker rarely fails to trick his targets into releasing sensitive information. The usefulness of the information and the difficulty of obtaining it depend on the individual security controls. If you are not incorporating social engineering into your assessment arsenal, you are ignoring a threat vector that may dramatically affect your risk exposure.

Categories of Attacks

A variety of attacks are evolving as users smartness is increasing. These attacks may be technical or non-technical in nature.

Phishing

A user may receive an email appearing to have come form a legitimate business, a bank, or credit card company requesting "verification" of information and warning of some dire consequences if it is not done. The letter usually contains a link to a fake Web page that looks authentic with company logos and content and has a form that may request username, passwords, card numbers or pin details.

Spam Mails

Some e-mails that offer friendships, entertainment, gifts and various free pictures, and information to take advantage of the anonymity and friendship of the internet or plant malicious code. The user opens e-mails and attachments through which may have Trojans, viruses, and worms and other uninvited programs find their way into systems and networks. User is motivated to open the message because it appears to offer useful information, such as security notices or verification of a purchase, promises an entertainment, such as jokes, scandal, cartoons or photographs, give away something for nothing, such as music, videos, or software downloads. The outcome can range in severity from nuisance to system slowdown, destruction of entire communication system or corruption of records.

Overt Social Engineering

The fast growing internet based communication attracted hackers to use social engineering tactics to exploit users. It may be initiated as a believable story to gain users trust, but will often include a factor of fear to persuade user to act quickly. The story itself will appeal to one of the basic human instincts. It will offer you money for nothing (greed); it will ask for gentle aid either for a friend in trouble or a suffering population (sympathy); or it will be threatening to persuade you to pay up or face the consequences (fear). This may include

Advance Fee Fraud—user pays a little now to get a lot more lately, which never materializes.
Auction Fraud—You bid for a bargain, pay the money, but never get the goods.
Disaster appeals—Fake requests that follow all natural disasters etc.

These allurements are made in such a way that user may be convinced with the requests and itself indulge in jeopardy.

Covert Social Engineering

In the same fashion as in overt social engineering, covert social engineering also begins from an emotional story. In covert social engineering, attackers do not openly ask for money; their purpose is to unknowingly steal your financial details.

Attacks on Medical Security

Attacks on Medical security are best characterized by viewing the function of the computer system as a provision of information. In general, normal communication is represented as a flow of information from source to destination.

There are four categories of attacks:

Interruption: An attack on availability. Information is destroyed or becomes unavailable or unusable.

Interception: An attack on confidentiality. An unauthorized party gains access to information.
Modification: An attack on integrity. An unauthorized party not only gains access to, but also tampers with information.
Fabrication: An attack on authenticity. An unauthorized party inserts counterfeit objects into the system.

These attacks can be divided further into two categories, according to the nature of the attacks:

Active Attacks

These attacks involve modification of the data stream or the creation of a false stream and can be subdivided into four categories:

Masquerade: One entity pretends to be a different entity.
Replay: The passive capture of a data unit and its subsequent retransmission to produce an unauthorised effect.
Modification of messages: Some portion of a legitimate message is altered, or messages are delayed or recorded to produce an unauthorised effect.
Denial of service: One prevents or inhibits the normal use or management of communications facilities.

Passive Attacks

These attacks involve eavesdropping on, or monitoring of, transmission and can be subdivided into two categories:

Release of message contents: An unauthorised party obtains information that is being transmitted.
Traffic analysis: An unauthorised party obtains information useful in guessing the nature of communication by observing the pattern of masked message transmissions. The modification and fabrication attacks on medical images can be secured by Watermarking, Reversible watermarking.

For most people, going to the doctor means thinking about co-pays and when they will feel better. For me though, it means thinking about those plus the cyber security of the computer systems being used by the medical professionals. Data security is becoming a real concern. Your medical records, now being converted to electronic media, can easily be stolen, lost and compromised. Digital data, all adheres to the same rules. It can be erased, modified, and easily stole—no matter what laws are in place.

How to Defend?

Social Engineering attacks are hardest threats to defend because it involves humans as an alternative of firewalls, routers, Web servers or database. They are relatively unpredictable. Yet, there are some measures which can definitely bring the risk of social engineering attacks to tolerable levels.

Clearly defined objectives are a must for a useful social engineering safeguard. "Obtain sensitive information" is usually too vague, and presents opportunities for blame, hurt feelings, and lawsuits. Consider tying your goals to the controls in your security program.

For example:

- The security awareness presentation explains how to identify phishing scams. Test what percentage of targeted peoples will click on a link in a phishing-like email you send out.
- Helpdesk training materials outline procedures for resetting a caller's forgotten password. Test whether helpdesk personnel follow protocol when you call impersonating a colleague who cannot log in.
- The security policy warns employees against strangers walking into the building behind an employee who swiped his badge at the entrance. Test how employees will react when you try to follow them through the door they opened. Without specific goals, the social engineering test might conjure some war stories, but it will not produce actionable recommendations for improving the people's security posture.

Integrating Social Engineering into Your Security Consideration

- People empathize with those in trouble: "Please reset my password. My boss will kill me if I don't submit the time sheet in time!"
- People reciprocate a favor: You picked up the papers the person dropped; he holds the door to let you in.
- Your scenario should specify the individuals or groups designated for social engineering, timing of the test, location, and persuasion tactics. Account for laws, contractual commitments, policies, and the company's culture. Also consider the possibility of something going wrong, and define back-out and escalation procedures.

A Word of Caution

Consider how targeted individuals will react to being deceived. If you have to work with them afterward, the good will you may lose could cost you. For this reason, companies tend to err on the side of caution, often selecting impersonal email-based scenarios in place of confrontations by phone or in person. You can easily get into trouble without a written approval for the scenario from your manager or client, and preferably from their manager as well. If you are a consultant, you will be wise to seek a lawyer's perspective before accepting the project.

Arm Yourself with Knowledge

Employees ARE your biggest security threat. Many employees are unaware that certain actions are not safe. Others may know the actions are unsafe, but are willing to take the chance to avoid what seems like a burdensome security procedure. These training courses do not stop at simply describing why certain actions are unsafe. They also discuss how to detect and prevent future information leakage.

Prevention from Social Engineering Attacks

The best combat strategy against social engineering is user awareness that these attacks do happen. Examples of social engineering exploit:

- A confused and befuddled person will call a clerk and meekly request a password change.
- Seemingly powerful and hurried people, identifying themselves as executives, will telephone a new system administrator and demand access to their account IMMEDIATELY!
- At an airport, somebody will look over a shoulder ("shoulder surfing") as telephone credit card numbers or ATM PINs (sometimes even using binoculars or camcorders) are keyed.
- A visitor, incognito, will watch as you enter a login-ID and password at your keyboard.
- Somebody will call and confidently instruct a computer operator to type in a few lines of instruction at the console.
- An attacker will sift through your paper trash (also known as "dumpster diving"), looking for clues to unlock your IT treasures or financial life.
- Here are some good practices:

- Train yourself never to give out passwords or confidential information over the phone.
- Update your security policy to address social engineering attacks.
- Update your incident-handling procedures to include social engineering attacks.
- Keep all trash in secured, monitored areas.
- Shred important and sensitive data.
- Attend periodic security awareness training programs.

Conclusion

Yet Social Engineering Threats are hardest to counter, they can be moderated in acceptable levels by adapting suggested safeguards. Concentrating on your protection, do not give more access to others than necessary. Minimizing the number of people who have access to confidential files like confidential patient records can help to reduce the risk but will not eliminate it. Ultimately, social engineers can be best thwarted by educating yourself. These days risk is in all places. You simply need to be alive to the risks and stay watchful.

References

1. The human element in cyber security: the worm in front of the screen robert larose, telecommunication, information studies, and media
2. Robert D The role of the community college in educating the cyber security workforce. Campbell
3. Keizer G How common is phishing?
4. Barber R Social engineering: a peoples problem. Articon Integralis
5. Social engineering: a thaper
6. Weir GRS, Toolan F, Smeed D The threats of social networking old wine in new bottles

Fixed and Mobile Infrastructure-Based Routing Protocol in Opportunistic Networks

Sanjay K. Dhurandher, Deepak Kumar Sharma, Aseem Garg and Diksha Khatri

Abstract In Opportunistic Networks (OppNets), network partition and disconnections are very common as nodes may move out of the radio range of each other. So, routing and forwarding in these networks is a very challenging task. However, with the introduction of some infrastructure it is still possible to create a fully connected network. This infrastructure is generally composed of some special nodes that are more powerful in terms of energy, transmission range, buffer space, etc., as compared to the normal nodes. The routing protocol proposed in this paper uses the combination of both static as well as mobile infrastructure for message passing between the nodes. The fixed infrastructure is used in form of infostations (IS) and the mobile infrastructure in form message ferry (MF). This new protocol is energy efficient, robust, and expected to reduce the routing overheads seen in the previous protocols.

Keywords OppNets · Infostation · Message ferry · Infrastructure-based protocols · Network partition · Routing in OppNets

S. K. Dhurandher (✉)
CAITFS, Division of Information Technology, Netaji Subas Institute of Technology, University of Delhi, New Delhi, India
e-mail: dhurandher@gmail.com

D. K. Sharma
Division of Computer Engineering, Netaji Subas Institute of Technology, University of Delhi, New Delhi, India
e-mail: dk.sharma1982@yahoo.com

A. Garg · D. Khatri
Division of Information Technology, Netaji Subas Institute of Technology, University of Delhi, New Delhi, India
e-mail: ase.aseem@gmail.com

D. Khatri
e-mail: dksh.khatri@gmail.com

V. Kumar and M. Bhatele (eds.), *Proceedings of All India Seminar on Biomedical Engineering 2012 (AISOBE 2012)*, Lecture Notes in Bioengineering,
DOI: 10.1007/978-81-322-0970-6_28,

Introduction

Opportunistic Networks (OppNets) [1] are considered as the most recent evolutions of mobile ad hoc networks (MANETs) in present times. They have all the challenges and issues similar to MANETs and the research in this area is mainly focused on MANETs application areas. They are also considered as the subclass of *Delay Tolerant Networks* (DTNs) [2–4]. In such type of networks, it is assumed that a continuous end-to-end path between the sender and the receiver rarely exists or is highly unstable as it can exist only for a very short unpredictable time period. Thus, the existing ad hoc network and internet routing protocols fail to deliver messages in OppNets since they presume a fixed end-to-end path between the sender and the receiver node before the delivery of the message. The network topology is dynamic and nodes do not have any prior knowledge about the network configuration and topology [5, 6].

OppNets facilitate communication between heterogeneous devices in network environments where disconnections and reconnections are very frequent due to short radio range and low power of nodes. Network connectivity is poor due to the high mobility of nodes and the intermittent links between them. Network partition and intermittent connectivity are considered as characteristics of OppNets rather than a problem, and thus the source to destination reliable message delivery is not guaranteed in such networks. Due to these issues OppNets are emerging as a very interesting research area among the research community [6, 7].

The routing and forwarding of messages in OppNets can be classified as infrastructure based and infrastructure less on the basis of the infrastructure used in the network [8]. This chapter mainly focuses on developing a routing protocol for infrastructure-based OppNets. The network architecture considered and the protocol proposed in this paper uses both fixed as well as mobile infrastructure for the communication.

The rest of the chapter is organized as follows. Background and related work presents the background and related works carried out in the area of routing protocols for infrastructure-based OppNets. The protocol gives the detailed description about the working of the proposed protocol's algorithm. Conclusion and future work gives the final conclusive remarks and provides some insight on future work.

Background and Related Work

As routing is one of the major areas of concern in OppNets, various routing protocols such as Infostation Model [9], SWIM [10], Data-MULE [11], MF [12] to name a few have been proposed. A brief literature survey of these existing routing protocols in infrastructure-based OppNets has been discussed in this section.

In the *Infostation model* [9] nodes communicate with each other with the help of static infrastructure elements called infostations. They are permanently connected, and provide a high bandwidth service in a specified area. The sender node has to move close to a nearby infostation and upload it with its message. It is then the responsibility of the infostation to deliver this message to the final destination node, which is always outside the considered opportunistic network. In this approach, messages experience very high delays.

The *Shared Wireless Infostation Model* (*SWIM*) [10] extends the technique used in the infostation model. In this model, both node-to-node and node-to-base-station forwarding is allowed for communications. Thus, the sender node can either deliver the message directly to the base station, if it is within communication range; or it delivers the message to a near neighboring node that will take it to the base station whenever encountered. The message routing between the nodes follows an epidemic model [13]. Instead of aiming at a specific destination, any of the infostations may act as the termination node for any given message. The SWIM model, simulation results shows that there is a decrease in the delivery delays by 1.6–3.5 times as compared to infostation model.

The *Mobile Ubiquitous LAN Extensions* (*Data-MULE*) system [11] is a method that is used to retrieve data from sparse wireless sensor networks. It is designed as a three-tier architecture. The first level consists of sensor nodes that periodically collect data from the surrounding environment. The second level consists of mobile agents, named MULEs, which move randomly in the area covered by sensors. These MULEs collect the data gathered by the sensor nodes. The third level consists of access points and data repositories which receive information from the MULEs. These access points are connected to a data warehouse where the received data is stored for further processing.

In the *Message-ferrying approach* [12], some extra mobile agents called ferries are employed in the network which offers a message relaying service. These agents have high energy, speed, and buffer space as compared to the normal nodes. These ferries move around in the network and collect messages from source nodes. Once a message is given to the ferry, then it becomes the responsibility of the ferry node to deliver it to the destination node. Message collection can take place in two ways:

- *Node-initiated message ferrying*: The ferry node moves in the network following a predefined and known path. Every node in the network knows the path that is taken by ferries. The sender node wishing to send a message moves closer to the path followed by the ferry. After meeting with the ferry it transfers the message to the ferry for delivery to the destination.
- *Ferry-initiated message ferrying*: The ferry node roams in the network following a fixed predetermined path. Any node wishing to communicate with other nodes in the network sends a service request to the ferry, which also includes its current position. After receiving the service request from the source node, the ferry changes its path to meet the source node.

The Protocol

This section presents the detailed description of the proposed routing protocol. It exploits the advantages of both infostation and MF-based routing techniques to create an infrastructure based routing mechanism for OppNets. The architecture of the proposed protocol is discussed first, then list of assumptions made while designing the algorithm, followed by the detailed explanation of the algorithm.

Architecture

Figure 1 shows the architecture used for the proposed protocol.

The entire network area is geographically divided into square grids as shown in the Fig. 1. In Fig. 1, IS represents the infostations. The size of the smallest block depends upon the radio range and the power of the nodes and the ferries. The smallest block is called a *Level* 1 *zone*. A combination of four *Level N zones* forms a *Level* $(N + 1)$ *zone*. The intersection point of four *Level N* zones forms a *Level N Junction*. A *Level N* infostation is placed at a *Level N junction*. The nodes are spread and can move throughout the network in a random manner. The functions and responsibilities of various components used in this system are listed below.

Node: It can be any static or mobile networking device capable of sending and receiving messages and can move between zones. It can transfer and receive messages from the ferry. Nodes can communicate neither with each other nor with the infostation.

Ferry: It is a high power mobile node responsible for carrying out communication in a zone. It communicates with nodes and infostation to deliver and receive messages. It also tells the infostation to which all nodes is communicated with during its one round in the zone. A ferry can move only in a *Level* 1 zone.

Infostation: It is a very high power device present at the junction of four same level zones. The IS is not mobile i.e., it is static and fixed. It has a large buffer to store messages received from the ferries. It keeps a record of the location of various nodes present in the four zones connected to it. It also communicates with ferries to facilitate interzone communication. Each *Level N* infostation is directly connected to one *Level* $N + 1$ Infostation that is its parent infostation and four *Level* $N - 1$ infostations that are its children infostations.

Assumptions

The various assumption made in the design of the algorithm are listed below.

- Nodes can exchange messages only with the corresponding zone ferry. There is no communication between the node and the infostation.

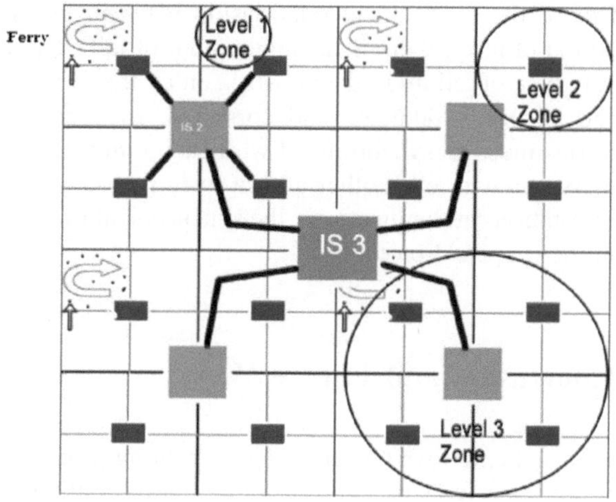

Fig. 1 Architecture of the protocol

- If a node does not meet a ferry during its movement, it will stay at a point and wait for the arrival of the ferry.
- The buffer of a ferry is limited.
- The ferry gathers every node's location information present in its zone and transfers it to the corresponding infostation.

The Algorithm

The basic steps involved in the routing process are as follows:

1. A sender node waits for a ferry.
2. When in contact it transfers its own ID, the message and the receiver details to the ferry.
3. If the receiver is in the same zone, the ferry delivers the message, and acknowledges the infostation and the sender.
4. Else the ferry transfers the message and receiver details to the infostation.
5. The infostation either forwards the message to some other ferry (in case of adjacent zone) or it forwards the message to its parent infostation (in case of non-adjacent zone).
6. The message climbs up the hierarchy of infostations until it encounters an infostation which has the receiver registered in its buffer.
7. Now, the message descends the hierarchy to *Level* 1 infostation to the ferry and finally to the receiver.

The proposed protocol has advantages over the *Infostation model* and the *Message-ferrying approach.* The *Infostation model* based routing has a single point of failure. If the head infostation fails, the whole network will become dead.

Due to the hierarchical relationship between the infostations and the fixed time period of ferry, there is no single point of failure present in the proposed protocol. Any type of failure in the network, either the ferry failure or the infostation failure, can be easily detected and corrected. In *Message-ferrying approach*, multiple ferries must be synchronized with each other so that they can meet and exchange messages with each other after a fixed period of time. Due to the presence of the infostations at the junctions, the synchronization between the ferries is not required in the proposed protocol.

Conclusion and Future Work

In this chapter, we presented a new routing protocol for Oppnets which is a hybrid of message ferrying and infostation based routing protocols. This protocol proves to be energy efficient as substantial energy is saved because the sender node communicates over a short range. When a node has to transfer a message it can either keep on moving till it encounters the ferry or wait at its place for ferry to arrive. The architecture of the protocol is easily scalable as deployment of new infostations or ferries requires no network reconfiguration. An infostation can be made to serve more than four *Level* 1 zones (for simplicity we have taken only four zones under each infostation). Without configuring existing architecture a new level can be added. It also tries to reduce the average delays and to improve message delivery rate. Future work includes a refined analytical and experimental study for reinforcing our results. Comparison of the proposed protocol with already existing protocols will be done to analyze how it performs in comparison to them in terms of average message delay, number of messages delivered, etc.

References

1. Lilien L, Kamal ZH, Bhuse V, Gupta A (2006) Opportunistic networks: The concept and research challenges in privacy and security. In: Proceedings of NSF International workshop on research challenges in security and privacy for mobile andf wireless networks (WSPWN 2006), pp 134–147
2. Zhang Z (2006) Routing in intermittently connected mobile ad hoc networks and delay tolerant networks: overview and challenges. In: IEEE communications surveys and tutorials, first quarter 8(1):24–37
3. Fall K (2003) A delay-tolerant network architecture for challenged internets. In: ACM SIGCOMM, pp 27–34
4. Jain S, Fall K, Patra R (2004) Routing in a delay tolerant network. In: Proceeding of ACM SIGCOMM, pp 145–158
5. Chen L-J, Hung Yu C, Tseng C, Chu H, Chou C (2008) A content-centric framework for effective data dissemination in opportunistic networks. IEEE J Sel Areas Commun 26(5):761–772

6. Dhurandher SK, Sharma DK, Woungang I, Chao HC (2011) Performance evaluation of various routing protocols in opportunistic networks. In: IEEE GLOBECOM 2011, joint workshop of SCPA 2011 and SaCoNAS 2011, 5–9 Dec 2011, Houston, Texas, USA, pp 761–772
7. Huang C-M, Lan K-C, Tsai C-Z (2008) A survey of opportunistic networks. In: Proceedings of the 22nd International conference on advanced information networking and applications (WAINA), Biopolis, 25–28 March, Okinawa, Japan, pp 1672–1677
8. Pelusi L, Passarella A, Conti M (2006) Opportunistic networking: data forwarding in disconnected mobile ad hoc networks. IEEE Commun Mag 44(11):134–141
9. Goodman DJ, Borras J, Mandayam NB, Yates RD (1997) Infostations: a new system model for data and messaging services. In: IEEE VTC'97 2:969–973
10. Small T, Haas ZJ (2003) The shared wireless infostation model—a new ad hoc networking paradigm (or where there is a whale, there is a way). In: Proceedings of 4th ACM international symposium mobile ad hoc networking and computing (MobiHoc 2003), Annapolis, MD, June 1–3 2003, pp 233–244
11. Jain S, Shah RC, Bbrunette W, Borriello G, Roy S (2006) Exploiting mobility for energy efficient data collection in wireless sensor networks. In: ACM/Kluwer mobile networks and applications (MONET) 11(3):327–339
12. Zhao W, Ammar M, Zegura E (2004) A message ferrying approach for data delivery in sparse mobile ad hoc networks. In: Proceedings of 5th ACM international symposium mobile ad hoc networking and computing (Mobihoc), ACM Press, pp 187–198
13. Vahdat A, Becker D (2000) Epidemic routing for partially connected ad hoc networks, technical report CS-2000-06, Department of Computer Science, Duke University, Durham, NC

An Innovation in Education Through Cloud Computing

Vishal Paranjape and Vimmi Pandey

Abstract Today most of the learning activities are concerned on Web-based learning environment and it has become a major area on researching for remote education. The technique of cloud computing has got great recognition in many organizations with its dynamic scalability and usage of virtualized resources as a service through the Internet. Cloud computing is changing the way industries and enterprises do their businesses in that dynamically scalable and virtualized resources are provided as a service over the Internet. In this chapter, we discuss the use of cloud computing in the educational and learning arena, to be called "education and learning as a service" (ELaaS), emphasizing its possible benefits and offerings that will have a significant impact on the educational environment in the future. The concept of cloud computing is an excellent alternative for educational institutions which are constrained to a limited budget in order to operate their information systems effectively without spending any more capital for the computers and network devices. Universities take advantage of available cloud-based applications offered by service providers and enable their own users/students to perform business and academic tasks. In this chapter, we will review what the cloud computing infrastructure will provide in the educational sector, especially in the universities where the use of computers are more intensive and what can be done to increase the benefits of common applications for students and teachers.

Keywords Cloud computing · Virtualization · SaaS

V. Paranjape (✉)
CTA, CS Deptt, Gyan Ganga College of Technology, Jabalpur, India
e-mail: vishalparanjape@rediffmail.com

V. Pandey
Department of Information Technology, Gyan Ganga College of Technology, Jabalpur, India
e-mail: vimmipandey@ggits.org

V. Kumar and M. Bhatele (eds.), *Proceedings of All India Seminar on Biomedical Engineering 2012 (AISOBE 2012)*, Lecture Notes in Bioengineering,
DOI: 10.1007/978-81-322-0970-6_29,

Introduction

Cloud computing has emerged as an important factor for fulfilling educational computing needs. The term includes both the applications delivered as services over the Internet and the hardware and systems software in the datacenters that provide those services [1]. Another definition is given in (Cloud Computing, retrieved [2]): Cloud computing uses the Internet and central remote servers to maintain data and applications which is broken down into three segments: "applications", "platforms", and "infrastructure". The cloud is the term for networked computers that distribute processing power, applications, and large systems among many machines. The concept of cloud computing offers the educational sector a way to increase IT capacity and add on the fly capabilities without investing in new infrastructure, new training, or licensing new software. There is no need to setup, configure, and manage large physical installations of hardware and networks. This technology allows much more efficient computing by centralizing storage, memory, processing, and bandwidth. It reduces/eliminates problems associated with software version installation, control, and updates.

Approaches to E-Learning Services

E-learning services have evolved since computers were first used in education. There is a trend to move toward blended learning services, where computer-based activities are integrated with practical or classroom-based situations.

Computer-based learning:

Computer-based learning (CBL), sometimes abbreviated to CBL, refers to the use of computers as a key component of the educational environment. While this can refer to the use of computers in a classroom, the term more broadly refers to a structured environment in which computers are used for teaching purposes.

Computer-based training:

Computer-based trainings (CBTs) are self-paced learning activities accessible via a computer or handheld device. CBTs typically present content in a linear fashion, much like reading an online book or manual. For this reason they are often used to teach static processes, such as using software or completing mathematical equations. CBTs provide learning stimulus beyond traditional learning methodology from textbook, manual, or classroom-based instruction. For example, CBTs offer user-friendly solutions for satisfying continuing education requirements. Instead of limiting students to attending courses or reading printed manuals, students are able to acquire knowledge and skills through methods that are much more conducive to individual learning preferences. For example, CBTs offer visual learning benefits through animation or video, not typically offered by any other means and certificate programs via the Internet at a wide range of levels and in a wide range of disciplines. In addition, several universities offer online student support services, such as online advising and registration, e-counseling, online textbook purchase, student governments, and student newspapers.

Educational Usage of Cloud Computing

The recent trend in the E-Learning sector is screencasting. There are many screencasting tools available but the latest buzz is all about the web-based screencasting tools which allow the users to create screencasts directly from their browser and make the video available online so that the viewers can stream the video directly. The advantage of such tools is that it gives the presenter the ability to show his ideas and flow of thoughts rather than simply explain them, which may be more confusing when delivered via simple text instructions. With the combination of video and audio, the expert can mimic the one on one experience of the classroom and deliver clear, complete instructions. From the learner's point of view this provides the ability to pause and rewind and gives the learner the advantage of moving at their own pace, something a classroom cannot always offer.

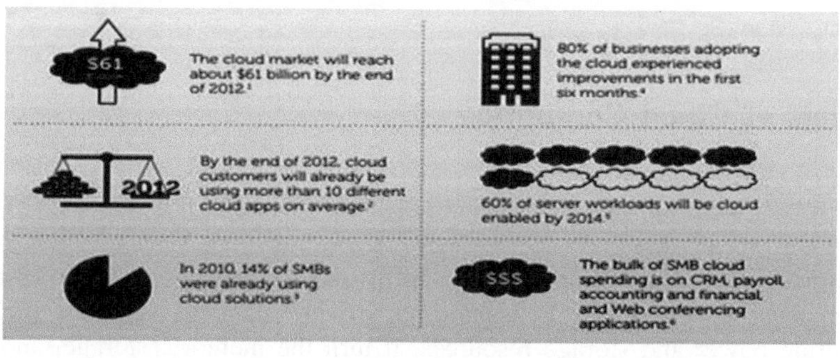

Cloud computing is a new business model wrapped around new technologies like virtualization, SaaS, and broadband internet. The cloud delivers computing and storage resources to its users/customers. It works as a service on demand policy. Recent interests offered new applications and elastic scalability with higher computing parameters. So that, these positive effects have shifted to outsourcing of not only equipment setup, but also the ongoing IT administration of the resources as well. The results of a survey that have been completed in 2009 by Gartner analysts (Fig. 1) about the IT trends (especially cloud computing) show that it is being used more in the areas of finance and business when compared to other sectors [3]. Results are shown as a pie chart and the labels on each different slice represent different industrial sectors and services. The "/" is used to separate different sectors with the same percentage.

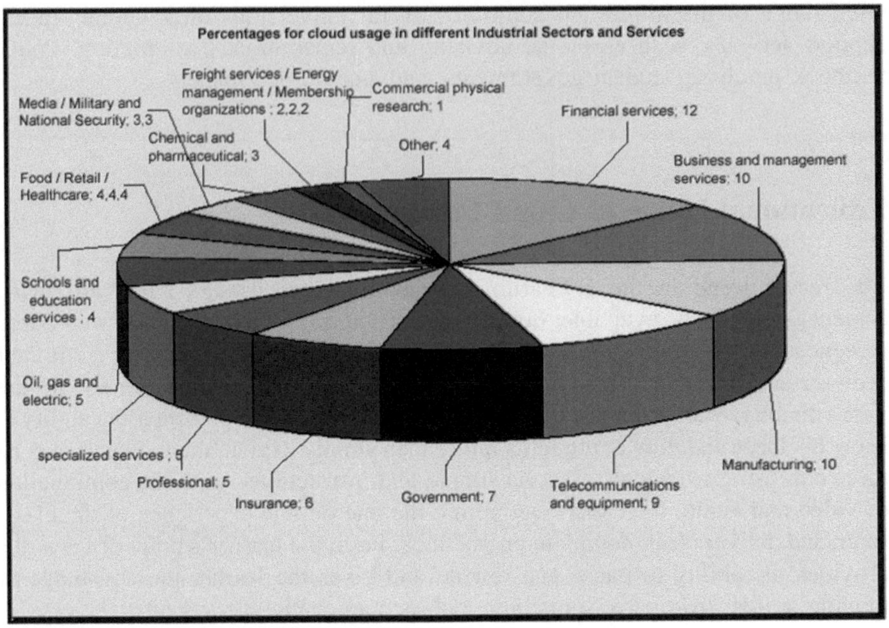

Fig. 1 Cloud usage

Services of Cloud Computing

IaaS

Infrastructure layer corresponds to IaaS infrastructure services, is the lowest layer of the network. Users can household to provide standard services, including computing power and storage resources. It turn the memory, storage, and computing power into a virtual whole resource pool for the entire industry to provide the required computing power and storage resources.

PaaS

Platform layer corresponds to platform as a service (PaaS) that made a higher level of abstraction on the base of Iaas layer to provide a development environment, test environment, server platforms, and other services, users can develop applications based on Internet and other servers service providers infrastructure, then share it to other users.

SaaS

Software as a service (SaaS) is a software distribution model, designed for web delivery, user can deploy and access through the Internet hosting. SaaS providers need to build information for all network infrastructure, software, hardware, operating platform, and is responsible for the implementation of all post-maintenance and other services. Compared with the traditional method of service, SaaS not only reduces the cost of traditional software licensing, and vendors deploy application software on a unified server, eliminating the end-user's server hardware, network security devices and software upgrade, and maintenance expenses, the customer does not need other IT investment in addition personal computers and Internet connections to obtain the required software and services.

Framework for Cloud-Based E-Learning

The Base Layer of E-Learning Cloud

The base layer of e-learning cloud shares IT infrastructure resources and connects the huge system pool together to provide services. Cloud computing allows the hardware layer to run more like the internet, to make the hardware resources shared and accessed as data resources in secure and scalable way. Virtualization technology separates the physical hardware from operating system, which on one hand can make computing and storage capacity of the existing server into smaller size and re-integration, to improve the utilization and flexibility of IT resource; on the other hand, can provide a common interface for large-scale cloud computing integration that enables the publication of calculation. The base layer can provide the basic hardware resources for the platform layer, and the users can also make use of it the same as using a local device.

The Platform Layer of E-Learning Cloud

With the support of the powerful hardware, platform layer carries out the tasks of data storage, computing, and software development, and it can even achieve the tasks of completion of the original mass data storage, business intelligence processing, and so on which have been difficult to complete. Users can choose the devices and the number of devices according to the complexity of dealing with the content. Virtualization technology enables the platform to show a strong level of flexibility.

The Application Layer of E-Learning Cloud

The application softwares or services provided by a school or university, the students to pay in the similar way of on-demand access, according to the amount to calculate the cost, complete the production, marketing, trading, and management. E-Learning cloud environment provides user-oriented ubiquitous adaptive hardware resources, computing environment, and software services. In e-learning cloud space, users can access to digital services transparently at any time in anywhere. The users can obtain the necessary network and computing services very naturally at any position. The information space and physical space will be integrated because of ubiquitous computing capability. And the ubiquitous information terminals together with the embedded system equipment will be the vehicles of e-commerce in the future.

E-Learning Application Model Based on Cloud Computing

With the progress and application of technology, the emergence of cloud computing offers e-learning good opportunity to develop, so we are convinced that it also can resolve the problem mentioned above properly. School or the enterprise neither needs to worry about the construction of the environment of e-learning software and hardware nor invest enormous capital and human and material resources to construct the system. All those issues can be handed to service providers of e-learning cloud, who can customize for users. In e-learning cloud model, data storage is highly distributed, data management is highly centralized, and data service is highly virtualized, all of which offer a much safer data service. Intelligent business policy-making. E-leaning cloud environment provides large data center with mass data storage and high-speed computation. This architecture for the cloud platform provides a variety of user interface forms, such as Web Service interfaces, Java interfaces, C interfaces, Shell interface, etc. Cloud computing platform provides resource services to teachers and students in the form of rental. A module is designed which is based on the consumption billing to ensure that users only pay for the resources they have used.

A promise of the cloud computing is the virtualization which reduces the number of servers required. Therefore, the key is to identify the user to meet the expected demand for the infrastructure needed to balance the amount of cloud: too few computing resources, the request from the user must wait for the release of resources or reject those requests until more hardware is added to the environment. Too much computing resources, hardware costs, and other expenses will be denied cost-cutting promises of cloud computing. In the cloud platform, teachers and administrators enter their requests for IT resources website (server, software, storage, etc.), immediately know whether these resources are available. If resources are available, submit a request immediately and automatically routed to the cloud administrator for approval. This process is automated, so it can be met in a very short period of time. Resource use planning and management are important activities of the cloud. Handled properly, the plan will provide needed capacity computing resources to create new solutions and to meet application performance goals, promote teaching, and researching goals.

Conclusions

Cloud computing as an exciting development is a significant alternative today's in educational perspective. Students and administrative personnel have the opportunity to quickly and economically access various application platforms and resources through the web pages on-demand. The gradually removal of software license costs, hardware costs, and maintenance costs, respectively provides great flexibility to the university/corporate management. From the points of advantages provided by cloud, there is a great advantage for university IT staff to take them away the responsibility of the maintenance burden in the university. Through the research we believe that, we can create an e-learning application model based on cloud computing by means of cloud computing's mass data storage, high-speed computing capabilities, as well as its ideal allocation, and the sharing mode of resources. Some problems such as platform security, technical standards, regulatory, and other services are not well resolved yet in practice, pending further research and exploration. Either way, e-learning application model based on cloud computing will not stop its pace to proceed. As the cloud computing technologies become more sophisticated and the applications of cloud computing become increasingly widespread, e-learning will certainly usher in a new era of cloud computing.

Adopting cloud network redundancy eliminates disaster recovery risks and its high costs. There can always be new tools and applications to improve IT features. There are of course some disadvantages too. The cloud computing services needed to deliver the majority of IT services needed by customers do not yet exist. There are still problems and constraints with application offerings, service-level agreements, more importantly security issues. All of the cloud providers do not have the same capability for their technological levels.

References

1. Armbrust M, Fox A, Griffith R, Joseph AD, Katz R, Konwinski A, Lee G, Patterson D, Rabkin A, Stoica I, Zaharia M (2009) Above the clouds: a Berkeley view of cloud, computing, Technical report no. UCB/EECS-2009-28. http://www.eecs.berkeley.edu/Pubs/TechRpts/2009/EECS-2009-28.pdf
2. DeCoufle B (2009) The impact of cloud computing on schools, http://datacenterjournal.com/content/view/3032/40/Educause
3. Gartner (2009) Cloud Computing Inquiries at Gartner, http://blogs.gartner.com/thomas_bittman/2009/10/29/cloud-computing-inquiries-atgartner

Digital Image Processing for the Thermal Images to Find Land Cover and Vegetation Density

Pragyan Jain and D. Dutta

Abstract Land surface temperature (LST) on spatial and temporal domain controls vital physical, chemical, and biological processes on Earth-atmosphere system. It is also an important parameter at regional scale for energy budgeting and global circulation. Surface temperature at an instant is controlled by a large number of land surface and atmospheric phenomena viz., surface energy balance, atmospheric state, thermal properties of surface, and subsurface medium along with sensor calibration parameters. Hence, understanding the interaction of outgoing long wave radiation with each of these components is important to model LST precisely. The process of retrieval of LST from satellite data starts with radiometric calibration followed by correction for atmospheric water vapor, aerodynamic transfer function, surface emissivity as well as combined effects of viewing geometry, background, and fractional vegetative cover. Once the approximation of LST is done, it needs to be evaluated with respect to ground based measurement. In the present study, Landsat 7 ETM+ high gain thermal data was used to examine the relationship between different types of surface cover and vegetation density with sensible heat flux derived from inverse Planck's model. Seasonal dynamics of LST under the similar land cover and vegetation condition was also examined. Large dynamic range among different land cover types was found in August (59°K) in comparison to May (22°K). The LST is highest for salt affected and barren lands during May and August, respectively. In contrast, water body appears colder in both the seasons. The result shows that there is strong relationship with surface cover and LST. Vegetation density in the nonvegetated areas does not show any distinct pattern, however, it

P. Jain (✉)
Gyan Ganga Institute of Technology and Sciences Jabalpur, MP 482003, India
e-mail: pragyanjain@rediffmail.com

D. Dutta
RRSC (East), NRSC, Indian Space Research Organisation Rajarhat, New Town, Kolkata 700 156, India

V. Kumar and M. Bhatele (eds.), *Proceedings of All India Seminar on Biomedical Engineering 2012 (AISOBE 2012)*, Lecture Notes in Bioengineering,
DOI: 10.1007/978-81-322-0970-6_30, © Springer India 2013

shows similar distribution in both the seasons. On the other hand, LST decreases, in general, with increasing density of vegetated areas. Hence, the study reveals that emissivity of surface cover and vegetation density has strong influence on LST retrieval and needs to be studied vis-à-vis intrinsic soil properties, vegetation, and atmosphere condition. It would help to thermally characterize different land cover types, the convective flow, and effect on biophysical processes.

Keywords Landsat ETM+ · LST · Landuse · Vegetation density · Emissivity · Heat island

Introduction

Land surface temperature (LST) is one of the important factor controlling most of the physical, chemical, and biological processes on the Earth. LST is controlled by a large number of land surface and atmospheric phenomena viz., surface energy balance, atmospheric state, thermal properties of surface, and subsurface mediums in conjunction with sensor calibration parameters. Hence, understanding the complex interaction of thermal energy with each of these components is utmost important to model the actual ground temperature. The approximated LST after atmospheric, sensor, and emissivity correction serves as important parameter for land surface characterization, energy budgeting, and global circulation pattern in global scale. A large number of on board sensors with varying resolution and thermal bands are available for modeling various Earth processes but the challenge remains in retrieval of précised ground temperature from at-sensor brightness temperature. As the outgoing long wave thermal radiation while passing through the atmosphere interacts with water vapor and aerosols, and the return signals gets attenuated due to atmospheric water vapor absorption or gets scattered due to aerosols. Hence, sensing of LST from space platform required rigorous calibration for interfering components of atmosphere. Besides atmosphere intrinsic surface properties and surface vegetation cover also modifies the ground radiance due to differential thermal inertia of land cover complex which consists of materials, water, vegetation, etc. In the present study, major emphasis was given to understand how different land cover types and vegetation density affect LST seasonally along with thermal characterization of different land cover complexes. Effort has been made to validate the satellite derived LST with limited ground measured temperature.

Study Area

The study area consists of two Rayons (district) of western Oblast (state) of Republic of Kazakhstan (Fig. 1). The Rayons are Chingarlausky and Karatobinsky occupying area of 17,105 km^2. The landform is predominantly marine and littoral

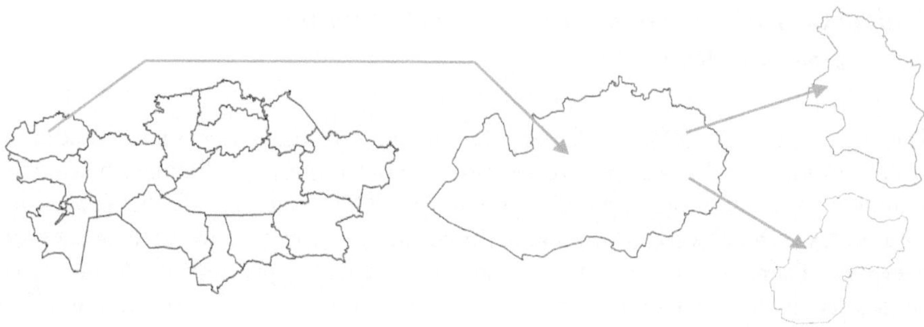

Fig. 1 Map of study area

plain along with traces of flat alluvium and dealluvium–proalluvium. The area is characterized by hot summer and very cold winter. During July to August, the average daily maximum temperature sores up to 40 °C in western Kazakhstan and in winter temperature falls below –6 °C. Average annual rainfall is less than 100 mm.

Materials and Methodology

Satellite Data Used

In the present study, Landsat7 ETM+ thermal band data of two different dates (29 May 2001 and 01 Aug 2001) of acquisition was used. The ETM+ includes new features that make it a more versatile and efficient instrument for global change studies, land cover monitoring, and assessment and large area mapping. The special feature of this sensor is its capability to provide thermal data in 60 m spatial resolution and in both high and low gain mode.

Landsat ETM+ thermal bandwidth is given below.

Band number	Spectral bandwidth (μm)	Ground resolution (m)
61 (low gain)	10.400–12.500	60
62 (high gain)	10.400–12.500	60

Landsat has 185 km swath, temporal resolution of 16 days, quantization of 8 bits, equatorial crossing time is 10:00 am.

Conversion of Thermal Band Digital Number into At-Sensor Radiance

The digital number (DN) has linear relationship with radiance. For calculation of radiance, upper and lower bounds of radiance are required to be known which is available in calibration parameter file (CPF). CPF contains all the processing parameters, which were downloaded from internet for specific date of satellite overpass. There are 15 radiometric and 11 geometric parameters. Radiometric parameters include detectors gain, bias, scaling parameters, etc. Conversion of DN into spectral radiance was performed using USGS [1] method as follows.

$$\text{Radiance }(L) = [(L_{\max} - - L_{\min})/255] * \text{DN} + L_{\min}$$

Conversion of Spectral Radiance to At-Sensor Temperature

At-sensor radiance was converted to a more useful variable namely the effective at-sensor temperature of viewed Earth-atmosphere system. The ETM+ thermal band data was converted from spectral radiance to at-sensor temperature assuming unity emissivity following the method given by Schott and Volchok [2], Wukelic et al. [3].

$$\mathrm{T_B}(^{\circ}\mathrm{K}) = K_2/\ln[(K_1 + L)/L].$$

Conversion of At-Sensor Brightness Temperature to LST

Estimation of LST from radiance directly does not represent a true surface temperature but a mixed signal or the sum of different fraction of energy. These fractions include energy emitted from the ground [4], upwelling radiance from the atmosphere, as well as downwelling radiance from the sky integrated over the hemisphere above the surface (Fig. 2).

Results and Discussion

Land Cover and Land Surface Temperature

Significant variation in near surface temperature exists among different land cover categories (Figs. 3 and 4) in both the seasons (May and August). Among different

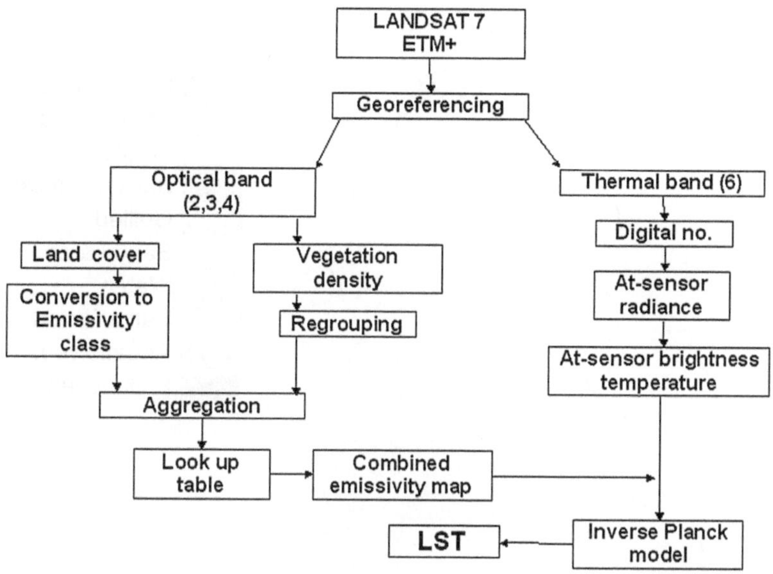

Fig. 2 Overall methodology for estimation of LST

land cover types, water body shows lowest surface temperature (Table 1) in both the seasons. The highest surface temperature was accounted for salt affected areas in May and over barren land during August. The results indicate effect of strong seasonal dependence on surface temperature under varying land cover types. The overall sequence of temperature (Fig. 5) under different land cover types from low to high, is as follows.

May: Water, Aquatic vegetation, Crop land, Fallow, Steppe, Eroded land, Built-up land, Barren, Sandy area, Salt affected area. Poor seperability is observed between fallow and steppe land, barren and sandy area.

August: Water, Aquatic vegetation, Crop land, Built-up land, Fallow, Salt affected area, Steppe land, Eroded land, Sandy area, Barren. Poor seperability was observed between fallow and steppe land, eroded, barren and sandy area, salt affected land and build-up land.

On the other hand, darker objects viz., barren land, rocks, etc., posses low albedo values and hence absorbs maximum solar radiation and emits more long wave thermal radiation during daytime and appears warmer. From the LST values, it is evident that during May the land cover classes which could be clearly identified are water, aquatic vegetation, crop, eroded land, salt affected land, and built-up land whereas during August only water, aquatic vegetation, and barren land could be identified. The class intermixing in thermal region was evident among built-up land, fallow, sandy area, and steppe land. The class intermixing of May and August are given in Tables 2 and 3, respectively.

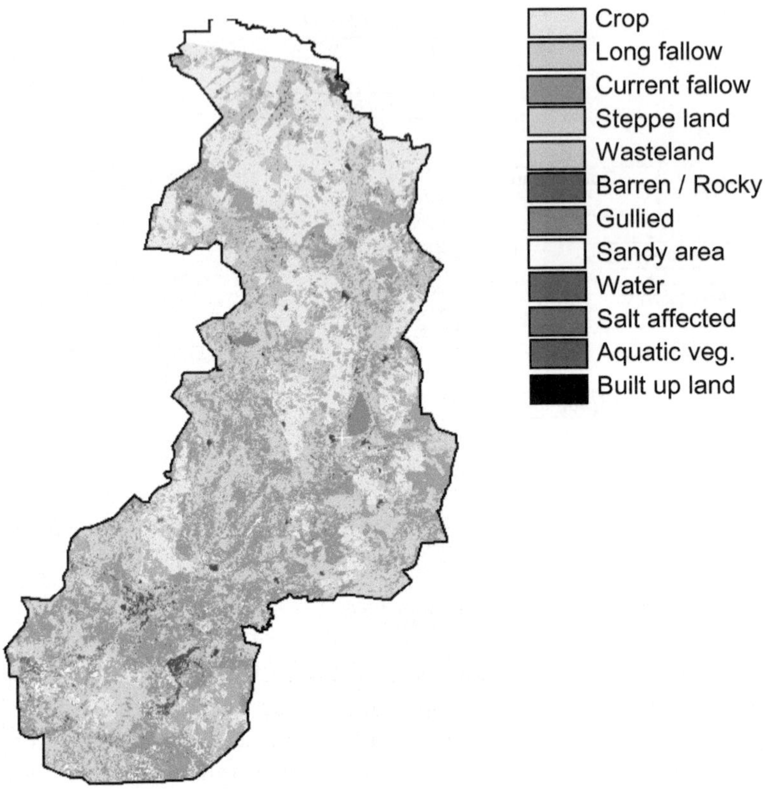

Fig. 3 Land cover map of May

Vegetation Density and Land Surface Temperature

The mean LST values under different vegetation density classes (Figs. 6 and 7) for nonvegetated and vegetated surfaces are given in Table 4.

Within vegetated surface (i.e. from VD8 to VD13) considerable difference in surface temperature exists (~4°K) in May due to differential crop growth and water balance. In general, surface temperature decreased with increased vegetation density, primarily due to low canopy air temperature difference as a result of high evaporative flux under unlimiting soil moisture. Similar trend is also observed in August except in higher vegetation density (VD12 and VD13) where the LST increases (Fig. 8), which indicates senescent vegetation with low evapotranspiration under limiting soil moisture. However, the dynamic range is ~4°K which is similar in both the dates of overpass.

The spatial variability of LST is higher over nonvegetated surface in both May (5.5°K) and August (9.8°K). The variation in August is more due to high air temperature induced large spatial dynamics of thermal inertia over water and bare

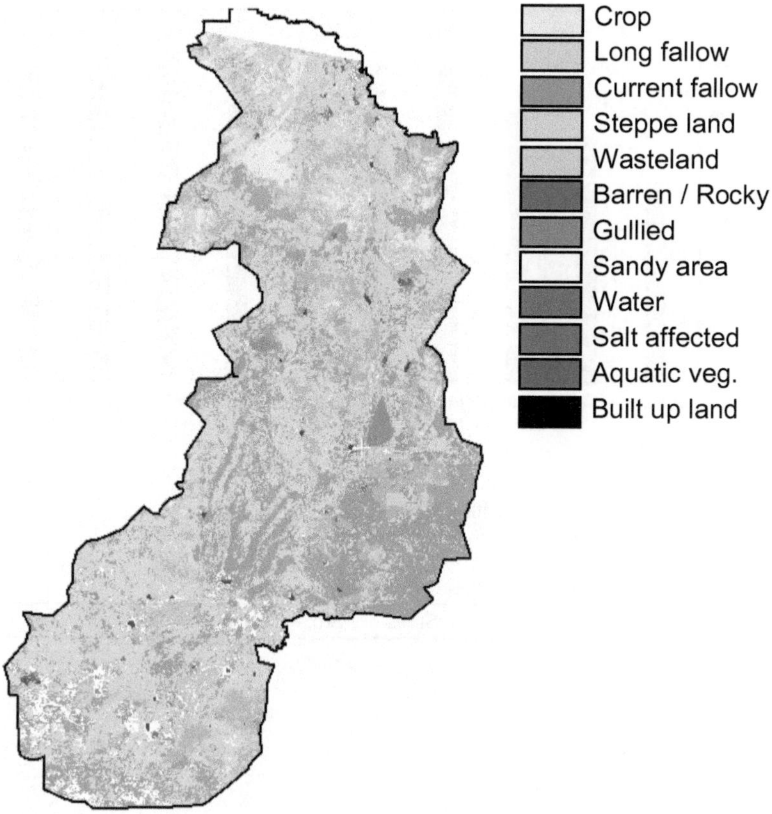

Fig. 4 Land cover map of August

Table 1 LST under different land cover classes

Land cover	May		August	
	Tmean	Tsd	Tmean	Tsd
Crop	294.69	1.31	305.38	1.33
Fallow	296.21	0.90	309.41	1.66
Steppe land	296.65	1.29	309.62	2.04
Barren	298.59	1.79	311.52	1.81
Eroded land	297.18	1.53	310.49	1.41
Sandy area	298.98	1.17	310.68	2.57
Water body	292.82	1.61	298.93	10.47
Salt affected	299.44	1.27	309.53	2.48
Aquatic vegetation	293.40	1.31	303.06	3.08
Built up land	297.58	1.39	309.16	1.42

Tmean mean LST, *Tsd* standard deviation within the cover type

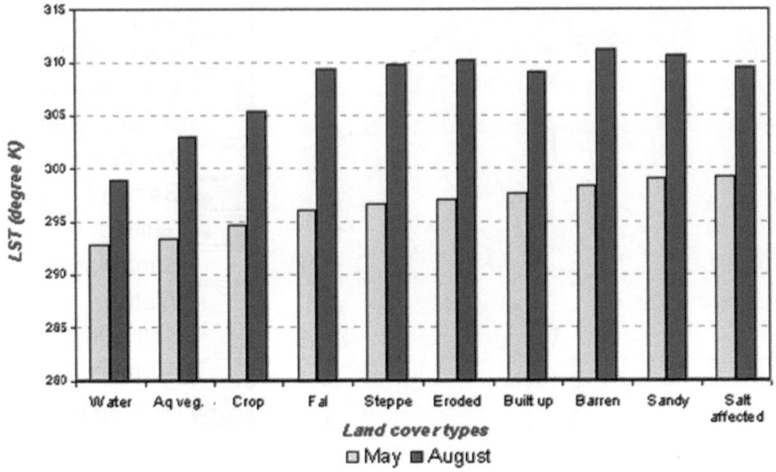

Fig. 5 Seasonal variation in LST with land cover

Table 2 Intermixing of land cover classes in thermal band (May)

	Aqv	Cro	Fal	Ste	Ero	Bul	Bar	San	Sal
Wat	x	x	x	x	x	x	x	x	x
Aqv		x	x	x	x	x	x	x	x
Cro			x	x	x	x	x	x	x
Fal					x	x	x	x	x
Ste					x	x	x	x	x
Ero						x	x	x	x
Bul							x	x	x
Bar									x
San									x

Table 3 Class intermixing during August

	Aqv	Cro	Fal	Ste	Ero	Bul	Bar	San	Sal
Wat	x	x	x	x	x	x	x	x	x
Aqv		x	x	x	x	x	x	x	x
Cro			x	x	x	x	x	x	x
Fal					x		x	x	
Ste					x		x	x	
Ero						x	x		x
Bul							x	x	
Bar								x	x
San									x

Wat water, *Aqv* aquatic vegetation, *Cro* crop land, *Fal* fallow, *Ste* steppe land, *Ero* eroded land, *Bul* buit-up land, *Bar* barren land, *San* sandy area, *Sal* saline area

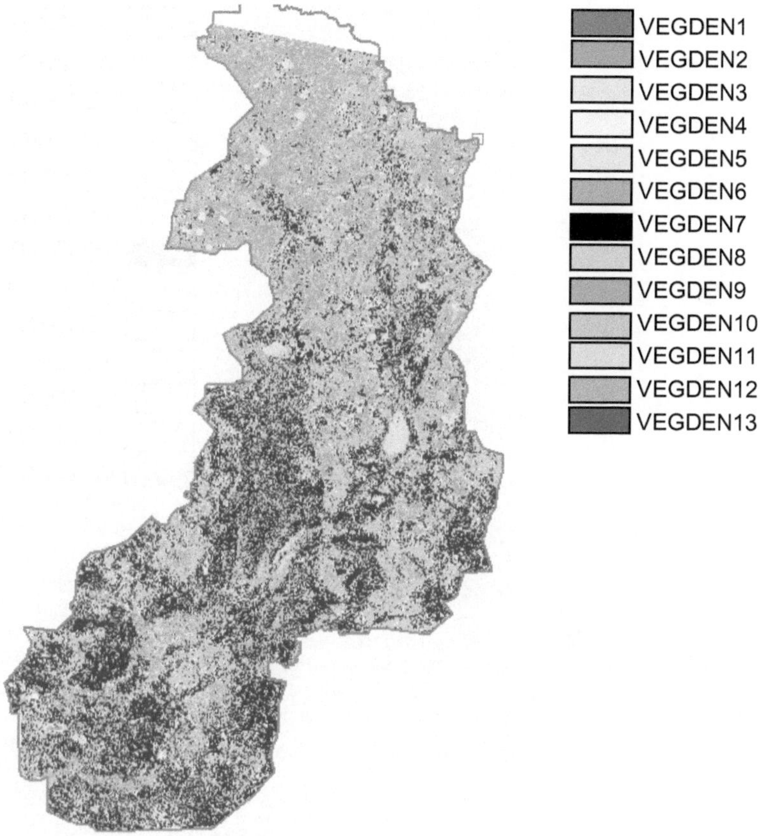

Fig. 6 Vegetation density map of May

land surface. In both the seasons, the distribution of NDVI and LST follows similar pattern except the standard deviation is more in August than May.

Seasonal Dynamics of Heat Island

Higher temperature (LST) is observed as a band recorded in central and scattered patches in south-west and eastern part of the study area during May (Fig. 9) whereas the heat islands move toward south-east and south i.e., in sandy and barren areas with higher intensity during August (Fig. 10). During August, the gradient is from south to north. Hence, it is probable that strong horizontal convection will take place during August and energy transfer would happen from south to north. On the other hand, the gradient is distributed in both south and

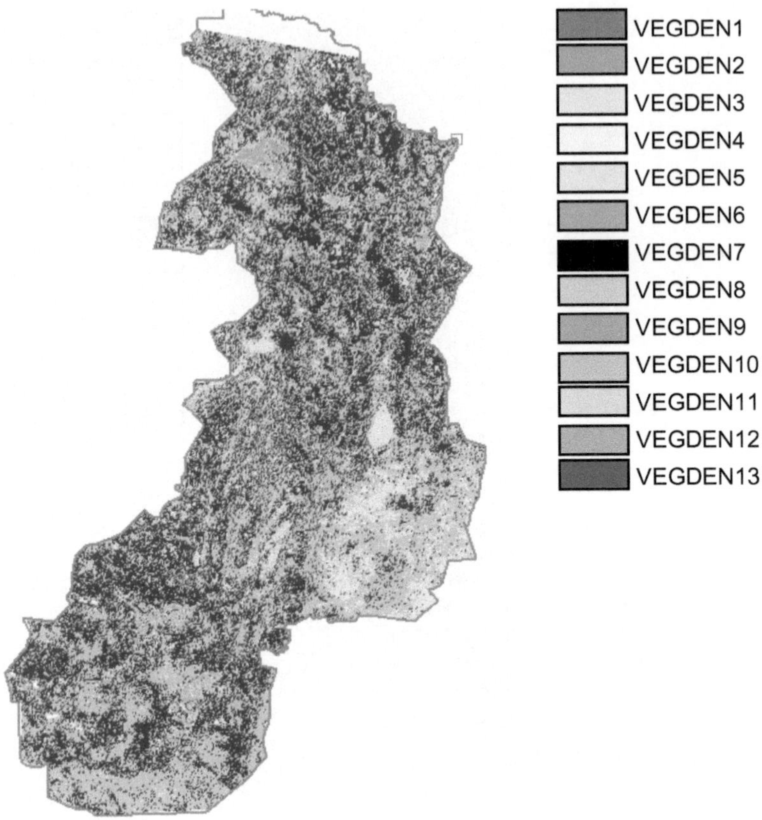

Fig. 7 Vegetation density map of August

Table 4 LST and vegetation density classes

Vegetation density classes	Mean LST (°K)	
	May	August
VD1	292.63	303.07
VD2	292.19	302.18
VD3	291.77	300.64
VD4	293.90	304.04
VD5	296.94	310.43
VD6	297.31	310.24
VD7	296.83	308.38
VD8	295.24	305.60
VD9	294.26	305.18
VD10	293.06	302.72
VD11	292.00	301.69
VD12	291.26	302.18
VD13	291.21	303.67

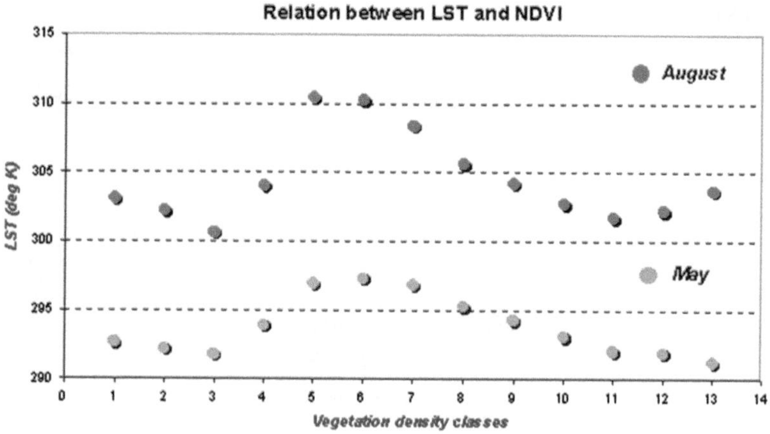

Fig. 8 Relation between LST and NDVI

Fig. 9 LST range during May

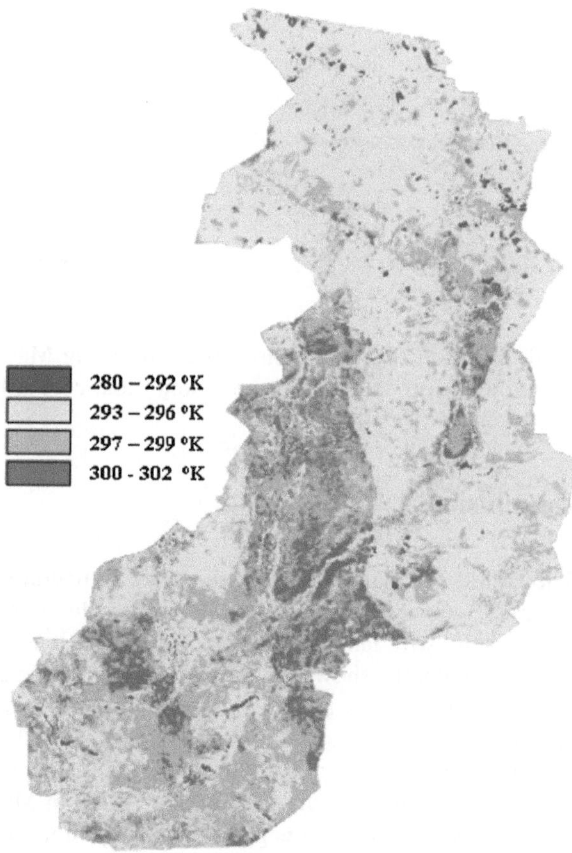

Fig. 10 LST range during August

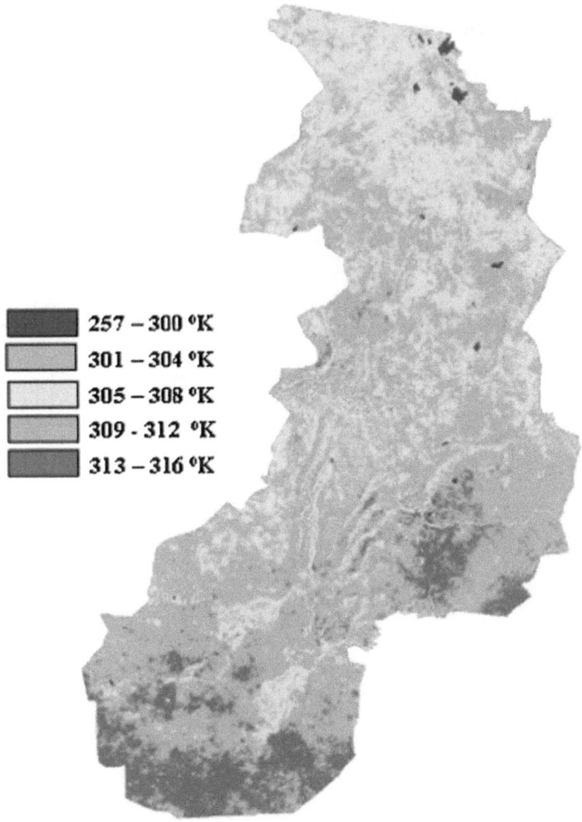

north direction from the central plateau during May, which would cause convective flow of low intensity in both south and northerly direction.

Conclusion

The ETM+ thermal band derived surface temperature provides more detailed and accurate temperature variation at microscale. Land surface temperature varies significantly with land cover types and vegetation density over the seasons. Water body consistently shows lowest brightness temperature and barren/salt affected area the highest due to low thermal inertia. During August, thermal characterization of some of the land cover class viz., fallow, steppe land, eroded land, barren, sandy, salt affected and built-up land becomes difficult due to considerable intermixing. However, the intermixing is less in May. In general, the LST follow the decreasing trend with vegetation density in the vegetated areas which is not so in barren areas. The shift of heat island is evident from central to southern part of the study area during May to August. This study of land cover complex–surface temperature relationship would help to understand the cause and dynamics of heat island.

References

1. USGS (2001) Landsat 7 Science data users handbook
2. Schott JR, Volchok WJ (1986) Thematic mapper thermal infrared calibration. Photogrammetric Eng Remote Sens 51(9):1351–1357
3. Wukelic GE, Gibbons DE, Martucci LM, Foote HP (1989) Radiometric calibration of landsat thematic mapper thermal band. Remote Sens Environ 28:339–347
4. Sutherland RS, Bartholic JR (1979) Emissivity correction for interpreting thermal radiation from a terrestrial surface. J Appl Meteorol 18:1165–1171

PID Controller Tuning Using Soft Computing Techniques

Nikhileshwar Prasad Adhikari and Amit Gupta

Abstract The aim of this paper is to design a position control of a DC motor by selection of a PID controller using genetic algorithm. This paper compares two kinds of tuning methods of parameter for PID controller. One is the controller design by the genetic algorithm, second is the controller design by the Ziegler and Nichols method. It was found that the proposed PID parameters adjustment by the genetic algorithm is better than the Ziegler and Nichols' method. This proposed method could be applied to the higher order system also.

Keywords DC shunt motor · PID controller · Ziegler Nichols method · Genetic algorithm

Introduction

DC drive systems are often used in many industrial applications, such as robotics, actuation, and manipulators. In the first two, a wide range of position control is required. Tuning method for PID controller is very important for the process industries. Proportional Integral Derivative (PID) controllers have the advantage of simple structure, good stability, and high reliability [1]. Accordingly, PID controllers are widely used to control system outputs, especially for systems with

N. P. Adhikari (✉)
Department of Electrical Engineering, Control System, Gyan Ganga College of Technology, Jabalpur, India

A. Gupta
Department of Electrical Engineering, Takshshila Institute of Engineering and Technology, Jabalpur, India

V. Kumar and M. Bhatele (eds.), *Proceedings of All India Seminar on Biomedical Engineering 2012 (AISOBE 2012)*, Lecture Notes in Bioengineering,
DOI: 10.1007/978-81-322-0970-6_31, © Springer India 2013

accurate mathematical models. The key issue for PID controllers is the accurate and efficient tuning of parameters. In practice, controlled systems usually have some features, such as nonlinearity, time-variability, and time delay, which make controller parameter tuning more complex. Moreover, in some cases, system parameters and even system structure can vary with time and environment. As a result, the traditional PID parameter tuning methods are not suitable for these difficult calculations.

As a popular optimization algorithm, the GA had been widely used to turn PID parameters. Soltoggio [2] proposed an improved GA for tuning controllers in classical, first and second order plants with actuator nonlinearities. Chen and Wang [3] used the population-based distribution GA to optimize a PID controller, and found that the search capability of the algorithm was improved by competition among distribution populations in order to reduce the search zone. The PID controllers based on GAs have good performance and have been applied in practice.

The aim of this paper is to design a plant using Genetic Algorithm. Genetic Algorithm or in short GA is a stochastic algorithm based on principles of natural selection and genetics. Genetic algorithms (GAs) are a stochastic global search method that mimics the process of natural evolution. Genetic algorithms have been shown to be capable of locating high performance areas in complex domains without experiencing the difficulties associated with high dimensionality or false optima may occur with normal PID techniques. Using genetic algorithms to perform the tuning of the controller will result in the optimum controller being evaluated for the system every time.

In order to solve this problem a PID controller under Genetic Algorithm with self-tuning is applied, which will perform high efficiency position control. The efficiency of Control Algorithm is presented through a simulation and compared with the quality of PID controller.

Mathematical Modeling of DC Motor

Modeling Scheme

As reference we consider a DC shunt motors as is shown in Fig. 1. DC shunt motors have the field coil in parallel (shunt) with the armature. The current in the field coil and the armature are independent of one another. As a result, these motors have excellent speed and position control [1]. Hence DC shunt motors are typically used applications that require five or more horse power.

The input voltage V is applied to the field winding which has a resistance and inductance of R and L, respectively. The armature current supplied to the armature is kept constant and thus the motor shaft is controlled by the input voltage. The field current produces a flux in the machine which in turn produces a torque at

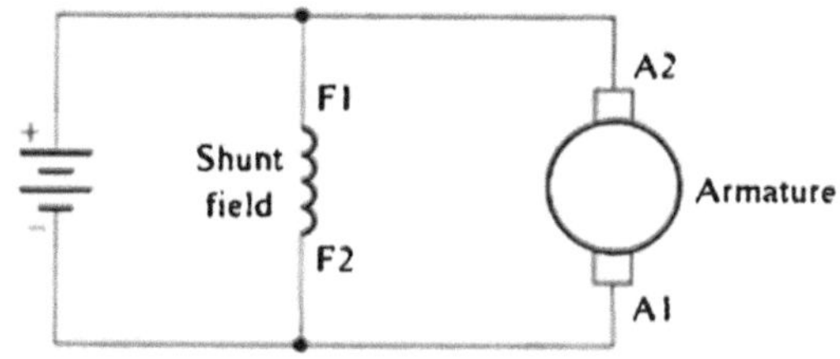

Fig. 1 Diagram of DC shunt motor

the motor shaft. The moment of inertia and the coefficient of viscous friction at the motor shaft are J_m and f_m, respectively. The angular shaft resulting in the motor shaft being θ_m and the corresponding angular velocity being ω_m.

System Equations

The armature current is kept constant and the relationship between the developed motor torque Tm and the field current is given by

$$T_m \alpha\, i_f \quad (1)$$

$$T_m = K_f i_f \quad (2)$$

The equations describing the dynamic behavior of the DC motor are given by the following equations;

$$V = R_i + L(\mathrm{d}i/(\mathrm{d}t)) + eb \quad (3)$$

$$T_m = K_t i_a \quad (4)$$

$$T_m = J_m(d\hat{}2\theta_m)/(\mathrm{d}t)\hat{}2 + f_m\,\mathrm{d}\theta_m/\mathrm{d}t \quad (5)$$

$$T_m = J_m(\mathrm{d}\omega_m)/\mathrm{d}t + f_m\omega_m \quad (6)$$

Simplification and taking the ratio of θ(s)/v(s) we will get the transfer function as below,

$$\Theta(s)/\ v(s) = K_b\ /\ [J\,L_a\ S3\ +\ (R_a\,J + B\,L_a)S2\ +\ (K_b2 + R_a\,B)S] \quad (7)$$

Where, R_a = Armature resistance in ohm, L_a = Armature inductance in Henry, i_a = Armature current in ampere, V_a = Armature voltage in volts, $e_b = e(t)$ = Back emf voltage in volts, K_b = back emf constant in volt/(rad/sec), K_t = torque constant in N-m/Ampere, T_m = torque developed by the motor in N-m, $\theta(t)$ = angular displacement of shaft in radians, J = moment of inertia of motor and load in Kg-m^2/rad, B = frictional constant of motor and load in N-m/(rad/sec)

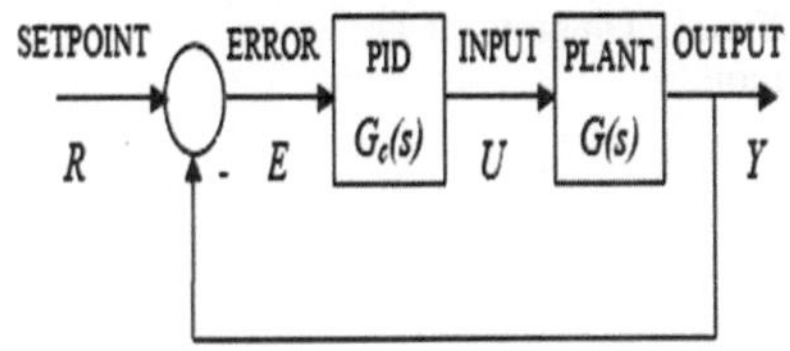

Fig. 2 PID control

Motor Specifications and Parameter

2hp, 230 v, 8.5 A, 1500 rpm;

$R_a = 2.45$ ohm, $L_a = 0.035$ H, $K_b = 1.0$ v/(rad/sec), $J = 0.022$ kg-m^2/rad, $B = 0.5 * 10^{-3}$ N-m/(rad/sec).

$$(\Theta(s))/(v(s)) = 1.0/(0.00077s\wedge 2\,0.0539s\wedge 1 + 1.441). \quad (8)$$

Tuning of PID Controller Using Ziegler–Nichols Approach

The block diagram shown in Fig. 2 illustrates a closed-loop system with a PID controller in the direct path, which is the usual connection. The system's output should follow as closely as possible the reference signal (set point) [4, 5].

The tuning of a PID controller consists of selecting gains K_p, K_i, and K_d so that performance specifications are satisfied (Table 1). By employing Ziegler–Nichols's method for PID tuning [6, 7] those gains are obtained through experiments with the process under control. Controller tuning involves the selection of the best values of K_p, K_i, and K_d. PID gain values after simulation is given in Table 2, (Fig. 3).

Tuning of PID Controller Using Genetic Algorithm Approach

Genetic algorithm (GA) is a heuristic mimicking the natural evolution process and is routinely used to generate useful solutions to optimization problems. In this paper, the genetic algorithm is used to derive the PID controller parameters. In GA [6, 7], a population of strings called chromosomes, encodes the possible solutions of an optimization problem and evolves for a better solution by process of reproduction (Fig. 4).

The process of evolution starts from a population of randomly generated individuals. Optimization is achieved in generations where in each generation, the fitness function evaluates each individual in the population and multiple individuals are selected stochastically based on their fitness. These selected individuals are modified to form a new population. The algorithm terminates when either a

Table 1 Recommended PID value setting

Types of controller	K_p (Ker)	T_i	T_d
P	0.5	0	0
PI	0.45	(1/1.2) Per	0
PID	0.6	0.5 Per	0.125 Per

Table 2 PID values

K_p	K_i	K_d
18	6.3223	12.811

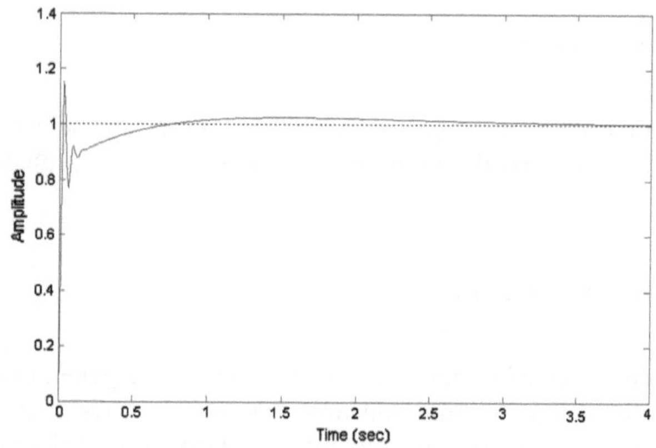

Fig. 3 Closed-loop step responses for DC shunt motor

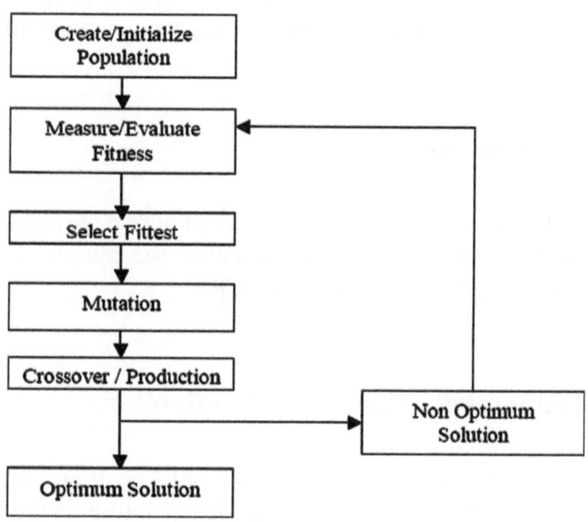

Fig. 4 Genetic algorithm process flowchart

maximum number of generations has been produced, or a satisfactory fitness level has been reached for the population [8]. The various steps in GA-based optimization are detailed below:

Initialization

From the initial population few individual solutions are generated. The population is generated randomly, covering the entire range of possible solutions.

Selection

In each generation, individual solutions are selected by evaluating the fitness function and the fitter solutions have a higher probability of selection.

Reproduction

Next set of population for the successive generation is generated by a process called reproduction and involves crossover (recombination) and mutation. These results in a new set of population derived from the fitter solutions of the previous population. Generally the average fitness of the population is heightened as compared to the population of the previous population.

Termination

The process of optimization is halted once a termination condition is achieved. The termination condition can be either the number of generations or the solution satisfying an optimum criterion [9].

Implementation of GA Controller

GA can be applied to the tuning of PID position controller gains to ensure optimal control performance at nominal operating conditions [10, 11]. The Genetic Algorithm parameters chosen for the tuning purpose (Table 3, Fig. 5).

Table 3 Parameters of GA

GA property	Value/method
Population size	80
Fitness function	MSE
Selection method	Geometric selection
Crossover method	Arithmetic
Number of crossover points	3
Mutation method	Uniform mutation
Mutation probability	0.01

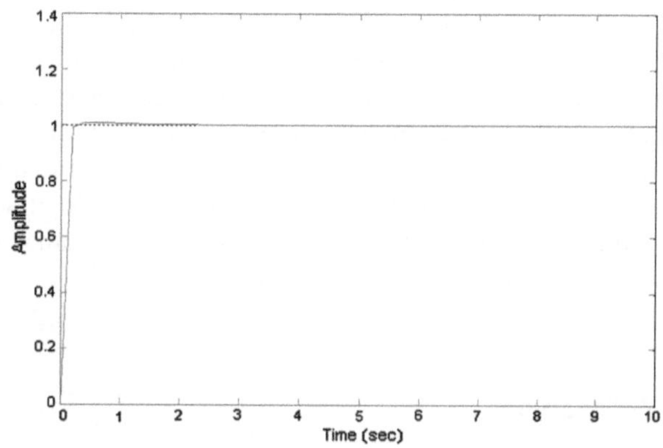

Fig. 5 Position control using genetic algorithm

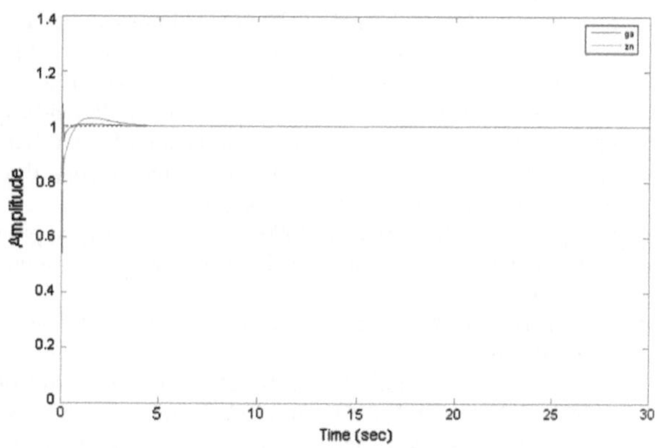

Fig. 6 Comparison of GA and ZN technique

Analysis of Result

All the conventional methods of controller tuning lead to a large settling time, overshoot, rise time, and steady-state error of the controlled system. Hence a soft computing techniques are introduced into the control loop. GA-based tuning methods have proved their excellence in giving better results by improving the steady-state characteristics and performance indices (Fig. 6, Table 4).

Table 4 Comparison of results

Tuning method	Rise time (s)	Maximum overshot	Settling time (s)
Ziegler Nichols	0.18	1.08	2.41
Genetic algorithm	0.161	1.01	0.7

Conclusion

The GA algorithm for PID controller tuning presented in this research offers several advantages. The errors resulting from model reduction are avoided. It is possible to consider several design criteria in a balanced and unified way. Approximations that are typical to classical tuning rules are not needed. Soft computing techniques are often criticized for two reasons: algorithms are computationally heavy and convergence to the optimal solution cannot be guaranteed. PID controller tuning is a small-scale problem and thus computational complexity is not really an issue here. It took only a couple of seconds to solve the problem. Compared to conventionally tuned system, GA tuned system has good steady-state response and performance indices.

References

1. Ogata K (1987) Discrete-time control systems. University of Minnesota, Prentice Hall
2. Soltoggio A (2005) An enhanced GA to improve the search process reliability in tuning of control systems. In: Proceedings of the 2005 conference genetic and evolutionary computation, GECCO'05, Washington, pp 2165–2172
3. Chen QG, Wang N (2005) The distribution population-based genetic algorithm for parameter optimization PID controller. Acta Automatica Sinica 31:646–650
4. Astrom K, Hagglund T (1995) PID controllers: theory, design and tuning. Instrument Society of America. Research triangle park, NC
5. Chowdhuri S, Mukherjee A (2000) An evolutionary approach to optimize speed controller of dc machines. In: Proceedings of IEEE international conference on industrial technology, Cilt 2, 682–687
6. Chambers L (1999) Practical handbook of genetic algorithms: complex coding systems. CRC, Boca Raton
7. Pelczewski PM, Kunz UH (1990) The optimal control of a constrained drive system with brushless dc motor. Ind Electron IEEE Trans on 37(5): 342–348
8. Goldberg DE (1989) Genetic algorithms in search, optimization and machine learning. Addison-Wesley Pub. Co, Boston
9. Chipperfield AJ, Fleming PJ, Pohlheim H, Fonseca CM (1994) A genetic algorithm toolbox for MATLAB. In: Proceedings international conference on systems engineering, coventry, UK, 6–8 Sept 1994
10. Kristinsson K, Dumont GA (1992) System identification and control using genetic algorithms. Syst Man Cybern IEEE Trans on 22(5): 1033–1046
11. Mahony TO, Downing CJ, Fatla K (2000) Genetic algorithm for PID parameter optimization: minimizing error criteria. Proc Control Instrum 2000: 26–28

Improvising the Ad hoc on Demand Distance Vector Routing Protocol When Nodes or Links Fails

Brijesh Soni, Biplab Kumar Sarkar and Arjun Rajput

Abstract Networks are being used in various areas and the demand of users' nowadays has motivated the emergence of the mobile ad-hoc network (MANET). MANET is a dynamic network without the fixed infrastructure due to their wireless nature and topology and changes due to their dynamic nature. Among various protocol used as routing protocol in the MANET the ad-hoc on-demand distance vector (AODV) is most popular and widely used due to their various beneficial characteristics. But its beneficial characteristics will degrades when nodes or links fails as it sends the error message back to the source and whole process is repeated again. In this chapter, we propose an method to carry forward the data packet when nodes or links fail from the last node it receives. This chapter will really improves the factors likes throughput, reliability, security, packet size, overheads, traffic congestion.

Keywords Reactive · Proactive · Hybrid protocol · Ad-hoc on-demand distance vector (AODV) routing · Mobile ad-hoc network (MANET) · Take another best route (TABR) · Acknowledgment to intermediate nodes (ACKI) · Acknowledgment to source nodes (ACKS) · Source (S) · Destination (d)

B. Soni (✉) · A. Rajput
CSE Department, T.I.T, Bhopal, India
e-mail: brijeshsoni91288@gmail.com

A. Rajput
e-mail: rajarjun07@gmail.com

B. K. Sarkar
CSE Department, T.I.T (Excellence), Bhopal, India
e-mail: dr.biplabkumarsarkar@yahoo.com

V. Kumar and M. Bhatele (eds.), *Proceedings of All India Seminar on Biomedical Engineering 2012 (AISOBE 2012)*, Lecture Notes in Bioengineering,
DOI: 10.1007/978-81-322-0970-6_32,

Introduction

Wireless networks can be broadly classified into infrastructure-based wireless network and infrastructure wireless networks or ad-hoc networks. In ad-hoc networks, the nodes are mobile and routing between source and destination node is achieved by intermediate nodes acting as routers if it not in radio range. As ad-hoc networks are highly dynamic, routing protocols play a crucial role to achieve quality of service. Other important factors to be considered in ad-hoc networks are dynamic networks topology, frequency of network updates, scalability, security, and energy required. Basically MANET [1] is a group of wireless computing devices like Laptop, mobile phone, personal digital assistant (PDA), or similar devices. In ad-hoc networks routing protocols are broadly classified into proactive (table driven) routing protocol, reactive (On-demand) routing protocols, and hybrid protocols.

In proactive routing each node in the ad-hoc network maintains a table or tables containing routing information of the network. Any node that needs to transmit data can start transmitting data using routes already present in the routing table enabling immediate data transmission. Popular proactive routing protocols include destination sequence distance vector (DSDV) [2] routing protocol, wireless routing protocol (WRP) [3], and optimized link state routing protocol (OLSR) [3]. The advantages of proactive routing protocols update its routing table irrespective of data traffic.

Unlike table-driven routing protocols, reactive protocols update routing information only when a route is required by a source node to transmit data. Reactive routing protocols reduce the control overhead which is advantageous in high mobility networks, whereas periodic updates in routing information leads to significant increase in networks overheads even when there is no data transmission between nodes in the networks. Some of the popular ad-hoc routing protocols falling in this category are dynamic source routing (DSR) [4], ad-hoc on-demand distance vector (AODV) [4, 5] routing and temporarily ordered routing protocols (TORA) [4].

In this chapter, our major objective is to build the ADOV routing protocol in such way that it can handle in a better way at the time of nodes or links failure. This chapter will avoid the procedure taken by the data packet in case of nodes or links fails in the AODV routing protocol thus they make it more efficient and faster and improves certain characteristics.

ADOV Routing Protocols

AODV is an adaptation of destination sequenced distance vector (DSDV) protocol used in wired networks and overcomes the shortcomings of DSDV in wireless environment. AODV eliminates the counting to infinity problem faced in other distance vector protocols by implementing a sequence number. Unlike DSR which carries the entire route between the source and destination in the packet, the nodes in AODV carry only the next hop information corresponding to each data flow. Being a reactive routing protocol route is discovered as when needed and the discovered routes are maintained as long as they are required.

A route discovery is initiated [4] when one of the nodes in the network wants to send a data packet to another node. If an active route is not available AODV initiates the route discovery process with the source node broadcasting a route request message (RREQ) to find a route to the destination. The route is found either with the RREQ reaching the destination or an intermediate node in the network which has "fresh enough" route to the destination with the sequence number equal to or greater than the sequence number contained in the RREQ. Once a valid route is found it is made available by a route reply (RREP) message back to the originator of the RREQ. Once the route is established the nodes monitor the state of the links continuously. If a link breaks in an active route, a route error message (RERR) is sent to the other nodes of the link breakage. This initiates a new route discovery process.

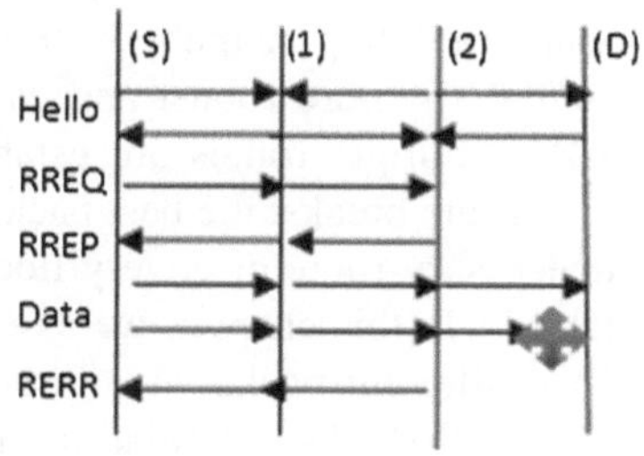

The advantages of AODV routing protocol are the selection of the least congested route instead of the shortest path. AODV supports both uncast and multicast data transmission. Performance is not drastically affected even if the topology changes continuously. Since source routing is not used, there are no additional overheads in the data.

Recent Work

There are so many developments that took place in an AODV routing protocols. They are as follows:

1. Corson et al. [6] have presented a loop-free, distributed routing protocol for mobile packet radio networks. The protocol was designed for networks, which does not change too fast or near-static networks. The objective of the routing algorithm was to build routes only when necessary and to build them quickly before topology changes. The proposed protocol maintains source-initiated,

loop-free multipath routing only to desired destinations. Thus, the overhead is reduced even in a varying topology.

2. Kim et al. [6] have proposed a reverse AODV (R-AODV) routing mechanism which attempts multiple route replies. In mobile ad-hoc networks, the nodes move autonomously due to which the topology of the network is highly dynamic. Ad-hoc routing protocols use single RREP along the reverse path. The proposed R-AODV addresses the problem by attempting multiple route replies. The proposed protocol introduces a novel aspect compared to other on-demand routing protocols on ad-hoc Networks: it reduces the path fail correction messages and obtains better performance than the AODV and other protocols have.
3. Tomar et al. [6] have proposed algorithm for selective flooding in place of broadcasting to overcome flooding problems in the network. The proposed algorithm reduces the routing packet overhead and can be incorporated in the AODV algorithm.
4. Tang et al. [6, 7], have proposed a robust AODV (RAODV) protocol for building routes on-demand and maintaining them. The proposed protocol is maintained by updating route information locally i.e., the active route information is broadcasted only to 1-hop neighbors, thus, the overhead due to updating is low. The RAODV is more robust and easily adapted to mobility than the traditional AODV. Multiple routes are established by the proposed protocol. Thus, when active route breaks, the best backup route can become the active route avoiding unnecessary route discovery flooding.
5. Zahian Ismail and Rosilah [8]. In this chapter, we assessed the performance of AODV routing protocol for different packet size in homogeneous and heterogeneous MANET through the OMNeT++ simulation. In the simulation, the size of the packets transmit has a high impact on throughput and PDR in wireless environment. Overall, the result shows as the size of packet increases, the throughput and PDR will also increase except for certain circumstances when the size of packets achieve certain limits as the large packet size keeps the transport layer channel busy and it affected the value.
6. Zongwei Zhou [2]. In this chapter, a set of novel security mechanisms based on the AODV are proposed. Three techniques, including digital signature, one-way hash function, and double one-way hash verification ensure the authentication, no repudiation, and integrity of important routing information in RREQ, RREP, and RERR packet of AODV.
7. Saleem. Sheik Aalam et al. [9] Mobile ad-Hoc networks pose a problem of finding stable multi-hop routes for communication between source to destination. This chapter proposes an adaptive routing protocol which extends ad-hoc on-demand multipath distance vector (AOMDV) routing. Specifically, the proposed approach (NP-AOMDV) focuses on the node prediction by using different approaches. Predicting the node movement can be done by avoiding the frequent link failures in ad-hoc environments. The performance of the

NP-AOMDV, throughput, End-To-End delay, routing control overhead compares with the well-known AOMDV.
8. Jyoti Jain et al. [10], MANET is a wireless self-organized distributed network. This chapter gives a general survey of research on local repair of link, if it is broken during communication for MANET and proposes a new local repair scheme in order to make up the deficiency of the existing local repair schemes. The improved local repair scheme concerns about the over head requirement and end-to-end delay in transmission. Nodes are required to keep the next two-hop node address for each route entry in routing table. During local repair, the repairing node uses Ant algorithm for finding new route for next-to-next node in the link considering that other part of the link is already in existence. Reduced size of F-ANT and B-ANT will give significant reduction in overhead. In this case, repairing node not only tries to discover the route to the destination node of data packet, but also attempts to establish the route to its downstream node (i.e., the next hop node). The proposed algorithm will be highly adaptive, scalable, and efficient and mainly reduces end-to-end delay in high mobility cases.

Problem Occurs

By all the recent work done by the researchers in field of the AODV routing protocols will increase the performance of the AODV routing protocols to a great extent. But despite of that if nodes or links fails then this performance will be going to suffer a lot [4]. There are several points that needs to be considered which degrades the performance of the AODV routing protocols when nodes or links fails they are [11]:

1. Suppose nodes or links fails then error message is sent back to the source this will activate the source nodes to resend the data back to destination and this will take too much time to perform the whole procedure again.
2. Time consuming [4].
3. Traffic congestion increases as same packet is send again and again.
4. The effect of traffic congestion will pay impact on the performance/throughput of AODV system due to resending of same packet will cause other nodes waited to send data.
5. The security [2] of AODV will be based on one-way hashed, two-hashed, and digital signature. All the three security procedure consist of several steps, several inbuilt functions that need to be applied, extensive procedure needs to be applied before sending and receiving the packet. Now suppose if nodes or links fails so all procedure, steps, inbuilt function needs to be applied again to same packet.

Solution Proposed

In this chapter, we propose to send the data packet from the last nodes it received when nodes or links fails instead of sending back. As if this has been done as suggested in this chapter will provide beneficial to AODV system like:

1. Network performance as well as throughput increases.
2. Less time consuming.
3. Traffic congestion will not occur.
4. Other nodes will not be going to wait for nodes that are sending.
5. We do not need to apply Security steps, procedure, and function again and again on the same data packet and hence security increases.
6. As AODV is dynamic in nature therefore its topology changes quickly so it helps to send the data quickly before changing its topology.

Algorithm Proposed

- In mobile ad-hoc network all nodes exchange periodic hello message to have information about its neighbors. Nodes also update its neighbors list periodically.
- If any node (source node) in the network wise to communicate with other node (Destination node) in the network, it look for required node in node list. If this is not available then source node will generate RREQ. Format for route request will be similar as in original AODV.
- When destination node or any node in the links have path up to destination receives route request, it generate RREP toward source node. RREP packet modifies routing table at each node. In our proposed algorithm, we used the methodology proposed by Kim, i.e., R-AODV routing mechanism which attempts multiple route replies. In mobile ad-hoc networks, the nodes move autonomously due to which the topology of the network is highly dynamic. The proposed R-AODV addresses the problem by attempting multiple route replies.
- When source node receives RREP, route for destination is available. Communication is possible from this node to required destination.
- During the communication liveliness of link is assured by periodic hello message. If link break is detected by missing two consecutive hello messages, proposed new algorithm is activated.
- In the case of link failure due to either node movement or power failure or any other reason an error message is generated to source (RERR). In our proposed algorithm the source now sends an another best route to last nodes in which data received (or RERR comes from) since it is having multiple route to destination (as Kim et al. R-AODV) under the Take another best route (TABR) packet.

- Now that intermediate nodes match location of it into new route and send data through that route to destination.
- Now when destination received data it first acknowledges that intermediate nodes under acknowledgment to intermediate nodes (ACKI).
- Last, the intermediate node acknowledges to source node under acknowledgment to source nodes (ACKS).

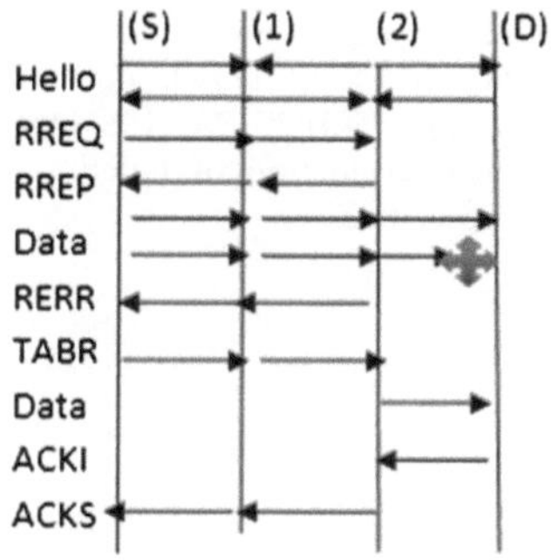

Conclusion

In this chapter, we will propose that in AODV routing protocols, the best way is to carry forward the data packet instead of sending back when nodes or links fails. This chapter will pose an great impact over the performance, security, traffic intensity, time consuming, and hence it will definitely increases throughput of AODV routing protocol system. As ADOV routing protocols are dynamic in nature it is necessary to send the data quickly to destination before any change in topology, that is the best way to send data from the last node which received instead of retransmission of whole sending procedure. This chapter will definitely help to improve the quality of sending data at the time of nodes or links fails.

References

1. Perkins C (2001) Ad-hoc networking. Addison-Wesley, Bostan
2. Zhou Z (2007) Security enhancement over ad-hoc AODV routing protocol, Tsinghua University, Beijing, zhou-zw02@mails.tsinghua.edu.cn
3. Aalam SS, Victorie TAA (2011) Node prediction—routing in mobile ad hoc networks © EuroJournals Publishing, Inc. http://www.europeanjournalofscientificresearch.com
4. Shastri A, Khatri P, Jain S (2010) Performance analysis of ad-hoc network under node failure. IJCTEE_0910 _32.pdf, vol 1(2)

5. Perkins CE, Royer EM (1999) ad-hoc on-demand distance vector routing. In: Proceedings of 2nd IEEE workshop mobile computing systems and applications (WMCSA'99), pp 90–100
6. Kuppuchamy NK, Manimegalai R (2012) A comprehensive survey of AODV routing protocol in MANET" © 2012 JCSE www.journalcse.co.uk
7. Zangeneh V, Mohammadi S (2006) New multipath node-disjoint routing based on AODV protocol, v76-116.pdf
8. Ismail Z, Hassan R (2011) Effects of packet size on AODV routing protocol implementation in homogeneous and heterogeneous MANET © 2011 IEEE doi:10.1109/CIMSim.2011.70
9. Aalam SS, Victorie TAA (2011) Node prediction—routing in mobile ad hoc networks © Euro Journals Publishing, Inc. 2011 http://www.europeanjournalofscientificresearch.com
10. Jyoti J, Roopam G, Bandhopadhyay TK (2011) On demand local link repair algorithm for AODV protocol. Int J Comput Appl 35(5):20–25. (ISSN:09758887)
11. Marandin D (2008) Performance evaluation of failed link detection in mobile ad hoc networks marandin@ifn.et.tu-dresden.de

Author Index

V. Kumar and M. Bhatele (eds.), *Proceedings of All India Seminar on Biomedical Engineering 2012 (AISOBE 2012)*, Lecture Notes in Bioengineering,
DOI: 10.1007/978-81-322-0970-6, © Springer India 2013